MENTAL HEALTH
IN EMERGENCY
CARE

MENTAL HEALTH
IN EMERGENCY CARE

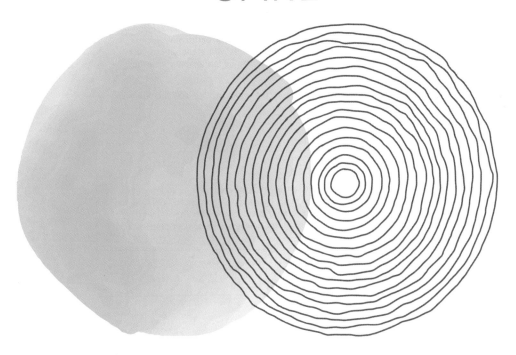

PETA MARKS

RN, BNurs, MPH, MCFT, CMHN, FACMHN
Chief Operating Officer
Australian Eating Disorders Research & Translation Centre
University of Sydney, NSW, Australia
National Programs Manager
InsideOut Institute, a collaboration between University of Sydney and
Sydney Local Health District, NSW, Australia

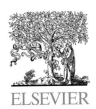

ELSEVIER

ELSEVIER

Elsevier Australia. ACN 001 002 357
(a division of Reed International Books Australia Pty Ltd)
Tower 2, 475 Victoria Avenue, Chatswood, NSW 2067

ISBN: 978-0-7295-4421-4

Notice

National Library of Australia Cataloguing-in-Publication Data

---

 A catalogue record for this book is available from the National Library of Australia

---

Content Strategist: Libby Houston
Content Project Manager: Shravan Kumar
Edited by Margaret Trudgeon
Proofread by Tim Learner
Permissions Processor: Naveen Raj R
Cover Designer: Georgette Hall
Index by Innodata
Typeset by GWTech
Printed in Singapore by KHL Printing Co Pte Ltd

Last digit is the print number: 9 8 7 6 5 4 3 2 1

Contents

About the Editor

Peta Marks is a credentialed mental health nurse and family therapist working in private practice, who specialises in working with people who have eating disorders and their families. She has extensive experience undertaking mental health project management at the national level, and as a mental health writer, and subject matter expert for online learning platforms – in particular, as lead writer for Mental Health Professionals Online Development (MHPOD). Peta is the Chief Operating Officer of the Australian Eating Disorders Research and Translation Centre and National Programs Manager at InsideOut Institute, at the University of Sydney. She is an author and co-editor of *Mental Health in Nursing: Theory and Practice for Clinical Settings*, 5th and 6th editions and a Fellow of the Australian College of Mental Health Nurses.

Contributors

Candace Angelo BNurs, GradCertNurs, GradCertChild&FamHlthNurs, GradDipIndigHProm, PhD

Program Director and Lecturer, Faculty of Medicine and Health, The University of Sydney, Sydney, NSW, Australia

Justin Chia BSci(Psych), BNurs, MMHN

Transitional Nurse Practitioner, Community Mental Health, Sydney Local Health District, Camperdown, NSW, Australia

Samantha Jane Clark DipHlthSt, DipDualDiagnosis

Dual Diagnosis Coordinator, Metro South Addiction and Mental Health Services, Metro South Health, Brisbane, QLD, Australia

Mathew Coleman BMBS, BA(Psych), MHSM, FRANZCP

Chair, Rural and Remote Mental Health Practice, The Rural Clinical School of WA, University of Western Australia, Albany, WA, Australia

Honorary Research Associate, Telethon Kids Institute, Nedlands, WA, Australia

Clinical Director, Great Southern Mental Health Service, WA Country Health Service, Albany WA, Australia

Catherine Daniel RPN, BPsychNurs, PGDipN(MtlHlth) MNurs, PhD, CMHN

Senior Lecturer, Department of Nursing, The University of Melbourne, Melbourne, Victoria, Australia

Consultation Liaison Psychiatry, The Royal Melbourne Hospital, Melbourne, Victoria, Australia

Madeline Ford BNurs(Sci), GradDipMid, GradCertEmergN, GradCertIntCareN, MNurs(Mgt&Lead)

Director of Nursing, Boulia Primary Health Service, Central West Hospital and Health Service, QLD, Australia

Kim Foster RN, PhD, Churchill Fellow, FACMHN

Professor of Mental Health Nursing, Mental Health Nursing Research Unit, School of Nursing, Midwifery & Paramedicine, Australian Catholic University & NorthWestern Mental Health, Parkville, Victoria, Australia

Fergus William Gardiner MBA, PhD Medicine, CHM, FACHSM

Director, RFDS National Emergency Response, Federation, Royal Flying Doctor Service of Australia, Canberra, ACT, Australia

Associate Professor, The Rural Clinical School of WA, University of Western Australia, Albany, WA, Australia

Brent A. Hayward RN, CMHN, PhD, MEd, PGDipAdvClinNurs(Psych), BNurs

Principal Behaviour Support Adviser, Department of Education and Training, East Melbourne, Victoria, Australia

Julia Hunt RN, BNurs, GradDipMHN, MANP, CMHN

Clinical Nurse Consultant – Consultation Liaison Psychiatry, Royal Hobart Hospital, Hobart Tasmania, Australia

Casual Academic, School of Nursing, University of Tasmania, Hobart Campus, Hobart, Tasmania, Australia

Fiona I'Anson BSc(Hons)(MentHlthNurs), MSc(SpecMentHlthCare), Accredited Person (under the NSW Mental Health Act 2007)

PACER Clinician (Mental Health Clinical Nurse Consultant), St George Hospital, Community Mental Health Service, South Eastern Sydney Local Health District, Kogarah, NSW, Australia

Sophie Isobel BNurs, GradCertCAFH, CAMH ResMeth, PhD

Clinical Senior Lecturer, Faculty of Medicine and Health, University of Sydney, Sydney, NSW, Australia

Senior Researcher, Mental Health, Sydney Local Health District, Sydney, NSW, Australia

Scott Lamont RMN, RN, MNurs (Hons), PhD

Clinical Nurse Consultant, Mental Health Liaison Nursing, Prince of Wales Hospital, Sydney, NSW, Australia

Casual Academic, School of Health & Social Sciences, Southern Cross University, NSW, Australia

Enara Louise Larcombe BSci(Psych), BNurs, GradCertInfecPreventionCont, GradCertDiabEdM, MMHN, MNurs(DiabEdM)

Tegan Louttit BNurs, GradDipMHN

Clinical Nurse Consultant, Queensland Eating Disorder Service- Metro North Mental Health, Brisbane, Australia

Peta Marks RN, BNurs, MPH, MCFT, CMHN, FACMHN

Chief Operating Officer, Australian Eating Disorders Research & Translation Centre, University of Sydney, Sydney, NSW, Australia

National Programs Manager, InsideOut Institute, a collaboration between University of Sydney and Sydney Local Health District, Sydney, NSW, Australia

Sally Matthews MPubHlth, BNursStud

Clinical Nurse Consultant, Mental Health, Community Mental Health, Sydney, NSW, Australia

Monica McEvoy BNurs, GradDipMHN, PhD

Nurse Practitioner, Child & Adolescent Mental Health, Women's & Children's Health Network, Adelaide, SA, Australia

Paul McNamara RGN (RAH), RPN(SAMHS), BNurs, MMHN, CertIMH, CMHN, FACMHN

Clinical Nurse Consultant, Consultation Liaison Psychiatry Service, Cairns Hospital, Cairns, Queensland, Australia

Bridget Anne Mulvey DipHSc(Nurs), MMHChild&Adole

Clinical Nurse Consultant, Child and Adolescent Mental Health, Sydney Children's Hospital Network, Randwick, NSW, Australia

Rea Nolan BNurs, BBehavStud(Hons), MMHN

Clinical Nurse Consultant, Queensland Eating Disorders Service, Statewide Service (RBWH), Brisbane, QLD, Australia

Anthony J O'Brien RN, PhD

Associate Professor, University of Waikato, Kirikiroa/Hamilton, New Zealand

Christine Parry Axten RMHN, BNurs, GradCertNursLead, FACMHN

Clinical Nurse Specialist, Consultation Liaison Psychiatry Service, Fiona Stanley Fremantle Hospital Group, Fremantle, WA, Australia

Leigh Peterson BNurs, PGDipMH – Adult, MMHN(NursPrac)

Mental Health Nurse Practitioner, Emergency Department, Royal Adelaide Hospital, Adelaide, SA, Australia

Jamie Ranse BNurs, GradCertClinEd, GradCertClinEp, MCritCarNurs, PhD

Associate Professor, Emergency Care, Menzies Health Institute Queensland, Griffith University, Gold Coast, QLD, Australia

Louise Roberts BHSc(Hons), BNurs, PhD

Lecturer, Research (Mental Health in the Prehospital Field), College of Medicine and Public Health, Flinders University, Adelaide, SA, Australia

Julie Sharrock RN, CertCritCare, CertPsychNurs, BEd, AdvDip(GestaltTher), MHSc(PsychNurs), PhD Candidate, FACMHN, MACN, MACSA

Mental Health Nurse Consultant, Private Practice, Ocean Grove, Victoria, Australia

Breeanna Spring Walsh BNurs, PGCertClinNurs(ICU), PGCertAeroRT, PGDipMid, PGDipAeroRT

Flight Nurse, Clinical, RFDSWO, Port Hedland, WA, Australia

Carla Trudgett BNurs, GCertPaedNurs, GradCertChildAdoleMHN, MNurs

Clinical Nurse Consultant, Child and Adolescent Mental Health, Sydney Children's Hospital, Randwick, NSW, Australia

Timothy Wand RN, NP, MNurs(Hons), PhD

Associate Professor, Sydney Nursing School, Faculty of Medicine and Health, University of Sydney, Sydney, NSW, Australia

Nurse Practitioner, Mental Health Liaison, Emergency Department, Royal Prince Alfred Hospital, Sydney, NSW, Australia

Kenton Winsley RN, RP, RAHP, BNurs, BHlthSc(Paramedic), DipPrimHlth, MACPara, CATSINaM

Regional Director Public Health, Emergency Management, Department of Health, Victoria Government, Melbourne, Victoria, Australia

Foreword

As many countries, including Australia, weigh up the costs of the unprecedented disruptions and dislocations caused by the COVID-19 pandemic and concurrently occurring natural disasters, such as bushfires and floods, it has become evident that these events have had serious impacts on people's mental health. We are already seeing significant increases in the rates of mental health conditions, and this is likely to continue well into the future. At the same time, the number of people with newly presenting, as well as pre-existing mental health conditions, has threatened to overwhelm already stretched and stressed health services.

These events have raised serious questions regarding how best to promote and protect mental health and how to respond to the needs of the increasing number of people living with mental health conditions. There is a clear need for transformative action to significantly improve all aspects of mental health care, and to do so through collaborative approaches that acknowledge and value of human rights and lived experience, and are free of stigma and discrimination. As stated in the World Health Organization's (WHO) *World Mental Health Report 2022*, 'Business as usual for mental health care simply will not do'.

Mental health in emergency care is a critically important area of consideration, if mental health systems are to be transformed in the ways envisaged by the WHO. There are increasing numbers of people experiencing mental health conditions presenting for emergency care. To sensitively, effectively and respectfully respond to the mental health needs of these individuals, emergency care practitioners need to have a strong grounding in mental health knowledge and skills; in short, emergency care practitioners need to build mental health 'know-how'. The chapters of this timely and informative text on mental health in emergency care provide exactly the kind of knowledge and skill base required by practitioners working in emergency care settings. The editor, Peta Marks, has assembled an impressive group of authors, who cover important topics within the mental health emergency care context. These include a range of clinical conditions and service types and locations – working with Aboriginal and Torres Strait Islander peoples presenting with mental health concerns, providing care for refugees and asylum seekers, mental health care provided in dedicated emergency departments, first responder work in disaster settings, paramedic intervention prior to transportation to hospital, and emergency care in remote locations; these are some of the areas addressed.

Especially noteworthy throughout the chapters of this impressive text is a focus on systems transformation, the social ecology of mental health, recovery-oriented and trauma-informed approaches to care, and, in most chapters, the inclusion of a lived experience commentary that provides poignant, insightful lessons on what it is like to live with a mental health condition and to interact with healthcare services and practitioners; to confront challenges and hurdles; to find hope, compassion and strength, despite adversity.

In Australia, as in other countries, there is a need for urgent action to reform mental health care. Such a transformation will necessarily involve careful consideration of how mental health care is provided in emergency situations, whether this be in an emergency department or in a community setting. The chapters in this impressive text have an authority and authenticity that accord well with the knowledge required by the practitioners who provide mental health care in emergency settings. The voice of lived experience that adds value to the theoretical and technical detail provided by the authors in each chapter is undoubtedly a key feature of the text. It is to be hoped that the production of professional texts in the mental health field has now reached a stage of development in which the inclusion of a substantive lived experience commentary is considered best practice and it will no longer be acceptable for such works to be undertaken without the inclusion of the voice of lived experience.

Conjoint Professor Mike Hazelton
RN, BA, MA, PhD, FACMHN (Life Member)
President, Australian College of Mental Health Nurses
August 2022

Preface

At a conference I heard a keynote speech by an incredibly inspiring and eloquent woman who was sharing her gender transition experience – the ups, the downs, her greatest fears and her biggest challenges. But the thing that touched me the most was her tender, heartfelt description of the impact of one particular nurse who had cared for her when she was in hospital during some of her darkest days, and who, according to the speaker, had saved her life – not physically, but in a spiritual and emotional sense, through their caring, acceptance and empathy. Don't all health professionals want to be *that* kind of clinician?

For nearly 30 years I have specialised in working with people who have eating disorders and their families. Over this time I have heard many clinicians from a range of disciplines say that they don't 'do' eating disorders. In the same way, I have heard mental health clinicians say they don't 'do' physical health, and generalist colleagues say that they don't 'do' mental health. This siloed way of thinking about the human experience is perplexing. People become nurses because they want to help other people … how can we claim to do that, or be 'holistic' practitioners without considering what is happening (or has happened) to the person as a whole? If someone experiences a physical illness or injury, shouldn't we consider the impact of that experience on their emotional wellbeing too? If someone develops a mental illness, shouldn't we make sure that their physical health is not adversely impacted, or is making things worse for them? If someone is presenting with symptoms which can be explained by or traced back to trauma, or disadvantage, or racism, or stigma, shouldn't we be cognisant of that and ensure our practice is informed by and responsive to that knowledge? To my mind, the best way to be *that* clinician, in any clinical situation or setting, regardless of discipline or area of specialisation, is to consider and connect with the human experience of the person in front of us – with all elements of their being – their unique identity, as well as their physical, emotional, psychological and social experiences. And to do that, we need to purposefully develop the required knowledge and skills in order to inform our practice; this text has been developed to help with that process.

There is nothing quite like the voice of lived experience – it is powerful, it is important and it helps to remind us why we do what we do as healthcare professionals. I've learnt so much from people's stories, and my practice as a mental health nurse and as a project manager has been enriched by listening to people speak about their healthcare journey or the healthcare journey of their loved one; about what has helped and what they have found lacking.

I feel very honoured that Bundjalung Elder Associate Professor Boe Rambaldini has shared his story in this text and that Helena Roennfeldt has so generously offered such insightful comment around each and every scenario chapter, informed by her lived experience and her knowledge of the lived experience of others with mental health concerns. I would also like to acknowledge Enara Larcombe and Paul McNamara, who used a true co-design approach to the development of their scenario chapter. I also feel incredibly appreciative that the nurses and other clinicians who have contributed to this text agreed to share their clinical knowledge, insights and experiences – their clinical expertise, demonstrated through their writing and what they have chosen to include here, adds a richness to the knowledge that can be gained from text books and journal articles.

The 2022 National Study of Mental Health and Wellbeing identified that nearly 44% of Australians have experienced a mental disorder at some point in their life – over 20% of people and nearly 40% of 16–24-year-olds in the previous 12 months. It is clear that now, more than ever, the mental health and social and emotional wellbeing of every patient seen in every clinical context must be considered, regardless of the person's presenting circumstances. While not every clinician needs to specialise in mental health, if we are to improve the mental health of Australians in general, First Nations people and young people in particular, all health professionals need to enhance mental health communication and observation skills, employ empathy and work in a culturally competent, collaborative and recovery-focused way.

In a post-COVID world, working in any healthcare setting is challenging. Clinical work can be exciting, interesting, exhausting, uplifting, upsetting, frustrating, humbling and hilarious – sometimes all in one day. It is my hope that the information and clinical scenarios shared in this text will support nurses and other health professionals to develop their mental health knowledge and skills, and more than anything, to connect (or re-connect) with the desire to be *'that'* clinician – to approach each patient as a person, and each person as unique, and not allow time pressures or staffing shortages, or the business of 'the system', to divert us from the need to be holistic, or to devalue the importance of the human-to-human interactions that make a difference to a person's wellbeing and their healthcare journey.

Peta Marks

August 2022

CHAPTER 1
INTRODUCTION TO MENTAL HEALTH IN EMERGENCY CARE

Peta Marks and Kim Foster

KEY POINTS

- People experiencing mental health issues, mental illness and mental distress are increasingly presenting to emergency settings.
- Health professionals working in emergency settings need to use fundamental mental health knowledge and skills to meet the holistic care needs of patients, relevant to their clinical setting and scope of practice.
- All clinicians and healthcare settings need to incorporate mental health recovery-focused and trauma-informed practice approaches to care.

LEARNING OUTCOMES

This chapter will assist you to:
- understand the holistic healthcare needs of patients presenting for emergency mental health care
- develop further understanding of the range of mental health presentations in emergency contexts
- gain further mental health knowledge that can be applied to holistic practice with patients presenting for emergency care.

INTRODUCTION

Emergency departments (EDs) are settings of 'high volume, urgent care' (Corscadden et al 2021) and are an essential service element of the Australian healthcare system. The ED is also a major portal of entry for mental health care. Demand on ED and emergency ambulance services for mental health care have increased significantly over time, particularly for youth and younger adults (Tran et al 2019), exceeding expected growth relative to the population (Andrew et al 2020). Since the 1980s, when mental health services were first integrated with general health services, in a process called 'mainstreaming' (Broadbent et al

2020), presentations to emergency departments with a mental health-related principal diagnosis in Australia have been growing exponentially: 273 439 presentations in 2016; 286 985 presentations across 2017–18; and 310 417 presentations in 2019–20 (AIHW 2016; AIHW 2021; Daniel et al 2021). This trend is likely to continue.

Drivers for increased emergency mental health presentations include changes to the way health services are delivered, improved health awareness and community expectations of healthcare, not knowing where to access mental health help (Hiscock et al 2018), as well as access issues with same-day or after-hours general practitioner (GP) services. Financial barriers, such as lack of availability of bulk-billing, an ageing population, living in rural and remote or lower socioeconomic areas, and difficulty accessing community-based mental health services, also impact on emergency mental healthcare presentations (Alarcon Manchego et al 2015; Andrew et al 2020; Kalucy et al 2005). The increased demand in EDs and difficulty accessing hospital beds (which for mental health presentations can be due to downstream bed blockages; e.g. an inability to discharge patients from an acute mental health unit who are experiencing housing instability), can lead to overcrowding and increased waiting times. These in turn are known to lead to suboptimal system performance (such as increased costs), increased patient morbidity and mortality, and negative impact on the health-seeking experience (Morley et al 2018; Opoku et al 2018; Perera et al 2018).

Within this growing demand for ED services, mental health, drug and alcohol and behavioural presentations to ED settings in Australia and overseas have been steadily increasing since 2010, especially for young people 10–19 years old (Perera et al 2018). These are not just in absolute numbers, but also as a proportion of all presentations (Tran et al 2020; Wand et al 2019), and occur despite significant efforts at system reforms for mental health (See Box 1.1 for some examples). In 2019–20, 3.8% of all presentations to emergency departments were related to mental health. The most common mental health presentations were related to psychoactive substance use (28.1% of all mental health-related ED presentations 2019–20); anxiety, stress-related (e.g. situational crisis) and somatoform disorders (where someone presents with physical concerns that have no medical cause) (27%); psychotic and delusional disorders (11.9%) and mood disorders (9.7%) (AIHW 2021). Deliberate self-harm and behaviour related to personality disorder are also relatively common mental health presentations to EDs, with an overall trend of increasing numbers over time. In 2016–17 there were more than 33 000 ED presentations for deliberate self-harm across Australia (Pointer 2019), making up 7% of all injury-related hospital presentations that year. However, it has been suggested that suicide and self-harm-related presentations to EDs are grossly underestimated due to a lack of a standardised approach to formulation and recording of them within ED datasets (Stapleberg et al 2020; Sveticic et al 2020).

When someone is in mental distress, where they are experiencing mental and emotional upset (e.g. when they have intentionally harmed themselves or are experiencing suicidal ideation or behaviour), the ED is often the first point of contact within the healthcare system. A NSW study found that about 60% of people presenting for a mental health concern in ED were triaged as experiencing urgent or potentially life-threatening conditions (Perera et al 2018), and nationally, 77% were assessed as being urgent or semi-urgent presentations

Box 1.1 System reform for mental health

Significant efforts at system reform in Australia include:

- *Policy:* state/territory and national policy focus on mental health, since the first National Mental Health Plan (1992): with the National Suicide Prevention Strategy 2020–23 (NSPS 2020): the National Aboriginal and Torres Strait Islander Suicide Prevention Strategy (2013) and the 5th National Mental Health and Suicide Prevention Plan (NMHC 2017) raising awareness of suicide risk and committing all governments to integrated mental health and suicide prevention action. More recently the National Mental Health and Wellbeing Pandemic Response Plan (NMHC 2020) responded to the significant negative impact on mental health from COVID-19 and the containment measures required (including lockdown).
- *Early intervention for young people:* the establishment and expansion of Headspace centres nationally since 2006 for 12–25-year-olds, to address the high incidence and prevalence of mental health problems among adolescents and young people, and their reported low level of mental health service use (Rickwood et al 2019).
- *Provision of psychological therapy through Medicare:* Medicare funding of mental health treatment in primary care through the Better Access scheme (2006) triggered a significant increase in the provision of mental health care by GPs, psychologists and allied health professions (Jorm 2018).

(AIHW 2021). This demonstrates an appropriate acuity of presentation to an ED environment. However, the significant numbers of people who re-present with suicidal ideation and suicidal behaviours, or who do not engage with community mental health services, as well as the high rate of suicide in Australia, suggest that there are 'deficiencies in current models of care, access to general practice follow-up, and community mental health resource provision' (Perera et al 2018, p. 351).

In a busy clinical environment, increases in presentations related to mental health and alcohol and other drugs create several challenges – the safety of patients and staff, timely access to care that is appropriate, the difficulty of responding to challenging behaviours within the ED environment, and the need for all clinicians to increase knowledge, skills and confidence in managing this patient population (Perera et al 2018) in order to provide holistic care.

MENTAL HEALTH AND MENTAL HEALTH PROBLEMS

All people experience a spectrum of mental health and illness, including a wide variety of complex states that are constantly variable and open to change. In the same way that any physically healthy person may become sick, or a physically sick person may become well, there is always the opportunity for a person who is mentally healthy to develop mental ill-health, or for a person who experiences mental illness to recover and regain mental health. People can move along the spectrum of mental health and illness and remain in various states for shorter or longer periods of time. Understanding the spectrum of mental health and illness is therefore crucial if nurses and other healthcare professionals are to effectively

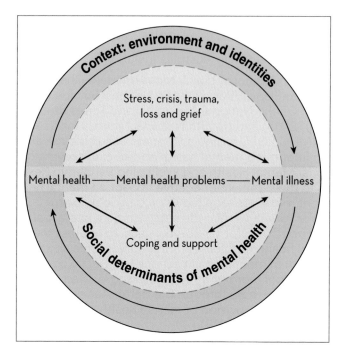

Fig. 1.1 The spectrum of mental health and illness.

assist people they are responsible for delivering care to. See Fig. 1.1 for the spectrum of health and illness.

Mental health cannot be separated from the concept of overall health, which is defined by the World Health Organization (WHO) as:

A state of complete, physical, mental and social wellbeing and not merely the absence of disease or injury (WHO 1946).

Unfortunately, mental health is often underemphasised by nurses and other health professionals, who often focus more on *assessing* people for mental illness than on *assisting* them towards recovery of their mental health. This may be compared to a football team that becomes focused on defence, forgetting to invest in training that supports them to score goals. Such service provision inevitably ends up in an ongoing cycle of assessment, diagnosis, treatment and discharge, resulting in poor outcomes for patients and families, with high rates of recidivism (Rosenberg & Hickie 2019).

The spectrum of mental health is heterogenous, meaning everyone experiences it differently, and it is important to acknowledge that a wide variety of words and concepts are used to explain various stages of the spectrum across health and illness states. The following section provides an overview of several major concepts in the spectrum of mental health and illness: mental health, stress, coping, crisis, mental health problems, and mental illness. People who present to ED will often be in states of crisis, experiencing mental health problems, or have acute mental illness.

Mental health

Perhaps the most widely accepted modern description of mental health is the one promoted by the WHO, which states that:

> *Mental health is defined as a state of well-being in which every individual realizes his or her own potential, can cope with the normal stresses of life, can work productively and fruitfully, and is able to make a contribution to her or his community (WHO 2001).*

A mentally healthy life is not an all-perfect, all-positive life. Most societies accept a wide range of diversity, and most human beings living a mentally healthy life present a wide range of personal and social characteristics. Mental health assists a person to live a life that is satisfying to them and the community they live in. It does not matter how this is achieved or what the person's life looks like – this is of no consequence at all – as long the person and the community they live in believe that their life is satisfying.

STRESS

Regular experiences of stress are a normal part of life. Stressors can include life events such as exams, a relationship breakdown, or running late for an important appointment. A person's response to these stressors is referred to as the 'stress response', where 'stress' involves the effects of something that might threaten a person's physical and psychological homeostasis, or constant state of being (Selye 1956). Emotional distress can occur in relation to personal and social difficulties created through a range of life stressors, a crisis, trauma, loss or bereavement. For the most part, a person presenting in mental and emotional distress needs empathy, understanding and emotional support, rather than a diagnosis, treatment and medication (Middleton & Shaw 2010).

Every person responds to stressors differently, depending on factors such as their appraisal of the stressor and their existing coping strategies. Stress may be acute or chronic, and is different to crisis, which is an acute state where the person's usual coping strategies and ability to manage a situation has been overwhelmed.

COPING

Coping refers to people's capacity to rebound after life stressors without experiencing ongoing problems and involves the use of cognitive and behavioural strategies to manage the demands of a situation that a person views as taxing their current resources, or to reduce negative emotions caused by stress (APA 2020). Our ability to cope is not only reliant on internal psychological attitudes; multiple external factors also contribute to each person's capacity to rebound after stressful events. There are a range of factors that can either protect or pose risks to a person's mental health. Protective factors commonly include things such as regular physical exercise and supportive relationships with family and/or friends. Risk factors include a lack of safe housing and biological stressors such as physical illness. People develop a range of coping strategies during their life that enable them to rebound from stressful situations. When a person's capacity to cope is exceeded, however, they can move into a state of crisis and/or mental distress.

CRISIS

Nurses see people who are experiencing crisis, trauma, loss and grief in all clinical settings.

A crisis is an acute, time-limited, difficult or dangerous situation that needs attention – associated with aspect(s) of a person's financial, social, environmental, political or personal life. Stressful events like job interviews or exams might be contrasted with experiences that the person perceives as threatening and which have the potential to trigger a state of acute crisis – for example, losing a loved one, a relationship or employment; or physical, emotional or sexual assault. All of us can experience a crisis state at some point in our life. With appropriate support and time to recover, most people resume their life without developing ongoing mental health problems.

In a crisis state, usual coping strategies can be seriously challenged, resulting in increasing feelings of vulnerability and rising levels of anxiety, distress and confusion. A person's usual ability to manage the demands of everyday life can be disrupted, resulting in disorganisation and disequilibrium. Without relief and support, such crisis may result in severe emotional, cognitive and behavioural dysfunction, leading to a person being a risk to themselves or others (James & Gilliland 2013).

Mental health problems

We are all capable of experiencing mental health problems. Mental health problems can be understood as social or emotional wounds that impact on a person's life, but not to the extent that they seriously disrupt the person's relationships or normal daily activities. For some, the chances of experiencing mental health problems may increase at times when they feel vulnerable – this may be heightened by anxiety or fear or perhaps by feeling that they have little or no control over a situation, or over what is about to happen.

Vulnerability to mental health problems may increase for groups in society who experience particular social or political issues needing solutions; for example, those who are homeless, people seeking refuge from domestic violence, or those in prison. Mental health problems may also increase for people at risk of physical abuse or violence, thus needing measures to be put in place to keep them safe. Importantly, mental health problems are not the same as diagnosable mental illness, although you may hear the two terms used interchangeably.

MENTAL ILLNESS

Many people who experience mental health problems never access a mental health professional for assistance and so never interpret their problems as mental ill health. Many people access the internet for advice, which may provide them with helpful advice on how to adapt and recover their mental health. However, research has also indicated that internet-based advice can lead to over-analysis of problems and self-diagnoses, which can lead people to have negative beliefs about their experience of problems and capacity to recover (Robertson et al 2014).

Definitions of mental illness vary considerably depending on the culture, language and interests of particular groups. The WHO definition, published in the International Classification of Diseases (ICD), 11th edition, defines mental illness as:

> *A syndrome characterized by clinically significant disturbance in an individual's cognition, emotion regulation, or behaviour that reflects a dysfunction in the psychological, biological or developmental processes underlying mental functioning. Mental disorders are usually associated with significant distress in social, occupational, or other important activities (APA 2013, p. 20).*

A person with mental illness often experiences such distress in their thoughts, feelings and behaviours that they lose the ability to meet the expectations they have for themselves and that society has for them. This can cause significant disruption in their relationships at home and in other areas of life, such as at school or work. In some instances, the person's experience of mental illness may cause such disruption to their pursuit of a satisfying life that they may be deemed to be 'disabled'. High prevalence mental illnesses include anxiety and depression. Low prevalence illnesses include schizophrenia and bipolar disorder.

It is often said that that no one experiences 'absolute health' or is 'completely normal'. However, often once a person has a diagnosis of mental illness, they are described as being either mentally ill or not. Such a concrete distinction between mental health and illness is overly simplistic, because it fails to address the range of human responses and limited states of mental distress that people can experience. It also does not account for the fact that many people do not have a mental illness forever. In the end, mental health and illness are complex social constructs that vary in each society and cultural group as we attempt to describe differences we perceive in life experiences.

These are important things to keep in mind in the emergency context, where people with previous diagnoses of mental illness may not necessarily be experiencing an episode of that illness at the time, but may instead present in a state of crisis or mental distress due to life events. It is important, as a clinician, not to make assumptions about a person's presentation based only on previous diagnoses.

A SOCIAL ECOLOGICAL APPROACH TO MENTAL HEALTH

A social ecological perspective refers to the dynamic interactions between a person and their environment that influence their health and wellbeing. This person–environment interaction involves several factors and processes. Mental health can be understood as involving a person's physical, mental, emotional and spiritual characteristics and the interactive processes that occur between them and their environment or ecology (including their social and family context) (see Fig. 1.2). This includes being able to access available resources that help sustain their mental health (Ungar 2011) and support their recovery, such as human resources and supports, including family and friends; healthcare resources, including nursing care and mental healthcare (hospital or community-based); and practical resources, such as financial support and housing.

A social ecological or holistic perspective is relevant because mental health problems can challenge people in every aspect of a person's life. Similarly, clinical practice is shaped by our personal characteristics and skills and the health service context we work in. This dynamic person–environment interaction involves personal and contextual factors that influence our practice and relationships with patients/consumers.

Social determinants

Social determinants of health are the social and economic circumstances within which we are born and live (WHO 2018). A range of social determinants impact on mental and emotional wellbeing – stigma, poverty, housing insecurity and homelessness, educational

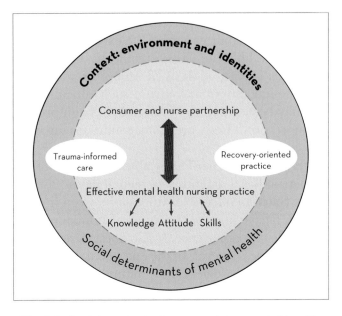

Fig. 1.2 Social ecological approach to mental health.

opportunities, employment, violence, social connection opportunities, financial stressors, forced migration, parenting and family issues (WHO 2018). As well, the impact of co-occurring drug and alcohol use and misuse, loss and grief and other critical events need to be considered. These are issues which impact on all of us at various times in our lives. Because mental ill health is strongly determined by these factors, mental health problems are not able to be improved by mental health treatments alone. The social factors that have contributed to these problems also need to be addressed and, wherever possible, eliminated.

An ecological approach to healthcare therefore requires that clinicians understand and address the social contexts within which people live. Healthcare professionals do not necessarily have the capacity to influence, prevent or intervene in all these factors, but it is vitally important that these factors are taken into consideration and identified as part of history taking and assessment. An ecological approach to practice also requires that clinicians understand the environments within which they practice. See Table 1.1 for the different social and cultural determinants that impact on people's mental health.

Contexts of mental health: environment and identities

It is important for clinicians to understand that the models of care and the health service approach within which they work directly influence their practice. Equally, practice can influence and shape the *environments* within which we work. People admitted to hospitals can pose unique ethical challenges to staff because they may experience episodes of mental ill health that are assessed as requiring restrictive care and/or compulsory admission under mental health legislation, removing part or all of their autonomy due to considerations of risk and safety. Working in such challenging environments means that clinicians need not

TABLE 1.1 Social and cultural determinants of mental disorders

Domain	Proximal	Distal
Demographic	Age Gender Ethnicity	Community diversity Population density Longevity Survival
Economic	Income Debt Assets Financial strain Relative deprivation Unemployment Food security	Economic recessions Economic inequality Macroeconomic
Neighbourhood	Safety and security Housing structure Overcrowding Recreation	Infrastructure Neighbourhood deprivation Built environment Setting Safety and security
Environmental	Natural disasters Industrial disasters War or conflict Climate change Forced migration	Trauma Distress
Social and cultural	Community social capital Social stability Cultural	Individual social capital Social participation Social support Education

Adapted from Lund et al 2018.

only have an up-to-date working knowledge of health conditions and interventions, but also need to be able to empathise with the difficulties patients face as they navigate their recovery from experiences of mental ill health, within what are often disconnected and under-resourced healthcare systems (Cleary et al 2018).

Identity can be thought of as an individual's enduring sense of themselves as a person. It is deeply influenced by belonging to, or difference from, significant social groups – for example, cultural groups, religious faiths and peer groups. By identifying with the values and beliefs of a social group we come to define our own unique sense of who we are. In the emergency context, it is relevant to understand that each patient will bring a unique identity that will influence their illness presentation and how they respond to treatment and care.

Some examples of identity are outlined in Box 1.2, but it is important to remember that individuals will have multiple identities and that these may change over the course of their lives. Clinicians should not presume to know what a patient's identities are, and should not expect individuals to conform to stereotyped ideas about a particular identity. Clinicians also need to reflect on their own identities and how they may influence their interactions with patients. We cannot be knowledgeable or skilled in all patients' identities, but it is

Box 1.2 Forms of identity

Cultural identity	• a person's sense of belonging to one or more cultural groups • culture may be the most important source of identity (e.g. for Indigenous Australians) • an important source of beliefs, values and practices • impact on mental health
Spiritual identity	• for some people, spirituality and religious faith are regarded as central to identity and to psychosocial functioning • often associated with religious faith, but many people have a non-religious worldview while still maintaining spiritual beliefs and values • while clinical support can help people manage distress and develop coping strategies, spirituality can provide a sense of hope and acceptance in the face of seemingly insurmountable life problems
Gender identity	• gender now seen as a fluid, socially constructed concept • should not be confused with sexual preference, which refers to an individual's gender preferences in intimate relationships • not necessarily fixed and can change in the course of psychosocial development • gender and sexuality can often be a source of distress due to stigma and prejudice

important that we respectfully acknowledge all cultural, sexual and spiritual identities and preferences.

Identity can be a source of stress for those whose identities are disvalued and subject to stigmatising views and prejudice. The term 'minority stress' (Spittlehouse et al 2020) refers to the experience of stigma and discrimination encountered by people in relation to their identity. This can relate to culture and ethnicity, religious affiliation, gender and sexuality and other aspects of identity. Discrimination can create a hostile environment in which minority stress leads to symptoms of mental illness, including depression, anxiety, suicidal ideation and harmful substance use. People who are subject to one form of marginalisation are more likely to also experience other forms of marginalisation, a concept referred to as 'intersectionality' (Grzanka & Brian 2019). Clinicians encounter many patients who experience one or more forms of marginalisation and need to be aware of how these experiences shape the person's health experience and the responses of clinicians.

Reflection

1. Reflect on your own individual identity. How might your identity and world view influence your clinical practice?
2. How might awareness of and attempts to understand a person's identity support a more positive clinical encounter?

RECOVERY-ORIENTED AND TRAUMA-INFORMED APPROACHES TO CARE

The concept of 'clinical recovery' (Slade et al 2015) considers mental illness as a health condition in need of clinical treatment. Working from this perspective involves the expectation that recovery should include a substantial reduction of symptoms and restoration of function in work and relationships. Conversely, people with lived experience have emphasised that recovery from mental illness is a personal journey (i.e. personal recovery) and that many people who are labelled or diagnosed with a mental illness have a substantial history of trauma. Recovery-oriented and trauma-informed care approaches have been developed to support people in their personal recovery from mental illness. These approaches are increasingly used in mental health care and can be used by clinicians in all settings to support people who are experiencing mental distress or illness.

Recovery-oriented care

There is no single definition of mental health recovery; however, one of the most commonly used explanations was written by Bill Anthony (1993, p. 15), who described it as:

> *A deeply personal, unique process of changing one's attitudes, values, feelings, goals, skills and/or roles. It is a way of living a satisfying, hopeful, and contributing life even with limitations caused by the illness. Recovery involves the development of new meaning and purpose in one's life as a person grows beyond the catastrophic effects of mental illness.*

Experiences commonly associated with personal recovery include connectedness; hope and optimism; identity; meaning in life; and empowerment (Leamy et al 2011). There are five key domains of recovery-oriented care that mental health professionals and services are expected to practise within:

1. Promoting a culture and language of hope and optimism.
2. Putting the person first and at the centre of practice and viewing their life holistically.
3. Supporting personal recovery and placing it at the heart of practice.
4. Organisational commitment and workforce development for skilled practitioners and an environment that is conducive to recovery.
5. Action on social inclusion and social determinants of health, mental health and well-being (Commonwealth of Australia 2013).

Trauma-informed care

The majority of people who use mental health services, and many people who experience mental health challenges, have a background of trauma. Research demonstrates clear links between trauma and the onset of a range of mental health problems (Green et al 2018). Box 1.3 outlines various elements that can define trauma.

Individual traumatic events (e.g. an unexpected death, a severe accident, a natural disaster) disrupt a person's life and create a period of destabilisation, but won't necessarily result in a state of crisis. After such events most people adjust and recover. Some people even describe positive effects – including enhanced ability to cope, personal growth and renewed appreciation for their life and the people they love – an experience understood as post-traumatic growth (van Weeghel et al 2019). However, for some people, depending on the

Box 1.3 Trauma

Trauma is the exposure to actual or threatened death, serious injury or sexual violence in one or more of the following ways:

- directly experiencing a traumatic event
- witnessing, in person, a traumatic event occurring to others
- learning that a traumatic event has happened to a close family member or friend
- experiencing repeated or extreme exposure to aversive details of a traumatic event.

American Psychiatric Association 2013.

nature of the trauma, their reaction to and perception of the event, the capacity to cope will be overwhelmed and result in an acute crisis state.

People who have experienced adverse childhood events, such as psychological, physical or sexual abuse; living in a situation of domestic violence with a mother who was being abused; or living in a household where people abused substances, were suffering from mental illness, were suicidal or had been in prison, are less likely to develop resilience and have a more than 50% increased risk of depression. The more of these adverse events a person experiences as a child, the higher the likelihood of developing physical illness (e.g. chronic obstructive pulmonary disease or heart disease) or mental illness (e.g. depression) as an adult (Felitti et al 1998; Jones et al 2018). Experiencing these events in childhood can also have longer-term impacts on a person's capacity to cope with future trauma or abuse.

A history of trauma has been associated with relapse of mental illness, increased substance misuse and reduced engagement with mental health services (Molloy et al 2020). Presenting to an emergency setting can be very challenging for people who have a history of trauma, because 'the environment and their experience of care can trigger traumatic memories' (Molloy et al 2020, p. 30) – including traumatic memories about past episodes of care, either in mental health or emergency settings. As such, it is imperative for clinicians to be sensitive to the vulnerabilities and potential triggers that may give rise to re-traumatisation and to be aware that this could impede their mental health recovery.

In this context it is important to consider that when people come into contact with an emergency setting, a sense of personal safety is an important basis for effective care. Often, people will be frightened; it is important to take time to find out how the person feels and what they need to feel safe and secure. It may require listening to them or helping them consider strategies they could use to increase feelings of safety – for example, calling for help if someone enters their room. Do not assume that the person experiencing mental distress will feel safe in the healthcare setting just because you feel comfortable in the environment as a clinician. The essentials of trauma-informed care therefore include recognising a number of key elements outlined in Box 1.4.

In summary, trauma-informed services are informed by three key principles to guide practice (Muskett 2014):

1. People need to feel connected, valued, informed and hopeful about their recovery from mental illness.

Box 1.4 Trauma-informed practice

Trauma-informed practice requires that clinicians:

- take a universal precaution approach that assumes all people who seek mental health care may have experienced trauma.
- help people feel safe and lower their distressing emotions – e.g. sit, listen; encourage basic breathing or relaxation techniques; and ensure a calm environment. When people feel calmer they are more likely to be able to engage their thinking brain and find ways that work for them to feel safe.
- understand how trauma and abuse may have shaped difficulties in relationships and affected therapeutic relationships.
- avoid coercive or restrictive interventions such as seclusion or restraint, which may re-traumatise people. Wherever possible, recognise the person's strengths and support them by collaboratively developing a care plan that affirms their preferences for care and how they can manage distress.
- avoid interventions that may be perceived as shaming and humiliating. Clinicians are responsible for maintaining the dignity and individual rights of the person at all times and providing services in ways that are flexible, individualised, culturally competent, respectful and based on best practice.
- focus on what happened to the person rather than pathologising the person as a result of their presenting symptoms (where the focus is on what is wrong with the person). Develop an understanding of presenting behaviour and symptoms in the context of past experiences.

Sweeney et al 2018.

2. Staff understand the connection between childhood trauma and adult mental health issues.
3. Staff practise in empowering ways with consumers and their family and friends and other services to promote autonomy.

While these principles focus on the needs of patients and their family and friends, a trauma-informed approach to care can also provide support for managing workplace stress (Isobel & Edwards 2017). Trauma-informed practice does not replace recovery-oriented practice, but is complementary and provides another perspective from which people (staff and consumers) may view recovery and therapeutic engagement.

SUMMARY

No matter which emergency setting health professionals choose to work in, be it a hospital ED, with police or emergency ambulance services, as part of a disaster response team, or with the Royal Flying Doctors Service, they will encounter people experiencing mental distress or mental illness, who present with acute physical or mental health concerns.

Clinicians need to be as competent in recognising and responding to emotional distress and the mental health needs of a person as they are in identifying signs of physical deterioration or a treatment side effect. This is the essence of a holistic approach to health care. We cannot profess to be 'experts' in health if we don't consider the person as a whole – their physical, psychological, social, cultural and spiritual wellbeing. Acknowledging the impact of a person's environment and experiences on their health and health outcomes is also an important part of understanding their overall health and providing holistic care. The interdependence between all aspects of personhood, including biological, psychological, social and spiritual dimensions requires that, regardless of the clinical setting, clinicians consider a person's mental health as part of their core business.

This text has been designed to support nurses and other health professionals working in emergency care settings to increase their knowledge about working with people who present with mental distress or mental illness and to meet some of the associated challenges. It is important to understand the context within which people develop mental illness or mental distress, and in which healthcare and mental health care is provided. This first chapter has provided an overview of the spectrum of mental health and illness, the considerations and context of mental health within the emergency care setting, and the foundations for holistic practice using a social ecological approach.

Chapter 2 introduces the key elements of mental health triage and assessment, and considers the importance of taking a strengths-based approach. In Chapter 3 scenarios developed by clinicians provide an overview of common mental health issues that people present to emergency care settings with; along with the key considerations, actions and interventions required. The scenarios reflect the clinical experiences of the authors and show how fundamental mental health knowledge and skills need to be applied. Chapter 4 explores the personal and professional challenges associated with working in an emergency care setting – the emotional labour, anxiety and stress inherent in this type of work and the importance of engaging with protective strategies that help develop resilience and maintain personal boundaries, including reflective practice and self-care.

Useful websites

Australian College of Mental Health Nurses: www.acmhn.org
Headspace: https://headspace.org.au/
Te Ao Maramatanga (New Zealand College of Mental Health Nurses): www.nzcmhn.org.nz/

References

Alarcon Manchego P, Knott J, Graudins A et al 2015. Management of mental health patients in Victorian emergency departments: A 10-year follow-up. Emergency Medicine Australasia 27:529–36.

American Psychiatric Association (APA) 2013. Diagnostic and statistical manual of mental disorders (DSM-5), 5th edition. APA, Arlington VA.

American Psychological Association 2020. APA Dictionary of psychology. Online. Available: https://dictionary.apa.org/coping

Andrew E, Nehme Z, Cameron P et al 2020. Drivers of increasing emergency ambulance demand. Prehospital Emergency Care 24(3):385.

Anthony WA 1993. Recovery from mental illness: The guiding vision of the mental health service system in the 1990s. Psychosocial Rehabilitation Journal 16(4):11–23.

Australian Institute of Health and Welfare (AIHW) 2021. Mental health services in Australia. Online. Available: www.aihw.gov.au/reports/mental-health-services/mental-health-services-in-australia/report-contents/hospital-emergency-services/patient-characteristics.

Australian Institute of Health and Welfare (AIHW) 2016. Mental health services provided in emergency departments. Online. Available: www.aihw.gov.au/getmedia/1ffc85db-f620-48e8-8d94-57a375e132fe/Mental-health-services-provided-in-emergency-departments.pdf.aspx.

Broadbent M, Moxham L, Dwyer T 2020. Understanding nurses' perspectives of acuity in the process of emergency mental health triage: a qualitative study. Contemporary Nurse 56(3): 280–95.

Cleary M, Raeburn T, West S et al 2018. Two approaches, one goal: How mental health registered nurses perceive their role and the role of peer support workers in facilitating consumer decision-making. International Journal of Mental Health Nursing 27(4):1212–18.

Commonwealth of Australia 2013. A national framework for recovery-oriented mental health services: Guide for practitioners and providers. Online. Available: www1.health.gov.au/internet/main/publishing.nsf/content/67D17065514CF8E8CA257C1D00017A90/$File/recovgde.pdf.

Corscadden L, Callander EJ, Topp SM et al 2021. Disparities in experiences of emergency department care for people with a mental health condition. Australasian Emergency Care 24:11–19.

Daniel C, Mukaro V, Yap C et al 2021. Characteristics and clinical outcomes for mental health patients admitted to a behavioural assessment unit: Implications for model of care and practice. International Journal of Mental Health Nursing 30:255–8.

Felitti VJ, Anda RF, Nordenberd D et al 1998. Relationship of childhood abuse and household dysfunction to many of the leading causes of death in adults. The Adverse Childhood Experiences (ACE) Study. American Journal of Preventative Medicine 14(4):245–58.

Green M, Linscott RJ, Laurens KR et al 2018. Latent profiles of developmental schizotypy in the general population: Associations with childhood trauma and familial mental illness. Schizophrenia Bulletin 44(Supp 1):S229.

Grzanka PR, Brian JD 2019. Clinical encounters: the social justice question in intersectional medicine. The American Journal of Bioethics 19(2):22–4.

Hiscock H, Neely RJ, Lei S et al 2018. Paediatric and physical health presentations to emergency departments, Victoria 2008–15. MJA 208(8):343–8.

Isobel S, Edwards C 2017. Using trauma informed care as a nursing model of care in an acute inpatient mental health unit: A practice development process. International Journal of Mental Health Nursing 26(1):88–94.

James RK, Gilliland BE 2013. Crisis intervention strategies, 7th edn. Brooks/Cole Cengage Learning, Belmont, CA.

Jones T, Nurius P, Song C et al 2018. Modeling life course pathways from adverse childhood experiences to adult mental health. Child Abuse and Neglect 80:32–40.

Jorm A 2018. Australia's 'Better Access scheme': Has it had an impact on population mental health? Australian and New Zealand Journal of Psychiatry 52(11):1057–62.

Kalucy R, Thomas L, King D 2005. Changing demand for mental health services in the emergency department of a public hospital. Australian and New Zealand Journal of Psychiatry 39(1–2):74–80.

Leamy M, Bird V, Le Boutillier C et al 2011. Conceptual framework for personal recovery in mental health: Systematic review and narrative synthesis. The British Journal of Psychiatry 199(6):445–52.

Lund C. Brooke-Sumner C, Baingana F et al 2018. Social determinants of mental disorders and the Sustainable Development Goals: A systematic review of reviews. Lancet Psychiatry 5(4):357–69.

Middleton H, Shaw I 2000. Distinguishing mental illness in primary care: We need to separate proper syndromes from generalised distress. British Medical Journal 320(7247): 1420–1.

Molloy L, Fields L, Trostian B et al 2020. Trauma-informed care for people presenting to the emergency department with mental health issues. Emergency Nurse 28(2):30–5.

Morley C, Stankovich J, Peterson G et al 2018. Planning for the future: Emergency department presentation patterns in Tasmania, Australia. International Emergency Nursing 38:34–40.

Muskett C 2014. Trauma-informed care in inpatient mental health settings: A review of the literature. International Journal of Mental Health Nursing 32(1):51–9.

National Aboriginal and Torres Strait Islander Suicide Prevention Strategy 2013. Australian Government Department of Health and Ageing. Online. Available: www1.health.gov.au/internet/publications/publishing.nsf/Content/mental-natsisps-strat-toc/$FILE/National%20Aboriginal%20and%20Torres%20Strait%20Islander%20Suicide%20Prevention%20Strategy%20May%202013.pdf.

National Mental Health Commission 2020. National mental health and wellbeing pandemic response plan 2020. Online. Available: www.mentalhealthcommission.gov.au/getmedia/1b7405ce-5d1a-44fc-b1e9-c00204614cb5/National-Mental-Health-and-Wellbeing-Pandemic-Response-Plan.

National Mental Health Commission 2017. The fifth national mental health and suicide prevention plan. National mental health strategy. Online. Available: www.mentalhealthcommission.gov.au/getmedia/0209d27b-1873-4245-b6e5-49e770084b81/Fifth-National-Mental-Health-and-Suicide-Prevention-Plan.

National Suicide Prevention Project Reference Group 2020. National suicide prevention strategy 2020–2023. Department of Health and Human Services, Victorian Government, COAG. Online. Available: www.coaghealthcouncil.gov.au/Portals/0/Reports/2001614_National%20Suicide%20Prevention%20Strategy-2020-2023%20FINAL.pdf.

Opoku ST, Apenteng BA, Akowuah EA et al 2018. Disparities in emergency department wait time among patients with mental health and substance-related disorders. Journal of Behavioral Health Services & Research 45(2):204–18.

Perera J, Wand T, Bein KJ et al 2018. Presentations to NSW emergency departments with self-harm, suicidal ideation, or intentional poisoning 2010–2014. The Medical Journal of Australia 208(8):348–53.

Pointer SC 2019. Trends in hospitalised injury, Australia 2007–08 to 2016–17. Injury research and statistics series no. 124. Cat. no. INJCAT 204. AIHW, Canberra.

Rickwood D, Paraskakis M, Quin D et al 2019. Australia's innovation in youth mental health care: The headspace centre model. Early Intervention in Psychiatry 13(1):159–66.

Robertson N, Polonsky M, McQuilken L 2014. Are my symptoms serious, Dr Google? A resource-based typology of value co-destruction in online self-diagnosis. Australasian Marketing Journal 22(3):246–56.

Rosenberg, S, Hickie I 2019. No gold medals: Assessing Australia's international mental health performance. Australasian Psychiatry 27(1):36–40.

Selye H 1956. The stress of life. McGraw-Hill, New York.

Slade M, Bird V, Clarke E et al 2015. Supporting recovery in patients with psychosis through care by community-based adult mental health teams (REFOCUS): A multisite, cluster, randomised, controlled trial. The Lancet Psychiatry 2(6):503–14.

Spittlehouse JK, Boden JM, Horwood LJ 2020. Sexual orientation and mental health over the life course in a birth cohort. Psychological Medicine 50(8):1348–55.

Stapleberg NJC, Sveticic J, Hughes I et al 2020. Suicidal presentations to emergency departments in a large Australian Public Health Service over 10 years. International Journal of Environmental Research and Public Health 17:5920.

Sveticic J, Stapelberg NC, Turner K 2020. Suicidal and self-harm presentations to Emergency Departments: The challenges of identification through diagnostic codes and presenting complaints. Health Information Management Journal 49(1):38–46.

Sweeney A, Filson B, Kennedy A et al 2018. A paradigm shift: Relationships in trauma-informed mental health services. BJ Psych Advances 24(5):319–33.

Tran QN, Lambeth LG, Sanderson K et al 2020. Emergency department presentations with a mental health diagnosis in Australia, by jurisdiction and by sex 2004–05 to 2016–17. Emergency Medicine Australia 32:383–92.

Tran QN, Lambeth LG, Sanderson K et al 2019. Trends of emergency department presentations with a mental health diagnosis by age, Australia 2004–05 to 2016–17: A secondary data analysis. Emergency Medicine Australasia 31:1064–72.

Ungar M 2011. The social ecology of resilience: Addressing contextual and cultural ambiguity of a nascent construct. American Journal of Orthopsychiatry 81(1):1–17.

van Weeghel J, van Zelst C, Boertien D et al 2019. Conceptualizations, assessments, and implications of personal recovery in mental illness: A scoping review of systematic reviews and meta-analyses. Psychiatric Rehabilitation Journal 42(2):169–81.

Wand T, Crawford C, Bell N et al 2019. Documenting the pre-implementation phase for a multi-site translational research project to test a new model Emergency Department-based mental health nursing care. International Emergency Nursing 45:10–16.

World Health Organization (WHO) 1946. Preamble to the Constitution of the World Health Organization as adopted by the International Health Conference, New York 19–22 June 1946. WHO, New York.

World Health Organization (WHO) 2018. Social determinants of health. WHO, Geneva. Online. Available: www.who.int/social_determinants/sdh_definition/en/.

World Health Organization (WHO) 2001. Strengthening mental health promotion. WHO, Geneva. (Fact sheet, No. 220). Online. Available: www.who.int/whr/2001/en/whr01_en.pdf.

CHAPTER 2
MENTAL HEALTH TRIAGE IN EMERGENCY SETTINGS

Leigh Peterson, Peta Marks and Cathy Daniel

KEY POINTS

- Triage systems for mental health presentations to emergency services.
- Determining the urgency of presentations amid mental health complexity and severity.
- Understanding safety in work and safety in care.
- Collaborative practices with emergency mental health liaison team.
- Assessing and responding to people presenting with acute mental illness deterioration and psychological distress.

LEARNING OUTCOMES

This chapter will assist you to:
- develop a more comprehensive overview of mental health triage in the emergency setting
- identify the factors that should be considered when undertaking a triage assessment of someone with a suspected mental health concern
- discuss why a review of triage category might occur
- develop confidence in determining risk and interventions required relevant to the triage category
- manage clients who demonstrate challenging behaviours during triage.

INTRODUCTION

As outlined in Chapter 1, the Emergency Department (ED) is considered the 'front door' of the healthcare system (ACEM 2018) and is frequently the first point of access to specialist mental health services (Wand et al 2021). Triage is an essential function of the ED. It is expected to take no longer than 2–5 minutes and determines the urgency of the presentation, including identification of the presenting problem, clinical history and pertinent physical observations (ACEM 2016). Triage is identified as the highest risk nursing activity for patient-related violence as patients have just arrived, may be acutely distressed and may be intoxicated with alcohol or other drugs (Pich et al 2017). The triage role is therefore carried out by an experienced registered nurse who is able to engage in agile decision making, anticipate the possibility of rapid deterioration, and determine how resource-intensive the person's condition is likely to be (Yancey 2020). Where someone presents with suspected mental health concerns, the initial triage can involve making sometimes difficult and complex decisions, and these often have to be made quickly and based on minimal information, to expedite appropriate intervention(s) and ensure patient safety and comfort (Varndell et al 2019).

Referral on for specialist mental health triage is a secondary triage process, where a mental health nurse will conduct a comprehensive mental health assessment and make further recommendations and referrals. The secondary mental health triage may take many hours (Broadbent et al 2020). Where mental health consultation liaison nurses work as part of the ED structure (at point of triage or in bespoke lower stimulus environments such as behaviour assessment units) rates of violence, behaviour disturbance and restrictive practices are reduced (Bost et al 2014; Daniel et al 2021; Wand 2021).

THE AUSTRALASIAN TRIAGE SCALE

In Australia and New Zealand, triage guidelines were developed first in 1994 (the National Triage Scale) and became known as the Australasian Triage Scale (ATS) in 2002, and used in EDs nationally since. Their purpose is to describe and grade clinical urgency, to determine priority needs and clarify appropriate actions (Procter et al 2016). Clinical urgency refers to the need for time-critical interventions and is not synonymous with severity or complexity.

The ATS includes five categories of acuity, from life-threatening to minor conditions, and includes timeframes within which a patient should receive care. Patients triaged to lower acuity categories may be safe to wait longer for assessment and treatment, but may still require hospital admission. The five categories are:
1. Resuscitation (see immediately)
2. Emergency (see within 10 minutes)
3. Urgent (see within 30 minutes)
4. Semi-urgent (see within 60 minutes)
5. Non-urgent (see within 120 minutes).

The ATS includes 79 clinical descriptors that relate to a person's presenting problem(s), appearance and pertinent physiological findings (Yancey 2021). The basic descriptors have been expanded to include more nuanced definitions relating to presentations where mental health is of key concern (Department of Health 2013). See Table 2.1 for detail of these descriptors.

Assessment of overall risk will influence the ED triage category selected for each individual.

Factors to be considered when determining a triage category for a person presenting with suspected mental health problems include:
- Has a physical/organic cause for the problem been excluded (e.g. head injury, dementia, delirium)?

- Has drug and /or alcohol intoxication been excluded as a cause?
- Is the person physically well enough (e.g. not sedated, intoxicated, vomiting or in pain) to undertake an interview with mental health staff?
- Is the person demonstrating behaviours of risk?

When triaging people who present with co-occurring conditions, the clinical symptom that is most life-threatening should guide the triage category.

While this chapter will focus on risks commonly considered in relation to mental health and the triage process, it is important to remember that there are many other issues relating to risk and safety in the context of a person's experience of mental ill-health, including (but not limited to):

- risk of being a victim of abuse, aggression and violence
- risk of homelessness and poverty
- risk of significant physical health problems (such as weight gain and metabolic syndrome) related to side effects from psychiatric medications
- risk of injury to the person associated with the use of restrictive interventions in health care settings
- risk of trauma or re-traumatisation experiences in healthcare settings relating to actions, attitudes or behaviours of others, including health professionals.

TRIAGE AND THE ISSUE OF 'RISK' AND SAFETY

Identifying whether or not a person is a risk to self or others is a core function of the triage process. Triage nurses use reported and observed information and determine risk based on clinical judgement (Daniel 2015). There is increasing evidence that brings into question the usefulness of risk assessments in mental health settings (Wand 2012). In an ED setting the best approach is to focus on collaboration with the person and explore the person's individual circumstances, risks and strengths. This includes considering:

- Why is the person presenting now? What are the recent triggers? (e.g. ask about interpersonal relationships)
- Does the person appear to pose an immediate risk to self, you or others?
- Does the person have any immediate (i.e. within the next few minutes or hours) intentions to harm self or others?
- Is the person displaying a high level of distressed behaviour that suggests psychosis and/or immediate risk?
- Does the person appear to be experiencing delusions or hallucinations?
- Is the person aggressive and/or threatening?
- Does the person have a history of violence?
- Is there any suggestion, or does it appear likely, that the person may try to abscond?
- Does the person have a history of self-harm?
- Is the person stating that they want to die? Do they feel that life is not worth living?
- Do they feel hopeless?
- Does the person have a history of mental health problems or psychiatric illness?
- What is the person's level of social support (i.e. partner/significant other, family members of friends), and are they in attendance in the ED?

TABLE 2.1 Australian Triage Scale (ATS) Emergency Department Triage Mental Health Descriptor

Category 1: Immediate	Category 2: Emergency (10 minutes)
Risk: • Definite danger to self/others' life/lives • Severe behavioural disorder with immediate threat of dangerous violence *Observed:* • Violent behaviour • Possession of a weapon • Self-harm in the ED • Extreme agitation/restlessness • Bizarre or disorientated behaviours *Reported:* • Command hallucinations – unable to resist commands to harm self/others • Recent actual violence *Supervision:* • Continuous 1:1 visual observation *Action:* Immediate alert: • Medical staff & MH triage nurse • Ensure safe environment for all • Provide adequate personnel to safely restrain/detain person – follow all policy/protocols *Consider:* • Security/police if required • AOD intoxication may escalate risk	*Risk:* • Probable danger to self/others • Patient requires/is physically restrained/contained • Violent/aggressive with immediate threat to self or others *Observed:* • Extreme agitation/restlessness • Physical/verbal aggression • Confused/can't cooperate • Hallucinating/delusional/paranoid • High risk of absconding/leaving prior to treatment *Reported:* • Attempted/threatened self-harm • Threatening harm to others • Cannot wait safely *Supervision:* • Continuous observation (visual) *Action:* • Immediate alert medical staff & MH triage nurse • Ensure safe environment for all • Defusing strategies – medication, low stimulus environment • Prepare for safe restraint if required • Assess promptly *Consider:* • Re-triage to Cat 1 if diffusion strategies ineffective • Security attend until patient treated • AOD intoxication may escalate risk

Commonwealth of Australia 2009.

Category 3: Urgent (30 minutes)	Category 4: Semi-Urgent (60 minutes)	Category 5: Non-Urgent (120 minutes)
Risk: • Possible danger to self/others • Moderately disturbed behaviour • Severely distressed • Risk of/actual self-harm • Acute psychosis/thought disorder • Situational crisis *Observed:* • Agitated/restless/withdrawn • Intrusive • Confused • Ambivalent about treatment/staying • Unlikely to wait *Reported:* • Suicidal thoughts • Situational crisis • Presence of psychotic symptoms • Presence of severe mood disturbance *Supervision:* • Regular close observation (10 mins) • Needs support person if in waiting room *Action:* • Alert MH triage nurse • Provide safe environment for all *Consider:* • Inform security • Re-triage if behavioural disturbance increases • AOD intoxication may escalate risk	*Risk:* • No immediate risk to self/others • Under observation *Observed:* • Not agitated/restless • Irritable but not aggressive • Cooperative with staff • Provides coherent history *Reported:* • Pre-existing mental health condition • Anxiety/depression symptoms without suicidal thoughts/behaviours • Prepared to wait *Supervision:* • Intermittent observation (30 mins) *Action:* • Discuss with MH triage nurse *Consider:* • Re-triage if behavioural disturbance increases • AOD intoxication may escalate risk	*Risk:* • No danger to self/others • Not acutely distressed/disturbed behaviour • Known PT, chronic symptoms • Social crisis, clinically well *Observed:* • Cooperative • Can discuss concerns • Follows instructions • Communicative • Participates in management planning *Reported:* • Known patient, chronic symptoms/unexplained somatic symptoms • Pre-existing non-acute mental health condition • Request medication/minor adverse side effects • Psychosocial stressors – finance, housing, social, relational *Supervision:* • General observation (1 hour) *Action:* • Discuss with MH triage nurse • Contact case manager/treating team

Observe a person's appearance and behaviour:

- Does the person appear obviously distressed, markedly anxious or highly aroused?
- Is the person's behaviour consistent with the situation?
- Is the person quiet and withdrawn, or loud and demanding?
- Is the person attentive and cooperative?

SAFETY IN CARE, SAFETY AT WORK

Interpreting, understanding and responding to high levels of distress are important skills for all nurses and other health professionals working in emergency settings. Understanding the social context within which safe care and work occurs is essential for identifying the numerous factors that precede and influence safety. A range of factors are in play (see Table 2.2):

Underlying principles

It is important to understand some general principles in creating safety in care and work (McAllister et al 2019).

TABLE 2.2 Factors that impact on safety in care, safety at work

Factors	Description
Staff	• Knowledge, skills, attitudes and subsequent behaviours are an important aspect of preventing, mitigating and managing how we deliver care • Engaging with people in a person-centred way, showing respect and being courteous, actively listening to people's fears and frustrations, and responding in an empathic way and communicating a genuine desire to help, is required. • Clinicians who are unable or unwilling to facilitate effective therapeutic relationships are likely to encounter difficulties in delivering care (Stein-Parbury 2016)
Patient/ consumer	• Among other things, distress, overwhelm, previous negative experiences within healthcare settings, the experience of mental illness and disorder can influence a person's ability to engage purposefully in healthcare and can influence the likelihood of difficulties in safe care delivery
Environmental	• Physical environment (i.e. noisy, crowded, too hot/cold, no natural light, lack of privacy) • Policies, procedures and practices (e.g. coercive or restrictive processes that limit choice)
Cultural	• Behavioural and communication nuances, along with perceptions of health and ill-health, may be interpreted variously by people from different cultural backgrounds • The need for cultural awareness has significant implications for nurses in the context of safe care and work (Holand 2017).
Social	• Negative labels can influence how we as professionals engage with people, including our language, e.g. people with mental illness labelled as 'at risk', 'dangerous', 'difficult', 'manipulative', 'absconders' and/or 'frequent fliers' • When labels are attributed to people, they can consequently be adopted by them, and individuals may therefore engage in behaviour that perpetuates these labels (Brunero et al 2018).

Brunero & Lamont 2020, pp. 51–3.

VERBAL INTERACTIONS

How we say things can often be more important than *what* we say. Use an appropriate tone of voice; the rate at which you talk and the volume and pressure in your speech can influence how you engage with someone. Make adjustments to the 'how' of speaking. Ask yourself, 'Am I speaking loud enough?', 'Am I too loud, and am I sounding threatening?'

Fine-tune your tone of voice as the interaction with the person occurs, test and retest your approach. Linking your words with actions can convey a sense that you are interested and can help maintain therapeutic rapport. Alternatively, if you show incongruence between your words and actions, the person and others may interpret this as you being untrustworthy and lacking authenticity.

NON-VERBAL INTERACTIONS

Non-verbal communication, how you hold yourself or behave, is important to engagement. Through body language we constantly (and sometimes unconsciously) send and receive non-verbal signals. Awareness of the non-verbal signals you are sending may be particularly useful. Your words might convey one message, but the movements and gestures you make might convey another, potentially creating confusion, misunderstanding and an array of negative feelings. The following are some ways of non-verbally responding:

- While you are talking, try to be aware of how you are sitting or standing, the expression on your face and what your hands and legs are doing.
- Let the person determine the distance between yourself and them. This may help them to feel some sense of control. Personal space or distance can vary according to cultural or personal nuances.
- Keep a relaxed open posture with your hands visible at either waist height or below to make yourself appear less threatening.
- It is helpful to make intermittent eye contact (avoid prolonged eye contact or staring).
- Use appropriate facial expressions for the situation– seek a balance between smiling and looking concerned. Expressions of warmth and acceptance can help. Be mindful that your position, movements and gestures may need to vary depending on the clinical situation.

Being flexible

Nursing requires the ability to be flexible and engage in different approaches. Nurses are often tempted to take control, when a more helpful approach is to consider how you can help the person to maintain or regain internal self-control – care versus control is a good mantra to keep in mind. You may be required to restructure requests and allow time for information to be processed. This requires qualities such as being patient and empathic, as well as skills in redirecting and negotiating.

Active listening

Active listening shows that we are attending to someone's needs. The act of active listening starts a process of being empathic and may give you more time to formulate your response. Reflecting on what the person is saying while taking a position of not offering advice, but expressing acceptance without agreeing may offer the person a more comfortable position to reflect on their behaviour. Active listening demonstrates the presence of empathy and helps people to acknowledge their emotions, enabling them to talk about their emotions as opposed to negatively acting upon them (Stein-Parbury 2016).

Empathy

A sense of openness can be developed by disclosing our concerns and issues with the person openly and honestly. Empathising with the person's feelings and trying to appreciate their point of view gives the person a sense that you are acknowledging their concerns and trying to connect with them (Gerace et al 2018). Respecting different points of view does not mean you agree with them; you can accept someone's experience, without the need to agree with it (Gerace et al 2018).

Assertiveness

Being assertive is a skill that requires careful consideration so as not to appear punitive or indeed aggressive. It may involve reflecting on your own experience while simultaneously setting expectations about behaviour from others. This approach involves displaying high levels of empathy while setting clear limits or boundaries. The following are examples of assertiveness statements that demonstrate showing empathy and setting limits in a way that is non-judgemental and therefore humanistic:

> 'You are speaking very loudly, and I am finding it hard to understand how I can help you.'

> 'You seem distressed and angry. Can we talk more when you are ready?'

Combining these assertiveness statements with statements such as, 'I realise you don't want to do this', 'I understand this is a stressful situation' and 'I appreciate you are trying', can also be helpful. It is important to avoid argument, conflicting advice and long-winded explanations.

Some situations may also require a firm and concise request about what needs to happen; for example:

> 'Can you please put down the syringe so I can help you with your injury.'

> 'I need you to spend some time in this area because your behaviour is upsetting some people.'

As you repeat your expectations your message is reinforced. Provided that your demeanour is not aggressive and your response is consistent, this offers the best opportunity for the person to modify their behaviour. Be mindful to acknowledge any satisfactory outcome; saying 'thank you' and showing humility are extremely powerful tools in any nurse–patient relationship.

ASSESSING AND MANAGING AGITATION AND DISTRESS

The word 'agitated' is often used to describe some of the behaviours seen in healthcare settings. Agitation is a signal that something is wrong. It can be the person's reaction to distress or an extremely abnormal situation (Renwick et al 2016). Aggression or aggressive behaviour is frequently perceived to be hostile, injurious or destructive, and is often caused by frustration. Sometimes, despite our best attempts at being empathic and actively listening, people become frustrated and agitated. While the anger may be directed towards you as the nurse, it is not directed towards you as a person. Although this difference appears subtle, the implications can be significant. By not personalising the behaviour, but rather seeing it through the eyes of your professional role, this will help you remain objective (Brunero & Lamont 2020, p. 57).

In emergencies, it can be difficult to differentiate between an acute behavioural disturbance resulting from acute drug intoxication, drug-induced psychosis, extreme distress relating to overwhelming emotions, organic disorders mimicking mental health deterioration or exacerbation of a pre-existing mental disorder or illness (Muir-Cochrane et al 2019). There are many causes for agitated behaviour that are *not* related to a person's mental health (see Box 2.1). As such, it is always important to consider whether a person's agitated behaviour is related to an underlying serious and possibly life-threatening condition which requires urgent medical intervention.

As each person presents, it is important for the triage nurse to consider:
- Can I safely interview this person on my own or do I need backup?
- Is the person going to be safe where they are?
- Can the person be left alone and/or with others (e.g. in the waiting room) safely?
- What degree of observation does the person need and can it be provided safely in the ED?
- Where is the most appropriate place to interview the person, given their level of arousal and agitation? (Procter et al 2016, p. 1038)

De-escalation strategies

Where a person is becoming agitated, is verbally aggressive, or there are concerns about the potential for behaviour to escalate, strategies that support de-escalation are required.

Box 2.1 Examples of possible underlying causes of acute behavioural disturbance

Non-medical	General medical	Intoxication or withdrawal
<ul><li>Relationship conflict</li><li>Anniversaries of past traumatic events</li><li>Interactions with police or security staff</li><li>Distress experienced by people with intellectual disability or autism</li><li>Family violence</li></ul>	<ul><li>Head trauma</li><li>Encephalitis, meningitis or other infection</li><li>Encephalopathy, particularly from liver or renal failure</li><li>Toxins, including prescription medication</li><li>Metabolic derangement</li><li>Thyroid disease</li><li>Seizure or post-ictal state</li><li>Pain, especially in people with intellectual disability or autism</li></ul>	<ul><li>Alcohol</li><li>Marijuana</li><li>Nicotine</li><li>CNS stimulants e.g. cocaine, methamphetamine</li><li>CNS depressants e.g. GHB, opioids, benzodiazepines, THC</li><li>Hallucinogens and dissociatives, e.g. LSD, magic mushrooms</li><li>Novel psychoactive substances, e.g. synthetic cannabinoids</li></ul>

CNS = central nervous system; GHB = gamma hydroxybutyrate; THC = tetrahydrocannabinol (marijuana); LSD = lysergic acid diethylamide

Safer Care Victoria 2021.

De-escalation aims to bring about resolution through effective communication techniques (not force) and its success is underpinned by an empathic, respectful and collaborative approach by the nurse (Price et al 2018). The goal is to ensure the safety of the patient, staff and others, to assist the patient to gain control of their emotional state, to avoid physical or mechanical restraint, and avoid coercive interventions (Richmond et al 2012). De-escalation involves understanding common signs of escalating behaviours (see Box 2.2) and an ability to use communication skills to purposefully engage anxious, emotionally aroused or agitated people (see Table 2.3) (Brunero & Lamont 2020, pp. 57–8). It is important to remember that 'risk is reduced when people feel respected, consulted, listened to and valued (Commonwealth of Australia 2013)' (Wand 2015, p. 1).

In situations where de-escalation techniques are unsuccessful or inappropriate, many health services have adopted a tiered approach to pharmacological management. This enables medical and nursing staff to escalate or reduce interventions, depending on response to treatment or sedation, to minimise the use of restrictive interventions. The most significant risk is prolonged sedation requiring respiratory support (Muir-Cohrane et al 2019). The sedation assessment tool (SAT) (see Table 2.4 for details) can be used to measure and describe a person's level of distress throughout the care episode, and support an appropriate response to deterioration in mental state (Calver et al 2011).

Box 2.2 The STAMP Framework

The STAMP framework identifies behaviours that can indicate a person's distress is increasing and which may increase the potential for behavioural escalation (i.e. violence or aggression) – particularly where frequency or intensity of the behaviours is increasing.

Staring and eye-contact
- Prolonged glaring at staff
- Absence of eye contact (culture and disability dependent)

Tone and volume of voice
- Sharp retorts
- Sarcasm
- Increased volume
- Demeaning inflection

Anxiety
- Flushed appearance
- Hyperventilation
- Rapid speech
- Expressed lack of understanding about care processes

Mumbling
- Talking under their breath
- Criticising care just loud enough to be heard
- Repetition of same or similar phrases

Pacing
- Walking around confined areas
- Walking back and forth to staff station
- Flailing around in bed

Adapted from Luck et al 2007.

Table 2.3 De-escalation: Principles, attributes and interventions

Communication	
Establish contact early in escalation	One person engages in a calm and measured way; use the person's name, and yours, use language tactfully
Non-provocative engagement	Relax your body, a calm demeanour, intermittent eye contact and non-threatening posture. Use an appropriate tone of voice and engage assertively.
Focus on person's current needs and experiences	Violent behaviour is a primitive form of communicating that something is wrong or a need is not being met. *"We're here to help you. How best can we do that?"*
Active listening	Ask open ended questions. Convey that you are interested and check you understand. *"Am I correct in saying…?"*
Display empathy	Empathy in verbal and non-verbal communication. Listen, offer understanding. *"I can appreciate how this is affecting you."*
Be concise	Concentration is compromised when emotionally aroused. Speak clearly, slowly, avoid medical terminology. *"We're concerned about your health and your safety."*
Agree or accept	Validate concerns and concentrate on opportunities for agreement. *"I would feel angry too if I had to wait this long."*
Offer choices and optimism	Offer choice where relevant. Perceived acts of kindness and comfort (e.g. food, blanket, pain relief) can help *"I'm sorry I can't do that, but I can help you with…"*
Self-regulation	
Self-control/remain calm	Use an appropriate tone of voice; engage assertively not emotively or confrontationally. Breathe and count to 3 before engaging.
Non-judgemental approach	Avoid making judgements, don't personalise challenging behaviour; separate feelings about the person and the problem. *"I don't think that about you at all."*
Self-reflection	Consider and make sense of what went well or not so well. Ask yourself and colleagues, *"Could I have done anything differently?"*
Assessment	
Is it safe to intervene?	Assess risk associated with intervention. What would happen if you did nothing, or waited for support? *"I need you to put that blade down before I can help."*
Here and now	Assess the person's emotional state or the immediate situation in relation to safety for all. Other aspects of assessment and intervention can wait.
Escalating aggression	Observe and recognise known early warning signs.
Actions	
Positional imitation	Stand if the person is standing, sit if they are sitting. Successful de-escalation requires a sense of equity. *'Do you mind if I sit down?"*
Reduce stimuli; create a safe space	Decrease environmental stimuli and encourage private interaction. *"Can we move over here and talk in private?"*
Distraction	Re-direct the person's attention from escalating behaviour. *"Is there anyone you'd like me to call to let them know you are safe?" "Can I get you a drink?"*

Continued

Table 2.3 De-escalation: Principles, attributes and interventions—cont'd

Set limits	Ensure limits can be consistently applied. Be clear about what you would like to happen and that you want to help. Be non-confrontational and respectful. *"When you're shouting, I find it hard to understand how I can help."*
Therapeutic treatment	Identify and alleviate causes of escalating behaviour where possible e.g. pain, confusion *"Can I give you something to help with the pain?"*
Maintain safety	
Situational awareness	Remain vigilant. Keep exits clear and accessible. Remove or moderate potential weapons, dangers and triggers. *"If you could put the syringe down, I'll attend to that."*
Situational support	Communication with colleagues is essential. Be mindful an excessive show of force can escalate a person's behaviour. *"No one's in trouble. The police are here for everyone's safety."*
Approach with caution	Approach in a measured way, avoid sudden movements. Maintain distance until you feel it is safe for close proximity *"Can we take a look at that injury?"*
Respect personal space	More personal space than usual may be required; be mindful not to appear fearful or disinterested *"I won't come any closer, I just want to talk."*
Debrief all involved	Post-incident support for the person: *"That must have been stressful. We did that because…"*, bystanders: *"That must have been difficult to watch. Are you ok?"* and colleagues: *"Are you ok? How do you think that went?"*

Adapted from Brunero & Lamont 2020, pp. 59–61.

TABLE 2.4 The Sedation Assessment Tool (SAT)

Sedation Assessment Tool	Responsiveness and speech	Visual observations	Strategies	Restrictive practice
+3	Severe behavioural disorder with immediate threat of dangerous violence High levels of physical activity, may demonstrate markedly increased levels of verbal abuse Cannot control signs of agitation if requested to do so	Requires continuous (special) nursing care/supervision and may require physical restraint	Imminent risk – Emergency code for personal threat Call team huddle Decide team response to deterioration Decide if police assistance is required	Consider mechanical restraint until emergency chemical sedation reaches efficacy Document interventions per local hospital instructions Restraint should be used as *last resort* when comprehensive de-escalation strategies have proved ineffective

TABLE 2.4 The Sedation Assessment Tool (SAT)—cont'd

Sedation Assessment Tool	Responsiveness and speech	Visual observations	Strategies	Restrictive practice
+2	Moderate levels of physical activity, Increased levels of verbal abuse May be verbally threatening to self or others Increased risk of violence or aggression	May require increase from regular hourly observation by nursing staff to continuous (special) nursing care/supervision	Implement MDT review within next hour Review identified calming strategies Contact mental health liaison team	Ongoing review of the need for restraint Restraint is a traumatic and distressing experience for patients and may inadvertently escalate agitated behaviour
+1	Slightly increased levels of physical activity May raise his or her voice volume, Is not threatening or violent Distressed, risk of self-harm Acutely psychotic or thought disordered	Requires regular nursing care/supervision 60/60	Utilise consumer's advance care plan or ED management plan, focus on de-escalation strategies and offer debrief for patient	Does not require physical, mechanical or chemical restraint
0	Normal levels of physical activity, Normal levels of verbal expression, awake with eyes continuously open Under observation and/or no immediate risk to self or others Known patient with chronic symptoms	Requires regular nursing care/supervision 60/60	Utilise consumer's advance care plan or ED management plan, focus on de-escalation strategies and underlying principles of creating safety in care and work	Does not require physical, mechanical or chemical restraint
−1	Slightly reduced levels of verbal and physical activity Eyes intermittently open Asleep but rouses to voice Remains awake when stimulus removed	Requires regular nursing care/supervision 60/60	Utilise consumer's advance care plan or ED management plan, focus on underlying principles of creating safety in care and work	Does not require physical, mechanical or chemical restraint

Continued

TABLE 2.4 The Sedation Assessment Tool (SAT)—cont'd

Sedation Assessment Tool	Responsiveness and speech	Visual observations	Strategies	Restrictive practice
−2	Sleeping deeply, aroused by moderate verbal (calling name) or physical stimulation (shaking shoulders) Returns to sleep immediately when stimulus is removed	Consideration should be given to upgrading level of observation from regular 60/60 to continuous the more sedated the person	Implement team huddle within an hour Review/ documentation of interventions If post overdose discuss with specialist team	Mechanical restraint in this patient is considered dangerous
−3	Sleeping deeply, cannot be aroused by either vigorous verbal or physical stimulation (sternal rub)	Continuous (special) observations are required in a cardiac monitored bed. Consider transfer to Resus/Resus step down	Medical emergency response code Decide medical response to deterioration	Restraint in this patient is considered dangerous, owing to risk of aspiration, difficulty to attend to airway management and inability to assess medical status

MDT = multidisciplinary team

Adapted from Calver, Stokes & Isbister 2011

It is important to remember that no pharmacological protocol is 100% safe, and sedation should only be used when all other simpler, safer, less restrictive measures have failed, and the patient is deemed to be a significant risk to self or others. As such, the approach to pharmacological management should always be part of an overall management plan that includes appropriate nursing care and de-escalation techniques.

The scenarios below describe two different situations and demonstrate the ATS category and SAT rating that would be applied in the circumstances. You will be asked to reflect on how you feel about these scenarios and what thoughts and attitudes might impact on your practice in such situations.

Practice Example

Boris is a 43-year-old single male of European background, with a known diagnosis of schizoaffective disorder. He is routinely seen by the community mental health team on a community treatment order. He has previously experienced relapses in relation to poor adherence with recommended treatment, and/or illicit substance use.

Boris has been brought into the ED by police after presenting to the police station to file a complaint about his neighbours. He stated they were controlling him by remote control switches, poisoning his coffee and cigarettes, and raping him overnight. He became very combative at the police station – he kicked in the windscreen of a police car with his bare feet and was involved in a tussle with a police officer, attempting to dislodge and discharge her firearm. Boris was pepper sprayed at the scene and is bleeding from his feet and legs. In the ED, Boris is shouting and kicking out at staff. He is experiencing pain from the pepper spray in his eyes, being handcuffed by police and the wounds to his legs and feet. He is understandably distressed at being held and controlled by a large group of people, which is contributing to his escalating paranoia.

In circumstances such as these, it can be difficult to consider how to offer comfort to the person and ensure a safe environment for all. Asking yourself the following questions might help you to determine your approach:
- What ATS category would you apply and why?
- What SAT rating would you apply and what rating would you aim for?
- What management or interventions would you initiate?
- What other information would you need?
- What category of risk does the person meet?
- What risk would you identify first?

It will also be important to reflect on how you feel in this type of situation, and how your practice might be impacted.

Reflection

1. Have you ever looked after a patient like Boris?
2. What emotions does this scenario evoke for you?
3. Why do you think it is important for staff to acknowledge that caring for people such as Boris can cause distress or difficult emotions?

Caring for Boris may result in fear, anger or frustration, as well as generating strong negative emotions within teams about how some staff approach the patient. For example, some staff may believe that Boris should not have been brought to the ED and staff should not have to care for people who are acutely agitated. It is important to be aware of our own emotions, so that we do not react in ways that are punitive or overly restrictive towards the person. And, where restrictive practices *are* used, ensure that they are removed as soon as possible.

ATS AND SAT RATING

The situation is assessed as requiring immediate intervention due to evidence of extreme risk relating to violent behaviour. It is recognised that a team response is required to ensure safety for patient, staff and others. ATS Category 1 and SAT +3. See Table 2.5 for the ATS assessment relating to Boris.

SOMATIC COMPLAINTS AND PSYCHOLOGICAL DISTRESS

Some people present to the ED with physical (somatic) symptoms that occur as the result of psychological distress – for example, pain (commonly chest pain or abdominal pain) or neurological symptoms not explained by a medical condition (e.g. sudden onset blindness), or preoccupation with concern about a serious medical problem where no problem exists

TABLE 2.5 ATS assessment for Boris

Observed	Ongoing aggression and violence, including spitting at staff and attempting to smear blood on staff, verbal abuse; requiring physical restraint. Marked volatility, property damage, threats to others. Observed to be responding to auditory hallucinations.
Reported	Bruno is expressing delusional ideas with bizarre themes - stating that he is the "father of the world's armies" and will "control staff DNA by transmission of (his) blood". At the police station, Bruno demonstrated significant paranoid and persecutory ideas – about his neighbours – and aggressive behaviour towards police and property.
Supervision	Bruno requires team response and physical and possibly mechanical restraint for his safety and the safety of others. Ongoing 1:1 observation required while restrictive measures are in place.
Action	Call emergency response code for immediate medical and mental health presence. Ensure adequate personnel to attend to restraint and ongoing safety of Bruno, staff and others. Police may assist in restraining Bruno in order for staff to attend to physical wounds, stem flow of blood and apply cold compresses to face to remove pepper spray. Allocate a clinician to be at Bruno's head. Attempt to reassure Bruno and explain what is happening, at each stage. He may not comprehend the reassurances at the time, but Bruno will remember the care he was offered when he returns to his baseline health. Provide goggles and or shields to protect staff from spitting Medication for sedation, for safety and to enable: • re-assessment after any acute effects of suspected illicit substance use have worn off • a more accurate differential diagnosis • assist in the provision of a safe environment. The aim of this intervention is to drop the SAT score to –1, where the patient is drowsy though rousable to voice and not necessarily sedated. The aim is to use restrictive practices sparingly and for our interventions to not worsen or delay appropriate treatment and assessment.
Consider	• Use of the mental health legislation applicable in your state for compulsory treatment • possibility of recent illicit drug use which may contribute to risk and aggression • possibility patient may be armed or have weapon on his person or in his possession

(Moukaddam et al 2015). People who have a low threshold for managing psychological distress can tend to experience pain and other physical symptoms more intensely, and often feel their symptoms and underlying problems are not validated or fully explored or treated. This can quickly lead to escalation in distress, frequent re-presentations to the ED, self-harm behaviours, feeling disgruntled and/or that their concerns have not been taken seriously. In such situations, there is potential for antagonistic relationships between staff and the person to develop. Judgemental terms such as 'attention seeking', 'manipulative', 'frequent flyer' persist in clinical practice and are unhelpful. It is more helpful to consider that the person's behaviour serves a function – identifying that function requires careful, professional assessment and collaborative advance planning to support patients in crisis (Anonymous 2021). Importantly, frequent presentations do not justify withholding medical or mental health assistance (Moukaddam et al 2015; Palombini et al 2021).

Where people with complex needs present frequently to the ED, an advance care plan is often formulated, recommending that physical examination of reported symptom(s)/pain is done by a senior registrar in the ED who will then determine the scope of intervention in liaison with an ED physician and perhaps the mental health liaison team. Generalist nurses working in emergency departments can expect the mental health liaison team to provide culture brokerage between two acute services that often have competing demands, and foster relationships that build confidence in a variety of presentations in the emergency department (Wand & Collett 2021). This collaborative arrangement is primarily about alleviating human suffering, preventing harm and optimising adequate holistic health assessment (Palombini et al 2021).

A thorough assessment of the somatic complaints to exclude an organic cause of symptoms and avoid potentially unwarranted and invasive diagnostic requests can lead to reduction in distress and improved patient care (Moukaddam et al 2015). Advance care planning for people who have attended EDs frequently should be co-produced and should never be used to exclude a person from treatment (Daniel 2021; Palombini et al 2021). ED physicians are tasked with determining imminent factors for medical instability that may be contributing to the behavioural presentation, to ensure organic disorders that pose an imminent threat are identified and minimise delays to disposition planning in the ED (Helman et al 2016; Kverno & Mangano 2021; Moukaddam et al 2015). When safe and appropriate, a detailed history, physical examination, set of vital signs (heart rate, blood pressure, temperature, conscious state) and blood sugar level should be obtained. Full medical clearance work-up is then relegated to patients with higher rates of disease, such as older adults, those with immunosuppression, new onset psychosis and acute substance abuse (Kverno et al 2021). Suggestions are included in Fig. 2.1.

Patients have reported that they value prompt attention, having a trusting relationship with healthcare providers, being active participants in decision-making, learning skills to empower themselves and receiving appropriate information for further supports (Nizum et al 2020). As described in Chapter 1, working from a trauma-informed lens can provide a focused response to help the person re-establish immediate coping skills, provide support, promote a sense of control and self-efficacy, restore pre-crisis functioning and provide access to further services and resources.

Practice Example

Amy is a 21-year-old single Caucasian female university student majoring in law. Amy presents frequently to the ED with unexplained medical symptoms of abdominal pain, which have been extensively investigated and determined to be psychogenically based.

Recently, Amy's presentations have been dominated by loud wailing, clutching her stomach, doubling over and lying on the floor, while she demands opiate administration, specifically fentanyl. Amy has stated that if she isn't given pain relief, she will kill herself. During the current presentation, Amy is accompanied by several friends who are also distressed, demanding urgent help and encouraging outrage from other people in the waiting room.

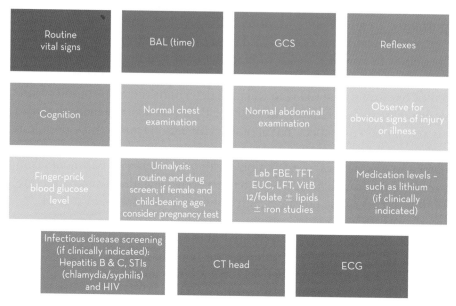

Fig. 2.1 A reckoner for full medical assessment for comorbid physical and mental illnesses. *BAL:* Blood alcohol level; *CT:* computed tomography scan; *ECG:* electrocardiogram; *EUC:* electrolytes (sodium, potassium and chloride), urea, creatinine; *FBE:* full blood examination; *GCS:* Glasgow Coma Scale; *LFT:* liver function test; *STIs:* sexually transmitted infections; *TFT:* thyroid function test; *VitB:* Vitamin B

Consider what clinical factors might mean that Amy was considered:
- ATS category 1
- ATS category 2
- ATS category 3
- ATS category 4
- ATS category 5?

If her SAT was considered a +1, what would be the likely intervention and would that correspond with the ATS?

For each of the above categories, what management or interventions would you initiate? In Table 2.6, you can see the triage nurses' assessment.

Looking at the risk factors and interventions associated with ATS categories in Table 2.1, it would be reasonable to consider that Amy meets criteria for ATS 3, based on her presentation. However, the triage nurse would also consider benefits of up-triaging her to ATS 2 due to the potential for deterioration in her mental state resulting in deliberate self-harm, heightened emotional expression and the possibility of agitating and distressing others in the waiting room.

Reflection

1. What additional information or other risks should staff be aware of, which may result in the revision of the original triage category?

TABLE 2.6 ATS assessment for Amy

Observed	• highly emotionally dysregulated, wailing loudly, disruptive and intrusive towards other patients in the department • any other clinical signs suggestive of an acute abdominal pain?
Reported	Known patient with chronic unexplained somatic symptoms
Supervision	Patient is in the company of people who are compounding her agitation, so they are not considered protective from a risk perspective.
Action	• Provide safe environment for patient and others. • Ensure communication utilises principles of de-escalation, non-verbal communication, verbal communication and environment (Table 2.5) • There is not always capacity within the ED setting to bring someone in quickly, however, if possible, move Amy to a quiet place away from other patients in the waiting room. • Ask Amy's friends to leave – one support person could be invited to stay if they are not themselves being disruptive. Security support may be required.
Consider	A young female, of reproductive age, can have abdominal pain for a variety of reasons, regardless of previous exclusion of acute diagnostics, a physical examination of reported pain is always recommended. Consider that she will not tolerate waiting, in absence of her friends and is likely to act on threats to deliberately self-harm in order to communicate her distress.

Amy is known to make repeated complaints, saying she is 'going to the media', or that she will take legal action against the health service. It is important to be mindful that filming and misreporting incidents on social media occurs without full context and can further inflame situations. However, Amy's propensity to provide negative feedback, in the absence of a change in acuity, would not be considered a reason to up-triage.

Reflection

1. What support could you give to someone who is stating that they will self-harm, to help them to reduce their distress?
2. How could you ensure that a person's expertise is included when drawing up a meaningful plan together to support them?

SUMMARY

Triage nurses are often the first contact point for people presenting to emergency settings experiencing emotional distress (for whatever reason) or mental illness. The triage role requires nurses to make a rapid assessment of risk and safety, consider and manage the complexities associated with the person's needs, balanced with the demands on, and capacity of, the department. Mental health knowledge and skills, particularly communication skills and the ability to identify and intervene with someone whose distress or challenging behaviour is escalating, is essential to the role. Where triage staff are cognisant of working in a person-centred, trauma-informed way, and are confident in providing interventions that maximise effective outcomes, length of stay will be reduced, aggression and critical incidents will be reduced, and the use of restrictive practices will be reduced. Consequently, people presenting with distress or mental illness, as well as staff and other patients, will have a better experience.

Useful websites

Australian College of Mental Health Nurses: https://acmhn.org/
College of Emergency Nurses Australia: www.cena.org.au/
Embrace Multicultural Mental Health Australia: www.embracementalhealth.org.au/
Flourish Australia: flourishaustralia.org.au
LGBTQI+ Australia: www.lgbtiqhealth.org.au/
Mental Health Commission: www.mentalhealthcommission.gov.au/getmedia/1871cc65-e51d-
    43fb-b2d5-7346a17248a9/Safe-in-Care-Safe-at-Work-Abridged-version
Mind Australia: mindaustralia.org.au
Orygen youth mental health: www.orygen.org.au/
Trauma-informed care implementation resource centre: www.traumainformedcare.chcs.org/what-
    is-trauma-informed-care/

References

Anonymous 2021. I am more than a body to stitch up and label. BMJ 373: n1003.
Australian Government, Department of Health and Ageing 2009. Emergency triage education kit. Commonwealth of Australia, Canberra. Online. Available: https://acem.org.au/getmedia/ c9ba86b7-c2ba-4701-9b4f-86a12ab91152/Triage-Education-Kit.aspx.
Bost N, Crilly J, Wallen K 2014. Characteristics and process outcomes of patients presenting to an Australian emergency department for mental health and non-mental health diagnoses. International Emergency Nursing 22(3):146–52.
Broadbent M, Moxham L, Dwyer T 2020. Understanding nurses perspectives of acuity in the process of emergency mental health triage: A qualitative study. Contemporary Nurse 56(3): 280–95.
Brunero S, Lamont S 2020. Safety in care, safety at work. In: Foster K, Marks P, O'Brien A et al (eds) Mental health in nursing: theory and practice for clinical settings, 5th edn. Elsevier Australia, Sydney.
Calver L, Stokes B, Isbister G 2011. Sedation assessment tool to score acute behavioural disturbance in the emergency department. Emergency Medicine Australasia 23:732–40.
Daniel, C 2015. Violence risk screening at ED Triage. Doctoral dissertation. The University of Melbourne, Melbourne.
Daniel C, Gerdtz M, Elsom S et al 2015. Feasibility and need for violence risk screening at triage: an exploration of clinical processes and public perceptions in one Australian emergency department. Emergency Medicine Journal 32(6):457–62.
Daniel C, Mukaro V, Yap C et al 2021. Characteristics and clinical outcomes for mental health patients admitted to a behavioural assessment unit: Implications for model of care and practice. International Journal of Mental Health Nursing 30:255–8.
Helman A, Ovens H, Steinhart B et al 2016. Medical clearance of the psychiatric patient. Emergency medicine cases. Podcast, episode 85. Online. Available: https:// emergencymedicinecases.com/medical-clearance-psychiatric-patient/.

Kverno K, Mangano M 2021. Psychiatric emergencies and the potential role of Psychiatric Mental Health Nurse Practitioners. Journal of Psychosocial Nursing 59(3):7–12.

Luck L, Jackson D, Usher K 2007. STAMP: Components of observable behaviour that indicate potential for patient violence in emergency departments. Journal of Advanced Nursing 59(1): 11–19.

Moukaddam N, AufderHeide E, Flores A et al 2015. Shift, interrupted: Strategies for managing difficult patients including those with personality disorders and somatic symptoms in the Emergency Department. Emergency Medicine Clinics of North America: Psychiatric and Behavioural Emergencies 33(4):797–810.

Muir-Cochrane E, Grimmer K, Gerace A et al 2019. Prevalence of the use of chemical restraint in the management of challenging behaviours associated with adult mental health conditions: A meta-synthesis. Journal of Psychiatric and Mental Health Nursing 27(4):425–45.

Nizum N, Yoon R, Ferreira-Legere L et al 2020. Nursing interventions for adults following a mental health crisis: A systematic review guided by trauma-informed principles. International Journal of Mental Health Nursing 29:351–60.

Palombini E, Richardson J, McAllister E et al 2021. When self-harm is about preventing harm: Emergency management of obsessive-compulsive disorder and associated self-harm. BJPsych Bulletin 45(2):109–14.

Pich JV, Kable A, Hazelton M 2017. Antecedents and precipitants of patient-related violence in the emergency department: Results from the Australian VENT Study (Violence in Emergency Nursing and Triage). Australasian Emergency Care 20(3):107–13.

Procter N, Ferguson M, Munro G et al 2016. Mental health emergencies. In: Curtis K, Ramsden C, Shaban RZ et al (eds) Emergency and trauma care, 2nd edn. Elsevier Australia, Sydney.

Safer Care Victoria 2021. Caring for people displaying acute behavioural disturbance Clinical guidance to improve care in emergency settings. Victorian Government, Melbourne. Online. Available: www.bettersafercare.vic.gov.au/sites/default/files/2020-04/Guidance_Acute%20behavioural%20disturbance.pdf.

Varndell W, Hodge A, Fry M 2019. Triage in Australian emergency departments: Results of a New South Wales survey. Australasian Emergency Care 22(2):81–6.

Wand T 2015. Recovery is about a focus on resilience and wellness, not a fixation with risk and illness. Australian and New Zealand Journal of Psychiatry 49(12):1083–4.

Wand T 2012. Investigating the evidence for the effectiveness of risk assessment in mental health care. Issues in Mental Health Nursing 33:2–7.

Wand T, Collett G, Cutten A et al 2021. Evaluating an emergency department-based mental health liaison nurse service: A multi-site translational research project. Emergency Medicine Australasia 33:74–81.

Yancey CC, O'Rourke MC 2021. Emergency department triage. In: StatPearls [Internet]. Treasure Island (FL): StatPearls PMID: 32491515.

PRACTICE SETTING SCENARIOS

Introduction to the practice-based scenarios

Peta Marks

KEY POINTS

- People experiencing mental health issues, mental illness and mental distress presenting to emergency care settings may, or may not, have a diagnosed mental illness.
- Mental health service delivery occurs across the service spectrum in a stepped care model that is person-centred and recovery-oriented – matching interventions with individual needs.
- All nurses need to develop their mental health nursing knowledge and skills relevant to their clinical setting and scope of practice; generalist and emergency nurses use fundamental mental health knowledge and skills, while mental health nurses use specialised mental health knowledge and skills.

LEARNING OUTCOMES

This chapter will assist you to:

- describe how mental health service delivery is integrated across the health service spectrum in Australia and New Zealand, and where emergency care settings and emergency nurses fit in
- develop further understanding of the elements of effective practice in emergency care settings
- orientate yourself to the framework of the clinical scenarios presented in Chapter 3, which describe how mental health nursing skills can be applied across a range of common presentations.

INTRODUCTION

As described in Chapter 1, our health, mental health and wellbeing are linked to biology, lifestyle, socio-economic and societal factors. Co-occurring drug and alcohol use, trauma, loss and grief, and other critical events also play a role. People's individual circumstances (e.g. social connections, parenting and family), their experience of a range of social determinants (such as housing, education, employment, income), their identity (cultural, spiritual, gender) and the environment all influence health and wellbeing. Importantly, people's beliefs, and the meanings they attribute to health, illness and wellbeing, are individually defined – by age, gender, education, personal experiences and cultural perspectives, which are diverse (McGough et al 2022).

As nurses, no matter which clinical setting we choose to work in, and particularly when working in emergency care settings, we will encounter people experiencing mental illness, or who are in crisis and experiencing mental distress. We will work with people who may be struggling with any number of issues related to the social determinants and other factors outlined above, or who have a life-changing experience as the result of physical or mental illness, who are gravely ill, or who die from disease or injury. We will interact with people's families and friends, and, if we are to practise in a holistic way, we will attempt to make meaning of and understand their experience, considering all the individual circumstances that have impacted on or influence the person's health and wellbeing.

The scenarios that follow have been written by clinicians and people with lived experience. They demonstrate common presentations relevant to the emergency care setting. They include an overview of the red flags that would highlight the possible presence of a mental health issue; and are designed to prompt you to consider the mental health needs of the individuals concerned and the mental health knowledge and skills *you* might need in order to provide comprehensive nursing care in similar situations. By getting you to think 'mental health' across a range of clinical scenarios within the emergency care setting, this chapter aims to support you to provide more holistic nursing care to *all* patients – whether they have a diagnosed mental illness or not.

As a starting point, it is useful to understand how mental health care is integrated across the healthcare system, how nurses provide mental health care in a stepped care model and how emergency care settings 'fit in'. Regardless of the setting, everyone has a role to play.

INTEGRATING MENTAL HEALTH ACROSS THE SERVICE SPECTRUM – STEPPED CARE

Mental health service delivery in Australia and New Zealand occurs in primary, community and hospital settings. While hospital and bed-based services dominated mental health care in the past, the process of deinstitutionalisation and a focus on recovery mean that the preference now is for contemporary mental health services to be delivered in community-based settings.

The co-location of mental health units into mainstream general hospitals has resulted in staff who are working in general hospitals and emergency departments (EDs) having increased contact with service users and clinicians from mental health services. People presenting to emergency care with physical illness or injury experience mental health impacts, and, of course, people with mental illness experience the same physical illnesses as the rest of the population and require medical treatment in emergency settings. In fact, they are at greater risk of physical health problems, such as cancer, cardiovascular disease and diabetes – and average life expectancy is significantly shorter. So, regardless of the reason for a person's presentation, it is essential to be alert to both their physical and mental health concerns.

At all times and in all settings, a 'least restrictive' model of care in relation to mental health is required; that is, one which enhances the person's autonomy, respects their rights, individual worth, dignity and privacy, and where any limitations placed on the person are the minimum necessary … enabling the person to participate as much as possible regarding all decisions that affect them. The philosophy of providing the least restrictive treatment option guides the choice of clinical setting and is one of the World Health Organization's Ten Basic Principles of Mental Health Care Law (1996). It requires that determining where a person will be treated includes consideration of the symptoms they are experiencing, the treatments available, their level of autonomy, acceptance and cooperation with treatment, and the potential for harm to be caused to themselves or to any others (WHO 1996).

In a person-centred healthcare system, services should be organised around the needs of people, rather than people having to organise themselves around the system. As a person's needs increase, the healthcare team should expand to include different support providers; and as people's needs decrease, the number of people involved will also decrease, with connection being maintained throughout by a general practice, the person's family, and other key supports.

A 'stepped care' model of matching an individual's needs with evidence-based, staged interventions (from least restrictive to most intensive), forms the framework of mental health service delivery nationally (see Table 3.1). In a stepped care approach, a person is matched to the intervention level that most suits their current need – they don't have to start at the lowest, least intensive level of intervention in order to progress to the next 'step'; rather, they enter the system and have their service level aligned with their requirements. As such, a person's first contact with mental health services may be through an emergency care setting.

You can see how the stepped care approach integrates well with a person-centred and least-restrictive model of care. The stepped mental health care model also aligns with providing a continuum of mental health care services – across primary, community, acute, subacute and extended care (rehabilitation) settings – all responding to the person's level of need. Table 3.0.1 demonstrates how these concepts integrate and the nurse's role regarding mental health care, and managing mental and emotional distress at each point in the mental health service continuum. Of course, these are not the only care settings or practitioners that need to respond to a person's mental health needs, they are merely some of the most common.

The emergency department is the key access point for health emergencies of all types, including psychiatric emergencies. People may present with mental health problems or mental illness which could be mild, moderate or severe. Those who require attention after self-harm, or who are suicidal, frequently present for care to EDs and may require ongoing care in a general hospital or acute mental health unit. Management will be in response to a triage process and respond to essential elements of care. As was explored in Chapter 2, during triage and assessment, clinicians may use a mental health screening or risk assessment tool, or identify the possibility that mental health symptoms are present and make the appropriate referral within their service context. The focus is on keeping people out of acute care (or getting them back to their community as rapidly as possible) by working with them to identify what it is they are experiencing and assisting in providing engagement with the level of mental health services and treatments that they need.

Table 3.0.1 Nursing, mental health and a stepped care response

Person's mental and emotional distress	Person's need for support	Elements of care	Care setting	Nurses involved
Severe distress	*Very high level of need* Risk to life; Severe self-neglect	Assessment Risk assessment Manage critical incidents Acute mental health care Medication Treatment	Acute mental health services Acute care teams	Mental health nurse practitioners Credentialled mental health nurses Mental health nurses
		Assessment Risk assessment Manage critical incidents Medication Arrange admission	Emergency departments	Consultation–liaison Mental health nurses Mental health nurse practitioners
				Emergency department nurses
Moderate to severe distress	*High level of need for support* Recurrent, atypical and those at significant risk, complex care needs	Assessment Risk assessment Brief psychological interventions Psychological therapy Medication education and management Social support and care coordination	Inpatient mental health Acute care teams Community mental health	Mental health nurse practitioners Credentialled mental health nurses Mental health nurses
			Primary health	Mental health nurse practitioners Credentialled mental health nurses
		Assessment Risk assessment Brief interventions Medication education and management Referral	Emergency departments	Consultation–Liaison mental health nurses Mental health nurse practitioners Emergency department nurses
			Acute alcohol and other drug services	Alcohol and other drug nurses

Person's mental and emotional distress	Person's need for support	Elements of care	Care setting	Nurses involved
Moderate distress	*Moderate level of need for support* Moderate or severe mental health problems	Brief psychological interventions Psychological therapy Medication education and management Rehabilitation services	Community mental health Primary health Forensic mental health	Mental health nurse practitioners Credentialled mental health nurses Mental health nurses Forensic mental health nurses
		Identifying distress Appropriate referral Social support	Medical settings Primary health General practice	Emergency department nurses Alcohol and other drug nurses Nurses working in chronic disease Nurses working in primary health General practice nurses
Mild to moderate distress	*Low level of need for support* Mild mental health problems	Guided self-help Brief psychological interventions	Primary health HeadSpace General practice	Mental health nurse practitioners Credentialled mental health nurses
		Identifying distress Raising awareness Flagging risk Watchful waiting	Medical settings Primary health General practice	Emergency department nurses Alcohol and other drug nurses Nurses working in chronic disease Nurses working in primary health General practice nurses
Minimal to mild distress	*Need for wellbeing and resilience promotion*	Recognition of risk and distress Mental health literacy Mental health promotion	All healthcare settings	All nurses in all settings

GREEN: Mental health nurses who use specialised mental health knowledge and skills

BLUE: Generalist nurses who use fundamental mental health knowledge and skills

Marks 2020, p. 396.

In some states and territories, consultation liaison (CL) mental health teams, including mental health nurses, psychiatrists, psychologists and/or mental health social workers, provide specialist assessment and treatment of people who present to EDs or who are admitted to general hospitals and who are experiencing mental health concerns. The ultimate goals of the CL team are to improve access to psychosocial care for people with medical illness, and to 'facilitate integrated, interdisciplinary service provision in the context of already complex medical management' (Gribble 2019, p. 559). Where CL mental health nurses are integrated with the ED as a specialist resource, the knowledge and confidence of ED nurses regarding mental health assessment and management is increased, workload is reduced, and the patient experience has been found to be more satisfying and beneficial (Wand et al 2020). Nurses working in emergency settings with integrated mental health nurses are encouraged to consider them as a professional development resource – not simply as a way of referring on people with mental health concerns.

EFFECTIVE PRACTICE IN EMERGENCY CARE SETTINGS

In Chapter 1 we identified the foundational concepts of recovery-oriented and trauma-informed approaches to working with people who present with mental health concerns. In Chapter 2 we described the underlying principles of safe and effective care for clinicians working in emergency care settings, including taking care with our verbal and non-verbal interactions, flexibility, active listening, developing empathy and assertiveness. In addition, we explored the assessment and management of agitation and distress, including de-escalation strategies. Effective practice in emergency care settings also requires culturally safe practice and interpersonal skills, such as being open to the belief systems of others, intuitiveness, being alert to the cues that tell us the things that matter to a person, self-awareness, spiritual awareness and reflective skills (Ramezani et al 2014). It also includes approaching people with compassion, focusing on strengths and promoting self-determination.

Compassion

Compassion underpins concepts of acceptance, a non-judgemental attitude, awareness, being present and listening. To be able to provide compassionate nursing care, we need to be able to imagine what it would be like to be in the person's situation, what it would be like to experience the world as they are experiencing it and to imagine what might help. Review Box 3.0.1 and reflect on how you might feel if you were presenting to an ED with any of the situations described.

FOCUS ON STRENGTHS

The strengths model proposes that all people have strengths, goals, talents and confidence, and that all environments contain resources, people and opportunities (Deane et al 2018). Focusing on strengths and personal values promotes a person's resilience, aspirations, talents and uniqueness. Focusing on what the person *can* do, rather than focusing on problems and perceived shortcomings, and how these strengths can be mobilised and built on to overcome current difficulties, is frequently a helpful approach.

Box 3.0.1 Reflection points

Consider how you might feel in the following situations, what you might be worried about and what you would need and expect from the healthcare professionals looking after you.

Imagine presenting with chest pain and having to wait ... How would you feel? What if you had also been sacked from your job that morning?

How might you feel if you presented with your child, only to discover they might have leukemia?

What would you need if you were experiencing intrusive thoughts of suicide for the first time?

What if your usually gentle grandfather became delirious, aggressive, and starts swearing in his residential aged care facility and has to be transferred to the emergency department for an assessment? How might you feel if you were the one experiencing those symptoms and behaviours?

How might you feel if you'd had unprotected sex with someone whose sexual history you weren't sure about? Or if you were a teenager who wasn't sure if they'd been sexually assaulted or not? Or if you were presenting with injuries as the result of domestic violence and worried about your children being removed?

What if you were so worried about an upcoming exam that you experienced a panic attack? Or you had a previous experience of depression and had just been dumped by your partner?

PROMOTE SELF-DETERMINATION

Self-determination is the basic human right to be able to make and participate in decisions about your life; having a choice in determining how you live your life; and having control over your life. These are fundamental tenets in all human rights declarations and conventions. Maintaining and promoting a person's right to be self-determining is a fundamental principle of mental health services standards and legislation (Australian Health Ministers Advisory Council 2013; Department of Health and Ageing 2013). It is important to remember that when we only interact with people during times of distress or challenge we may have a skewed view of their inherent capacities. Continually reflect on the assumptions you may be making about people to keep in check the capacity we all have to act 'as if' these assumptions are true.

CULTURAL SAFETY

Culture is shaped by intersecting factors and plays an important role in people's understanding of health and wellbeing, and how they experience health services. It also informs nursing practice and the structure and organisation of health care services.

The concept of cultural safety underpins a range of government health plans, frameworks, and standards in Australia. It is embedded in the Code of Conduct for Nurses and the Registered Nurse standards for practice (Nursing and Midwifery Board of Australia (NMBA)).

At an individual level, culturally safe practice extends beyond awareness of other people's cultural backgrounds, to reflecting on one's own cultural identity, privilege and relative power. Seek to minimise power differentials, engage with the person, and really listen, and make sure that your actions don't diminish, demean or disempower them (McGough et al 2022; Taylor & Guerin 2019). Cultural safety when working with Aboriginal and Torres Strait Islander peoples is discussed in more detail in the first scenario in this chapter (3.1). Among other things, this requires demonstrating your commitment to building a relationship that is trusting, includes an awareness of Aboriginal Australian history, keeping your promises, being humble and relinquishing control (Wilson et al 2020).

REFLECTIVE PRACTICE

Everyone develops biases that affect the way they view other people's behaviour. Self-awareness is about knowing how you are going to respond in specific situations, about your values, attitudes and biases towards people and situations, and about knowing how your human needs might manifest in your work. Lack of self-awareness can cause nurses to respond to a person's distress and behaviour in ways that may not be helpful. For example, it might cause nurses to use their power coercively in the belief that this is best for the patient. Lack of self-awareness can also lead to nurses being overly concerned, refusing to allow choice, or overwhelming a person with advice in an attempt to protect them. Alternatively, nurses may avoid contact with a particular patient, or fail to respond to their distress. Chapter 4 provides more detail on the role of reflective practice and the self-care required for working in emergency care settings.

ORIENTATION TO THE PRACTICE-BASED SCENARIOS

The scenarios in Chapter 3 have been written by clinicians and people with lived experience and have a practical rather than theoretical focus. They describe a person with common presenting circumstances who might be encountered in daily practice. The scenario developed may demonstrate the physical health needs of a person with mental illness (which are often overlooked and contribute to the poor physical health outcomes of people with mental illness), or the mental health needs of a person with a physical illness (which are often ignored and which impact on physical *and* mental health outcomes).

Each scenario is introduced by the authors who describe the mental health issues that are being discussed, the rates of presentation to emergency settings and the key considerations for all nurses and health professionals when working with this client group. The scenarios have been designed to provide some insight into how fundamental mental health nursing skills are required and can be used across emergency care settings, as well as to describe the specialist role that mental health nurses might take in a particular clinical situation.

At the end of each scenario, you will find a section outlining the 'red flags' that the scenario presents. These are elements of the person's background or clinical presentation that would highlight the possible presence of a mental health issue and should be explored. The mental health knowledge and skills you might need to provide comprehensive care in these situations is discussed, as are the important attitudinal concerns that relate to the presentation described.

You will notice that the authors all have different styles and while there are some commonalities across the scenarios (such as the importance of communication, for example), authors tend to highlight different elements of the scenario that they feel is particularly important. This probably reflects their own personal and professional experiences, and often, the type of setting they are working in. For example, some provide detailed descriptors of nursing interventions, particularly those who are working in highly specialised or technical areas, or where the patient's presentation is complex, whereas others provide more general, higher-level interventions for your consideration. Some authors have provided more detail on the relevant attitudinal issues that require attention, or the mental health knowledge and skills that are relevant to the scenario. And some have provided information relating to considerations for care that relate to the service that is offered within the setting, while others have included information that relates to therapies and treatments that might be relevant outside the emergency care setting.

As you read through these stories, identify any knowledge or skill gaps that you may have that relate to the scenarios presented – then consider how you might address your learning needs.

SUMMARY

The social ecological or holistic approach requires that emergency nurses are as competent in recognising and responding to emotional distress and the mental health needs of a person as they are in identifying signs of physical deterioration or a treatment side effect, and that acknowledging the impact of a person's environment and experiences on their health and health outcomes is an important part of understanding their overall health.

The interdependence between all aspects of personhood – including biological, psychological, cultural, social and spiritual dimensions – requires that all emergency nurses and other health professionals working in emergency care settings consider a person's mental health as part of their core business. In reading through the clinical scenarios that follow, it is hoped that you will develop a rich understanding of how you might incorporate mental health knowledge and skills into the care of all patients you work with, and why this is essential to a holistic person-centred approach.

Useful websites

Nursing and Midwifery Board of Australia: www.nursingmidwiferyboard.gov.au/

References

Australian Health Ministers Advisory Council 2013. A national framework for recovery-oriented mental health services: Policy and theory. Commonwealth of Australia, Canberra.

Deane F, Goff R, Pullman J. et al 2019. Changes in mental health providers' recovery attitudes and strengths model implementation following training and supervision. International Journal of Mental Health and Addiction 17(6):1417–31.

Department of Health and Ageing 2013. National mental health report: Tracking of mental health reform in Australia 1993–2011. Commonwealth of Australia, Canberra.

Gribble R 2019. Australia: Consultation–liaison psychiatry not psychosomatic medicine. In: Leigh H (ed.) Global psychosomatic medicine and consultation–liaison psychiatry. Springer, Cham.

Marks P 2020. Mental health in every setting. In: Foster K, Marks P, O'Brien A et al (eds), Mental health in nursing: Theory and practice for clinical settings, 5th edn. Elsevier Australia, Sydney.

McGough S, Wynaden D, Gower S et al 2022. There is no health without cultural safety: Why cultural safety matters. Contemporary Nurse 25:1–10.

Ramezani M, Ahmadi F, Mohammadi E et al 2014. Spiritual care in nursing: a concept analysis. International Nursing Review 61(2):211–19.

Taylor K, Guerin PT 2019. Health care and Indigenous Australians: Cultural safety in practice. Macmillan Education, South Yarra.

Wand T, Collett G, Cutten A et al 2020. Patient and clinician experiences with an emergency department-based mental health liaison nurse service in a metropolitan setting. International Journal of Mental Health Nursing 29(6):1202–17.

Wilson AM, Kelly J, Jones M et al 2020. Working together in Aboriginal health: A framework to guide health professional practice. BMC Health Services Research 20(601):1–11.

World Health Organization (WHO) 1996. Mental health care law: Ten basic principles. WHO, Geneva. Online. Available: www.who.int/mental_health/media/en/75.pdf.

CHAPTER 3.1

Supporting the social and emotional wellbeing of Aboriginal and Torres Strait Islander peoples presenting with mental health concerns

Candace Angelo and Madeline Ford

KEY POINTS

- The consequences of and traumas associated with colonisation have an ongoing impact on the health, mental health and wellbeing of Aboriginal and Torres Strait Islander peoples.
- Culturally safe and appropriate health services and the integration of social and emotional wellbeing (SEWB) concepts into care, enhances recovery for Aboriginal and Torres Strait Islander peoples.
- Access to appropriate mental health services is challenging in rural/regional/remote emergency settings, particularly for Aboriginal and Torres Strait Islander peoples.
- Nurses in rural/regional/remote areas are often the primary providers of holistic health care.
- Mental health assessment and promotion, including social and emotional wellbeing concepts, play an important role for practitioners in emergency settings.

LEARNING OUTCOMES

This chapter will assist you to:

- understand cultural safety when providing care for Aboriginal and Torres Strait Islander peoples presenting with mental and/or physical health concerns
- increase awareness of general mental health key concepts, assessment and mental health care approaches relevant to the rural geographical location and the emergency care setting
- appreciate the co-existence of multiple health issues and how these might be exacerbated by mental illness or mental distress and the intergenerational impacts of the traumas associated with colonisation
- apply holistic nursing care approaches, involving family, community members and kinship networks, wherever possible
- consider the impact of language and that the word 'mental' holds significant shame, stigma and fear for some people.

Lived experience comment
by Boe Rambaldini, Bundjalung Elder

MY WALK FROM THE TRAUMA OF THE PAST THROUGH THE TRAUMA OF TODAY TO THE OPTIMISM OF THE FUTURE

History has played some very devastating events to Aboriginal people, and my family and I were not excluded from the trauma of the past. Every state and territory government passed laws that allowed them to have complete control of our lives. With these laws, the authorities could do and did what ever they wanted to us, they also had full custody of Aboriginal children.

Having a brother removed simply for being Aboriginal caused some great painful emotions for our whole family, particularly my mother who, as a single parent, carried the hurt, pain, loss and guilt for not protecting her son. When my brother returned as an adult after many years separation it was clear that he had missed the kinship, love and cultural upbring that we were provided. My mother smothered him with love when he came home – she was so entrenched with guilt for not protecting him and did all she could to make up for the trauma of all those lost years of not knowing where he was or how he was.

On a personal level, I was deprived of a relationship with my brother and it was something that I could not comprehend. The kinship I had with my other siblings was so culturally rewarding and instilled the importance of cultural integrity with our strong values. I was provided with an understanding of our culture, customs, history and social positioning that laid the foundations of my being that allowed me to interact with others in a respectful way, valuing the interactions I have with Aboriginal and non-Aboriginal people.

During my early years my education suffered, and I was penalised from not having a proper education just because of being Aboriginal. Although I had a strong work ethic, the best opportunities were not offered to me and I was the subject of numerous floggings from the police. These traumatic events in my life led to difficult emotional feelings and questions, as well as struggles with my mental health and that of my wider family and friends. I still at times relive and suffer from the traumatic events in my past and there are many times when anxiety sets in, and I feel culturally unsafe. This and the racism I am constantly subjected to, impacts on my health. The trauma of the past has a huge impact on me and my family today and only truth-telling and allowing inclusion will work towards true reconciliation.

INTRODUCTION

As a consequence of the historical and ongoing intergenerational impacts of colonisation and its associated traumas, including racism embedded in our social systems and structures, there are vast disparities between the health and wellbeing outcomes of Aboriginal and Torres Strait Islanders and non-Indigenous people in Australia. Aboriginal and Torres Strait Islander people experience poorer physical and mental health and markedly higher levels of psychological distress, mental illness and comorbid mental disorder than the general population (Hepworth et al 2015; Priest et al 2011; Wilson & Waqanaviti 2021). As Sherwood (2021) identifies, 'First Nations health today is a story informed by history, policies, warfare, Western medicine and press bias' (p. 17). Simultaneously though, as the longest enduring culture in the world, Aboriginal and Torres Strait Islander peoples have also 'demonstrated an innate capacity to thrive despite such adverse conditions' (Wilson & Waqanaviti 2021, p. 282). Where nurses and other health professionals working in emergency care settings recognise and draw upon these strengths and align their practice with a social-ecological perspective, aimed at enhancing social and emotional wellbeing outcomes (for both the individual and their community), better outcomes can be achieved.

ABORIGINAL AND TORRES STRAIT ISLANDER SOCIAL AND EMOTIONAL WELLBEING

Aboriginal and Torres Strait Islander health and wellbeing does not just relate to a person's physical and mental health; it is viewed in a holistic context, which includes and is underpinned by the interconnection between the health and wellness of families, communities and the land, as well as cultural, psychological, spiritual, physical and emotional wellbeing. This perspective, described as social and emotional wellbeing (SEWB) (see Fig. 3.1.1), also acknowledges the relevant historical, political and social determinants – such as dispossession and the impacts of colonisation, collective and intergenerational trauma – and recognises the intimate connections between mental health and a person's background, culture, beliefs and experiences.

For First Nations people, 'SEWB is an expression of cultural and spiritual being and doing . . . it is experienced as an internalised sensation that is felt within the core of a person's humanity and is outwardly expressed through relationships between culture and lore in a continuous cycle of life and death' (Wilson & Waqanaviti 2021, p. 282).

Culture, self-determination and empowerment are powerful protective factors in providing a buffer to psychological distress for many Aboriginal and Torres Strait Islander peoples. Factors that have been identified as enhancing SEWB include connection to country, spirituality, ancestry and kinship networks, as well as strong community governance and cultural continuity (Zubrick et al 2014). Meaningful connections to people (kinship and

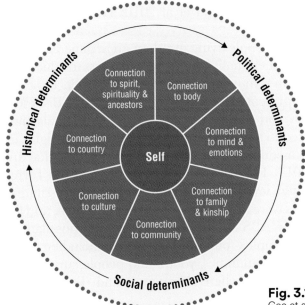

Fig. 3.1.1 Social and emotional wellbeing (SEWB).
Gee et al 2013.

community) and place (country) underpin the SEWB of many Aboriginal and Torres Strait Islander people (Wilson & Waqanaviti 2021); important considerations, especially when people live in urban areas or may be otherwise disconnected from their community or country.

In this chapter we share two clinical scenarios that describe Aboriginal and Torres Strait Islander people presenting with mental health issues – one to an urban emergency department (ED) setting and one to a remote area hospital. As you read through the background information below, which touches on just a few of the issues and health and wellbeing inequities experienced by Aboriginal and Torres Strait Islander people (relevant to the two different settings), please consider and reflect on how a shared understanding of social and emotional wellbeing will help support recovery for First Nations people you work with.

HEALTH, MENTAL HEALTH AND WHERE PEOPLE LIVE

Aboriginal and Torres Strait Islander peoples, who represent just 3.3% of the total Australian population (ABS 2018), are culturally, geographically and socially diverse, and are often an ambulatory population, with frequent interchange between and within urban, regional and remote areas (Brand et al 2016; Nasir et al 2018). While a range of factors shape and influence movement to urban areas (e.g. employment) and to regional and remote areas (e.g. to reconnect with country) (Memmott et al 2004), the urban population of Aboriginal and Torres Strait Islander people has been increasing since the mid-1960s and the majority (81%) of all Indigenous people (98% of non-Indigenous people) live in major cities, inner or outer regional areas. Even so, proportionally, Aboriginal and Torres Strait Islander people make up just 2.7% of the total metropolitan, inner and outer regional population (ABS 2018; Brand et al 2016; Ross 1996). For this and a range of other reasons – including 'colourism' and the commonly held stereotype that 'real' Aboriginal people live in remote communities – those who live in urban areas have been described as an 'invisible minority', exposing them to an increased risk of discrimination, inequality in service planning, access and provision, as well as segregation and isolation (Brand et al 2016; Priest et al 2011; Wilson & Waqanaviti 2021).

While Aboriginal and Torres Strait Islander people living in urban areas generally have similar lifestyles to other urban dwellers, and higher quality of life, better access to education and employment compared with those living in remote areas, they often experience racism on a daily basis and remain alarmingly overrepresented in relation to mental health disorders (Brand et al 2016, p. 13), as well as for injury and chronic disease. Urban Aboriginals have become accustomed to being constantly asked to affirm their identity, defend their rights as part of a marginalised group, and deal with assumptions of non-Aboriginal people that are grounded in stereotypes (Dudgeon & Ugle 2014). In 2018–19, 31% of Aboriginal and Torres Strait Islander adults identified high to very high levels of psychological distress necessitating a visit to a health professional. These numbers were higher for women than for men, and for those in non-remote compared to remote areas (ABS 2019). There are also sub-populations living in urban areas who have particularly complex (often unmet) needs, including those who are homeless, those visiting from remote communities, youth, and people currently in or recently discharged from correctional centres (where Aboriginal and Torres Strait Islanders are disproportionately represented).

Mental health in rural and remote areas

People living in regional, remote and very remote Australia experience similar prevalence of mental disorders to people living in metropolitan areas (AIHW 2019), but are at a higher risk of premature death and death by suicide (Roberts et al 2018; van Spijker et al 2019), and are less likely to seek mental health treatment (Commonwealth of Australia 2018). For Aboriginal and Torres Strait Islander peoples, the rate of suicide is almost double that of non-Indigenous people (Rouen et al 2019) and reported self-harm is also more prevalent and increases with remoteness. Physical family violence and sexual assault in remote settings is double the rate for urban areas (Smith 2016). Almost half (47%) of rural emergency presentations in Aboriginal and Torres Strait Islander communities include an interpersonal violence context, adding another level of complexity to consider in the provision of care. A higher prevalence of depression, trauma grief and loss contribute to illicit drug use, alcoholism and volatile substance use, which further exacerbate mental health issues. Violence experienced by Aboriginal and Torres Strait Islander women in remote settings is 45 times higher than for their non-Indigenous counterparts in urban settings (Lim et al 2020).

HEALTH AND MENTAL HEALTH SERVICE ACCESS IN RURAL AND REMOTE AREAS

In general, people living in regional and remote areas experience a variety of health disadvantages – poorer access to primary and acute care, poorer chronic disease management, social and geographic isolation, lack of consistent access to skilled healthcare providers, as well as long distances/travel times and costs associated with accessing services, poor service coordination and funding. Access to robust stepped care mental health services, mental health providers (such as psychiatrists, mental health nurses and psychologists) and effective models of care for both short and longer-term mental health issues/presentations, are also ongoing challenges (Beks et al 2018; van Spijker et al 2019). Lack of mental health services means early identification and intervention opportunities are missed. Mental health care models commonly service remote regions via an outreach approach from tertiary services in metropolitan areas, in the form of telehealth or a visiting individual in a fly-in fly-out model (Burke et al 2015). This approach often disrupts continuity of care, with designated staff changing frequently, shifting accountability and lack of opportunity to establish rapport, resulting in the person's healthcare journey being fractured (Byrne et al 2017).

It is widely accepted that emergency departments are not the ideal environment for treating people with mental health issues (Judkins et al 2019). However, lack of access to acute mental health care or after-hours mental health services in rural and remote areas means that people in mental health crisis *need* to present to ED settings as there is nowhere else to go (Sutarsa 2021). While people commonly present with several concerns, all requiring timely assessment and intervention (Smith 2016), rural and remote EDs often don't offer the resources needed to accommodate a holistic approach to complex physical and/or mental health concerns, so the primary focus will be on the acute presenting issue – which is often physical. For example, Haswell, Wargent and Hunter (2018) found examples of incomplete documentation and noted that some aspects of mental health care were often not addressed for Aboriginal and Torres Strait Islander people in rural and remote areas. This was attributed to a lack of mental health knowledge and skills of staff, and the focus on acute and physical health issues.

Physical health and mental health

It is important to remember that mental health disturbances could be manifesting and are sometimes the cause of an acute physical health presentation. For example, we know mental illness has a demonstrated reciprocal relationship between both intentional and non-intentional injury. Emergency presentations involving accidental injury are not uncommon in Australia; in fact, they account for 6% of all hospitalisations (a significantly higher number do not require hospitalisation) (Vallmuur & Pollard 2017). For many reasons, people in rural and remote areas face a higher probability of injury (e.g. higher risk-taking behaviour and less use of safety equipment) and a mental health crisis is known to further increase the likelihood of experiencing injury (Inder et al 2017). In the instance of an injury presentation where a person has a background of mental health issues, the acute physical injury perspective may be well managed, while the mental health issues are often poorly addressed or completely overlooked. It is essential for nurses to assess for and consider potential underlying mental health issues in all patients presenting to emergency care settings when assessing and treating any physical illness or injury.

The need for culturally safe and appropriate services

The problems outlined above impact on the health of all people in rural and remote communities. Aboriginal and Torres Strait Islander peoples living in rural and remote areas are therefore doubly jeopardised (Gynther et al 2019). For First Nations people across *all* geographic locations, any health service access issues are compounded by a range of barriers, including a lack of access to culturally appropriate health and mental health services (see Box 3.1.1) (Commonwealth of Australia 2018; Innes 2014; Wakerman & Humphreys 2019). Mainstream health services do not adequately address the complexity of many Aboriginal and Torres Strait Islander people's SEWB needs, are not culturally appropriate, culturally sensitive or culturally safe, and do not adequately address specific health problems that

Box 3.1.1 Barriers to mental health care for Aboriginal and Torres Strait Islander peoples

Barriers include:

- systemic and institutional factors – social exclusion, cultural dislocation, rapid urbanisation, socio-political disempowerment, disadvantage and marginalisation due to displacement, discrimination, forced removal and racism
- direct barriers, such as treatment costs
- indirect barriers, such as lack of transport
- opportunity costs, including lost wages and time away from family
- world view, conceptions of mental health, stigma
- lack of cultural training of healthcare staff
- lack of culturally appropriate assessment tools and treatments.

Page et al 2022.

require attention. For example, there is evidence to suggest Aboriginal and Torres Strait Islander people are more negatively affected by alcohol consumption and illicit drug use than non-Indigenous persons; however, it has also been reported they are less likely to access services for these issues than their non-Indigenous counterparts due to a lack of culturally appropriate programs (Berry & Crowe 2009).

CULTURALLY SAFE CARE

Unsafe cultural practice is 'any action which diminishes, demeans or disempowers the cultural identity and wellbeing of an individual' (Clear in Parker & Millroy 2014, p. 114). It leads to poor engagement and alienation from health services and health providers, misdiagnosis and poor health outcomes. Culturally safe practice is about providing care that takes people's unique needs into account – by challenging the status quo, by addressing the inequalities and power imbalances that are rooted in historical and structural violence and discrimination, through a continual process of learning and self-reflection, as well as empathy, shared respect, knowledge and experience. Cultural safety is essential to achieving equity and better health outcomes for Aboriginal and Torres Strait Islander peoples (McGough et al 2022).

To be able to provide culturally safe care, health professionals need to understand and acknowledge the impacts of colonisation and the intergenerational trauma that it has caused. Historically, discriminatory policies and practices (such as the forced removal of children from their families and country), as well as structural racism, have contributed significantly to the power imbalances that are embedded in institutions and systems, and contribute to fear and/or mistrust in government-run services – including healthcare services.

'Culturally valid understandings must shape the provision of services and guide assessment, care and management of Aboriginal and Torres Strait Islander people's health problems generally, and mental health problems in particular' (Commonwealth of Australia 2018, p. 3). While the statement that services should be shaped by culturally valid understandings is true, the terms 'mental health problems' and 'mental illness' have negative connotations for Aboriginal and Torres Strait Islander peoples – arising from shame, stigma and negative experiences with health and welfare services (Ward 2021). They imply a deficit approach and do not reflect all the factors that make up and influence SEWB. The concept of SEWB aligns with a more holistic and strengths-based approach – where the person's assortment of strengths (including their own, their loved ones and their community's) are identified and they are supported to recognise and draw from these strengths in their recovery (Wilson & Waqanaviti 2021). Similarly, trauma-informed care, where distress is seen as a symptom of underlying trauma(s), enables a standpoint from which a person is able to talk freely about their experiences, which might be sensitive, complex and difficult to speak about, without shame or embarrassment. In this way, trauma-informed care centres the person and their experience in an authentic relationship with the nurse and creates an environment where SEWB can be promoted (Wilson & Waqanaviti 2021). (See Chapter 1 for more information about a trauma-informed, strengths-based approach.)

Developing culturally safe practice is an essential journey which all nurses are responsible for undertaking. Box 3.1.2 outlines its key elements.

Box 3.1.2 The journey to cultural safety

Cultural awareness: Move towards understanding difference. Reflect on your own cultural background: what cultures and ethnicities do you identify with? How? Why? How does this shape your own identity, beliefs, values and attitudes?

Cultural sensitivity: Recognise the differences between yourself and Aboriginal and Torres Strait Islander people you work with. Seek out knowledge and better understand the ongoing impacts of colonial history. Acknowledge the profession of nursing has 'power' and 'whiteness' and that racism is inherent within the healthcare system, and that these impact on Aboriginal and Torres Strait Islander people.

Cultural safety: Cultural safety is achieved as the outcome of cultural awareness and cultural sensitivity, when an Aboriginal and Torres Strait Islander person experiences cultural safety in your care and in your service. When you value Aboriginal and Torres Strait Islander peoples and cultures and difference, commit to self-determination and build respectful partnerships.

Best 2021

Reflection

There are so many historic and contemporary threats to the social and emotional wellbeing of Aboriginal and Torres Strait Islander peoples.
1. How can you contribute through your nursing practice to improving the situation?
2. What do you need to learn?
3. What do you need to do?
4. How do you intend to be part of the solution and part of the change that is required?
5. How can you promote social and emotional wellbeing for all Aboriginal and Torres Strait Islander people you work with, including patients, their loved ones and your colleagues?

The two scenarios below explore the provision of culturally safe and competent care to Aboriginal and Torres Strait Islander consumers in urban and regional/remote emergency care settings. Example scenarios outline key details and information required to determine the appropriate nursing care approaches. Cultural considerations are examined to ensure that the needs of Aboriginal and Torres Strait Islander consumers are addressed, including specific gender business protocols, and the consideration of kinship and family roles.

SCENARIO 3.1.1
Matty

Matty is a 19-year-old Aboriginal man who presents to the emergency department clinic of a remote area hospital with a penetrating lower limb injury. Matty is accompanied by his aunty and several cousins, who carry him into the department. Matty says that he fell out of a large tree he climbed that morning.

On arrival, Matty's aunty says she thinks that he is 'buntha' (crazy) and says he is always injuring himself. She says that over the years he has had many occasions where he didn't 'seem himself', but his family weren't sure if he was 'gammin' (joking) or not. Most recently, he has been staying awake all night and talking quickly. His aunty says she asked Matty if he wanted her to take him to the city to see a doctor, but Matty expressed that he already felt shame that his brothers were calling him 'buntha' and didn't want the stigma.

On assessment
Matty reports he was followed and chased up a tree by 'warra wirrin' (bad spirits) and he lost his footing causing him to fall onto a fence below. Matty reports that he landed on his legs and there was no head strike. He had no cervical spine tenderness, his pupils were equal and reactive to light, he was alert and orientated to time, place and person. Matty is breathing independently with respirations 22 breaths per minute, his airway was patent and while talking rapidly, his blood pressure was 148/89. Matty was tachycardic with a regular heart rate of 130 beats per minute and afebrile 36.4 degrees. His lower left leg wound (14 cm × 3 cm) had defined wound edges, moderate swelling, was red and had localised pain. Matty's pain was 6/10 and described as 'throbbing'.

RED FLAGS

- Altered perceptions.
- Risk-taking behaviour resulting in physical harm.
- Reduced sleep.
- Painful physical injury to leg (will require medical intervention).
- Altered vital signs, e.g. tachycardia and hypertension.

PROTECTIVE FACTORS

- Family and kinship networks are reportedly strong.
- Matty has demonstrated awareness regarding his current situation, as he stated, 'Something isn't right'.
- Presented to hospital with his aunty, this can demonstrate his willingness to receive intervention.
- Currently not suicidal or engaging in self-harm.
- Orientated and Glasgow Coma Scale of 15.

KNOWLEDGE

- Many Aboriginal and Torres Strait Islander people have been impacted by discrimination and racism. There may be distrust in government-run organisations such as healthcare due to the impact and subsequent trauma of the Stolen Generations. This knowledge/understanding is foundational for culturally competent practice.
- Healthcare professionals have a tendency to assess Aboriginal and Torres Strait Islander people with non-Indigenous criteria and/or expose them to culturally insensitive environments. Consider your workplace; what adjustments for culturally appropriate care are required?
- Symptoms of a mental health crisis may be mistaken for spiritual or cultural traits, particularly where concepts of 'health' and 'illness' are integrated with culture and lore. For example, belief that illness is the result of individual punishment for a wrongdoing rather than poor adherence to treatment, or that delusions actually relate to 'spirits' (Hinton et al 2014).
- Involving family members and other kinship is a key factor in supporting the individual to remain connected to community. Health education and psychoeducation are as important for families as for the client (Sayers et al 2016).

- A genuine inquiry about connection to culture and land can help establish the therapeutic relationship. Determining the connection to land and kinship helps to establish a personal connection. Do this by asking the person's last name and if they are local to the area. If you recognise the last name from another client, then that may be used to form a connection (keeping confidentiality of course) (Ranzijn et al 2009).
- The impact of the social determinants of health on wellbeing outcomes, self-determination and empowerment can be powerful and should be considered by nurses and other health professionals when assessing and planning care.
- Access to definitive mental health care provision may require relocation to urban/tertiary facilities, i.e. taking people away from family, culture and other supportive factors. This should always be an approach of last resort.

ATTITUDES

- 'Reflective practice is a critical aspect of providing culturally safe care' (Cox & Taua quoted in Ward 2021, p. 158). Are you aware of your own biases? Do you subscribe to any stereotyping of Aboriginal and Torres Strait islander people in your life or work? Are your interactions culturally safe? Remember, racism can be subtle or intentional. How can you put practices in place so that you are not experienced as a 'racist nurse'? And what should you do if you discover cultural biases, assumptions or stereotypes in the care you provide? (Cox & Taua 2013).
- If you are a non-Indigenous person and you haven't done so already, undertaking cultural awareness training is an essential element of competent nursing practice.
- Reflect also on your own perceptions around mental health and illness to ensure these are not impacting on your practice in a negative way (reflective practice).
- Be open, respectful, empathetic, compassionate and transparent in your approach.

MENTAL HEALTH SKILLS

- Engage with the individual and their family or support network to develop a therapeutic rapport. Use culturally appropriate communication strategies. Direct eye contact can be seen as confrontational and rude, so should be kept to a minimum.
- Mental health care planning (short term and long term) should incorporate appropriate family and cultural supports into a mental health action plan. For example, asking Matty's aunty whether she thinks it is likely his agitated behaviour will escalate and how best to support him is important. Refer to medical records of previous presentations to identify any history of aggression or self-harm. Note previous interventions used to prevent escalation and replicate these as required, i.e. reduce stimuli, facilitate space and privacy, accommodate meals and personal hygiene.

CULTURAL SAFETY CONSIDERATIONS

- Provide access to cultural support (e.g. an Aboriginal and/or Torres Strait Islander mental health worker), family, Elder, community members; but try to avoid using family members as health interpreters, as the health issue may be viewed as 'shame' (Westerman 2004).
- Encourage the patient to maintain connection to country, spirituality and kinship networks.
- Remember that English may be the person's second, fourth or fifth language – ensure you speak in a clear, jargon-free way and remember Aboriginal and Torres Strait Islander people may speak in a circular way (Ramsay 2021).
- Cultural roles and understanding of women's vs men's business dynamics are important. Consider gender when providing care – it is culturally inappropriate to for men to discuss personal issues or 'men's business' with women, or for women to discuss 'women's business' with men. Facilitate another member of staff to attend if required.

- Ensure the assessment environment is a calm, inviting and culturally sensitive space; offer a comfortable place to sit and enough space for family and supports.
- Privilege Aboriginal and Torres Strait Islander culture and knowledge systems. This means listening to and respecting cultural knowledge, customs, values, feelings, religion/spirituality.

NURSING ACTIONS AND INTERVENTIONS

- Introduce yourself and explain what the assessment entails and its purpose.
- Consult with Matty and his kinship network – identify if he would feel more comfortable if an appropriate male Elder and/or male staff member were allocated and facilitate if requested.
- Gain consent from Matty and explain all procedures prior to performing them, maintaining privacy and dignity at all times. Validate and acknowledge any distress, and gently redirect the discussion to maintain safety as required.
- Assess current mental state and baseline mental state – include collateral information from Matty's aunty. What is Matty usually like? What has changed? See Box 3.1.3 for Matty's mental state assessment.
- Maintain awareness of cultural issues that may be relevant – if you aren't sure, ask.
- Note subjective and objective behaviours/experiences observed and voiced by Matty. Consider these in the context of cultural norms.
- Head-to-toe health assessment (primary survey) to determine other potential injuries from recent fall from tree – including, but not limited to, airway-breathing-circulation-disability, vital signs, pain score, neurovascular observations of affected limb and other investigations as indicated.
- Physical screen to rule out organic factor for behavioural disturbance, i.e. pathology, infection screening, imaging, therapeutic level testing. Once diagnostic screening is completed to eliminate any biological influences, refer to mental health or psychiatry team according to local policy.
- Promote independence and self-care wherever possible.
- Document findings, including interventions and outcomes.
- Liaise with medical officer for medical intervention, where appropriate.
- Invite a second staff member to assist/support with the assessment-taking if indicated. Remain conscious about personal safety, but avoid overcrowding. Note and ensure an exit strategy at all times during the assessment.
- Use opportunity for relevant education and health promotion – with Matty and his aunty.
- Collaborative care planning with extended teams as indicated, e.g. mental health community service, rehabilitation services, Aboriginal and Torres Strait Islander community controlled health services.

RELEVANT TREATMENT MODALITIES AND CONSIDERATIONS

Physical injury presentation of a penetrating leg injury
- A–G assessment/primary survey (systematic assessment approach to ensure a full physical assessment).
- Analgesia for pain relief.
- Check tetanus and immunisation status.
- Wound care and ongoing dressing management.
- Imaging and x-ray for unknown fracture status.

Mental health
- Provide access to treatment and care that is appropriate to, and consistent with, Aboriginal and Torres Strait Islander cultural and spiritual beliefs and practices.

BOX 3.1.3 Matty's mental state assessment

Appearance
- Age 19 years, alert, Aboriginal male of thin athletic build, with rigid posture. Avoids eye contact (culturally appropriate). Distinguishing features included multiple scars to torso and lower limbs, no tattoos, tobacco-stained fingers.
- Clothing choice was inappropriate for current conditions – wearing only footy shorts, no footwear or shirt.
- Manner was suspicious; appeared distracted.
- Prominent physical irregularity: profuse sweating
- Emotional facial expression: stressed, tense, screaming, furrowed brow

Motor/Behaviour
- Agitated, unable to lie still, excessive movement

Speech
- Rate rapid, pressured, hyper-talkative
- Volume appropriate and articulation clear

Mood/Affect
- Stable
- Intensity: exaggerated
- Affect: euphoric, pleasant

Thought Content
- No suicidal or homicidal ideations
- Expressed paranoid and magical ideation related to being chased by spirits
- Delusions: reports he is being followed

Thought Process
- Stream: flight of ideas

Perception
- Illusions (misinterpretation of actual external stimuli) frequently reports seeing 'warra wirrin' (bad spirits), but family say that it is just wild dogs.

Cognition
- Orientated to time, place and person
- Capacity to read and write, completed year 10 at high school
- Level of consciousness: alert and orientated Glasgow Coma Scale of 15

Insight/Judgement
- Awareness of illness – has insight that there is something 'not right', but fearful of bringing shame to his family.

- Assess and treat specific mental health symptoms.
- Therapeutic management.
- Use de-escalation strategies if required.
- Psychosocial interventions with individuals and families, i.e. holistic and social factors that contribute to ongoing care.

SCENARIO 3.1.2

Tahnee

Tahnee is a 21-year-old female who presents to the emergency department by ambulance with a police escort, called by Tahnee's sister Jess. Jess reported that Tahnee had moved from a regional town several hours away, to stay with her 18 months ago to look for employment. Jess said that about 2 weeks ago she noticed that Tahnee was talking 'rubbish' and she couldn't make sense of her, but she was in a rush to get to the train station for work and thought that Tahnee was just waking up and wasn't quite alert yet. She also reported that Tahnee has been increasingly disorganised, forgetting to pay her board, attend job interviews or social gatherings with her friends. Over the past week Jess noticed Tahnee has been talking increasingly about religion, which she has never previously done. Jess reported that when she returned home from work today, Tahnee had 'trashed' the house, she had smashed several photo frames and crockery, upturned furniture and was trying to light a book on fire. Jess said that Tahnee was screaming in 'some other language' and lunged at her when she tried to stop her from setting fire to the house. Tahnee identified herself as Aboriginal on the intake form.

RED FLAGS

- Altered perceptions.
- Relatively rapid deterioration in mental health.
- Destruction of property.
- Unpredictable behaviour and potential for aggression.
- Possible sense of disconnection from country.

PROTECTIVE FACTORS

- Strong family, friends and kinship networks in existence.
- Tahnee has presented to hospital with her sister in attendance and is accepting of being in the ED setting.
- Not suicidal or self-harming.

KNOWLEDGE

- For many Aboriginal and Torres Strait Islander people, connection to country, to the natural world, to culture and cultural practices, are intrinsic to SEWB. While many urban-dwelling First Nations people have a very strong connection to land and community, loss of connection to country (including living 'off-country' or relocating to an urban area where there is limited access to shared cultural practice) may cause cultural/spiritual trauma, compromising a person's resilience and impacting SEWB.
- Kinship carers, particularly siblings, are often not recognised, yet their role in supporting a loved one through a crisis is vital and their involvement during mental health assessment is part of culturally safe practice (Parker & Millroy 2014). A meaningful partnership between health services/providers and family and kinship networks will strike the balance between them being overlooked and under-utilised, and being exploited and abandoned to care for their loved one without support (Wright 2014).
- The experience of psychosis is a significant issue for Aboriginal and Torres Strait Islander people (Parker & Millroy 2014). While research is limited (another outcome of systemic racism), Australian findings indicate an extremely high prevalence of psychosis among Aboriginal people (five times higher for men and three times higher for women) in the

Northern Territory – higher than for Torres Strait Islander populations and for mood disorders, which are similar to the general population – and increasing over time (Gynther et al 2019).

- Vitamin B_{12} deficiency is a known cause of psychosis. HIV and systemic lupus erythematosus (SLE) can present like psychosis and there are considerably higher rates of both in Aboriginal and Torres Strait Islanders, along with higher rates of diabetes, anaemia and kidney disease than non-Indigenous Australians (Dorney & Murphy 2020).

- While Aboriginal and Torres Strait Islander people are more likely to present to EDs than non-Indigenous people (Chapman et al 2014), many people are not asked their Aboriginal status and do not reveal it to health services. They fear experiencing stigma or discrimination, fear not being believed (particularly if they don't 'look Indigenous' (Chapman et al 2014)), fear adverse consequences like having their children removed, fear not being taken seriously, and/or fear health professionals attributing health or mental health issues to the use of alcohol and other drugs.

CULTURAL SAFETY CONSIDERATIONS

- Recognising the influence of culture and working in collaboration with Aboriginal mental health workers is vital for those presenting with psychosis. This helps to create a shared meaning. For example, Parker and Millroy (2014) identify that it is common for First Nations people to hear their relatives' voices, and that where relevant cultural issues are not considered, this may be misinterpreted as a hallucination. They cite various authors who describe a range of meanings that relate to the words 'schizophrenia' and 'psychosis' – including Pintubi words relating to living in a 'world of their own' and having 'closed ears', and other explanations that relate psychosis to emotional stress, and relating delusions to sorcery against the person.

- The inclusion of identifiable cultural features, such as Aboriginal flags, artwork and symbols, as well as health promotion and illness prevention information available in waiting rooms and other areas, supports feelings of acceptance and welcome (Chapman et al 2014).

- Appreciating DSM-V criteria that guide diagnosis, while also recognising that signs and symptoms need to be considered through a patient-centred lens, which is inclusive of Aboriginal and Torres Strait Islander context. Always consider culture-bound syndromes when assessing patients.

ATTITUDES

- Reflecting on the beliefs, values and attitudes that we have formed about Aboriginal and Torres Strait Islander peoples – through our upbringing (family, socioeconomic status), our ethnicity, our education and the media (including social media), where Aboriginal people are often stereotyped, excluded or shown in a negative light – is an important part of practising in a culturally safe way (Best 2021).

- The clinical approach to mental health assessment is embedded in the Western biomedical model – the same place from which concepts of mental health and illness emanate. This approach generates expectations and ways of understanding symptoms, experiences, diagnoses and treatments. It is important for all nurses to understand and acknowledge the impact of this position on practice, and to challenge any pre-existing assumptions about Aboriginal and Torres Strait Islander people relating to assessment, diagnosis, experience and treatment of illness.

- Nursing as a profession is also entrenched within the biomedical model, which has typically excluded Aboriginal and Torres Strait Islander health knowledge. The goal of providing holistic care requires that we reflect on this and consider how to expand and facilitate our knowledge about Aboriginal and Torres Strait Islander approaches and practices in order to improve our cultural awareness and facilitate a more collaborative and culturally safe approach to recovery.

MENTAL HEALTH SKILLS

- Culturally appropriate mental health assessment includes the use of tools that have been developed, tested and validated for First Nations peoples wherever relevant. There are several mental health assessment scales and protocols that have been validated as culturally appropriate (e.g. the Kimberley Older Person Depression Scale and the Kimberley Deliberate Self Harm and Suicidal Behaviour protocols available through Australian Indigenous HealthInfoNet).
- Culturally appropriate mental health assessment also includes exploring cultural identity, seeking to understand cultural explanations of illness/symptoms/experiences, cultural factors that may impact or support psychosocial functioning, cultural factors that might influence the relationship between the person and the health professional, exploring individual and kinship strengths and supports. Considering threats to SEWB is also part of a comprehensive mental health assessment (Wilson & Waqanaviti 2021).
- There are a number of considerations that need to be taken into account when undertaking a Mental State Examination (MSE) with an Aboriginal and/or Torres Strait Islander person. Table 3.1.1 overleaf identifies some of these.
- Miscommunication and misinterpretation of symptoms is common and contribute to negative experiences for Aboriginal and Torres Strait Islander people in the emergency care setting. Interpersonal interactions that include empathetic responses, and support a person's sense of personal control, and which demonstrate that the nurse is advocating for the person, help to improve the experience of being in the ED (Chapman et al 2014).

NURSING ACTIONS AND INTERVENTIONS

- Attend to introductions. In addition to speaking with Tahnee, it may be helpful to speak to Jess separately if she wants to and if Tahnee is happy for that to occur.
- Gain consent and explain the rationale for any physical and neurological investigations that might be ordered to rule out organic causes for presenting symptoms (e.g. laboratory investigations, brain imaging, ECG, EEG) and monitor and record physical observations and vital signs.
- Mental health assessment and risk assessment should be conducted, keeping in mind relevant cultural factors. Facilitate another member of staff to attend if culturally inappropriate, i.e. male practitioner discussing women's business with female consumer.
- Offer a comfortable and relaxing sitting area in a calm, quiet space. Avoid information overload by allowing Tahnee to speak and give simple prompts to lead the discussion. Redirect topics that cause a distressed response, but if safe, acknowledge the distress and invite Tahnee to discuss when comfortable to do so.
- Model inviting body language, speak with a soft tone and avoid standing over Tahnee when communicating. Remain conscious about personal safety, but avoid agitating Tahnee with overcrowding and potentially feeling outnumbered.
- Note and ensure an exit strategy at all times. Be aware of duress alarms and how to engage them.
- Document findings, including interventions and outcomes.
- Liaise with medical officer for medical intervention where appropriate, consider early use of oral anti-psychotics to prevent escalation or physical intervention and use of intramuscular anti-psychotics.
- Respect Tahnee's right to refuse oral medications, ensuring education has been provided. However, consider having intramuscular anti-psychotics drawn up and ready. This ensures quick access, and the correct dosage is calculated without added pressure, if Tahnee becomes a danger to herself or others.
- If it is decided that Tahnee requires admission for her safety or the safety of others, and she refuses admission, ensure mental health orders are completed correctly and seek advice where required.

TABLE 3.1.1 Implications and considerations in mental state examinations

Appearance	• compare with usual self care and appearance • note changes that might indicate mental health issue • are there cultural influences and manifestations (e.g. grief) that need to be considered
Behaviour	• understand behaviour in the context of Aboriginal culture • behaviour (e.g. posture, gesture, touch and eye contact) can be culture-specific and have cultural interpretations that differ from one setting to the next.
Affect	• culture can influence affect e.g. the manifestation of anxiety and depression may be significantly different for Indigenous/non-indigenous persons • anger or resentment might be more historical than circumstantial.
Mood	• culture can influence mood expression • seek assistance of Aboriginal Mental Health Workers to identify thought disorder
Speech and thought form	• if English is the person's second language, it can be difficult to assess/detect thought disorder • seek assistance of Aboriginal Mental Health Workers to identify thought disorder
Thought content	• differentiating between delusions, culturally accepted ideas and Aboriginal spirituality can be complicated • identifying the time sequence can help – do the symptoms precede the culturally-based attributions or vice versa
Perception	• culture can influence perception, or it can be pathological • auditory hallucinations are not commonly culturally sited and may indicate a mental disorder • seeking advice from an Aboriginal Mental Health Worker is recommended
Cognition	• lack of culturally appropriate cognitive assessment tools • assessing a person's functioning and capacity to undertake activities of daily living aren't appropriate where a person lives in a remote community and lifestyle is more 'collective' in nature than individual • families seek help as a last resort

Sheldon 2010.

• Promoting self-determination and empowerment as much as possible in the care plan, and encouraging Tahnee to make informed choices in her care whenever possible, will help.

RELEVANT TREATMENT MODALITIES AND CONSIDERATIONS

• Use of illicit substances can precipitate psychosis and drug screening is part of routine practice. Substance use (including tobacco, alcohol, cannabis, methamphetamine, solvents and pain medications) is significantly higher in Aboriginal and Torres Strait Islander peoples and if present, needs to inform treatment planning (Dorney & Murphy 2020).

- Mental health treatment planning needs to focus on promoting SEWB, not just on the symptom treatment (Molloy et al 2021). Strategies that enhance and promote cultural practices prevent SEWB deterioration and reduce the burden of mental illness for Aboriginal and Torres Strait Islander people (Wilson & Waqanaviti 2021).
- Provision of clinically and culturally safe care and treatment is the responsibility of all health professionals. This 'requires a commitment to ongoing learning and unlearning, critical reflection and evaluation, which in turn requires the development of skills and knowledge, and changes in attitudes and behaviours' (West et al 2022, pp. 9–10).

SUMMARY

Regardless of whether living in urban, metropolitan areas or regional, remote or very remote areas, Aboriginal and Torres Strait Islander peoples have poorer physical health and mental health outcomes compared with non-Indigenous Australians. This is the result of the ongoing intergenerational impacts of the trauma associated with colonisation, limited access to culturally safe services, and a range of issues related to stigma and discrimination.

Aboriginal and Torres Strait Islander peoples living in urban areas, who form the majority of the Indigenous population in Australia, experience a range of issues associated with being a minority group and there is significant unmet needs relating to health and mental health. For those who live in regional, remote and very remote areas, where there is significant disparity in access to general healthcare resources relative to urban settings generally, Aboriginal and Torres Strait Islanders experience compounded health disadvantage.

Mental health disorders can be missed or mismanaged in settings where there is a lack of access to mental health specialist providers. Individuals in regional and remote communities commonly present to EDs with acute illness/injury and co-existing health and mental health issues. However, where combined acute health issues and a mental health issue exist, it is common that the person is treated for the acute health issue, with no consideration given for the impact of mental health factors or appropriate intervention. Given the increasing prevalence of mental health presentations to emergency settings and the need for nurses to practise in a holistic way, it is important that all nurses develop their mental health knowledge, skills and confidence in this area.

The term mental health has a significant stigma in Aboriginal and Torres Strait Islander culture. Mental health and mental illness are often described as medical terms that have a deficit approach and negative connotation. Additionally, they do not describe all the factors that make up and influence wellbeing. Because of this, most Aboriginal and Torres Strait Islander people prefer the term social and emotional wellbeing (SEWB) as it aligns more with a strengths-based approach and holistic view of health. Aboriginal and Torres Strait Islander culture, self-determination and empowerment can be powerful protective factors in providing a buffer to psychological distress. Factors that have been identified as enhancing SEWB include: maintaining connection to country, spirituality, ancestry and kinship networks, as well as strong community governance and cultural continuity (Zubrick et al 2014).

The two scenarios presented in this chapter demonstrate the relevant knowledge, mental health and nursing actions and interventions required to provide holistic, culturally safe care for the person and their family during the mental health crisis. Cultural safety is an integral aspect of care when providing support for Aboriginal and Torres Strait Islander consumers, with particular emphasis on family and community involvement. The nursing actions and interventions demonstrate the integrated healthcare and community approach required within the rural context.

| Reflection

Cultural awareness prompt

All individuals have varying world views depending on their experiences, culture, community input and family influence; this is known as your social schema. A crucial skill as a health practitioner is to practise cultural awareness when working with clients who come from different cultural backgrounds to your own. Reflect on your viewpoints, attitudes and belief system.

1. Where do they come from?
2. How are they different from other individuals, and what influences have made them different?
3. How might this influence your practice?
4. What additional training or learning do you need to ensure you provide culturally safe and competent practice to your community?

Mental health prompt

1. Would your attitude and approach differ if it was a member of your family or close friend who presented to the ED experiencing a mental health crisis?
2. Reflecting on your role as a health practitioner, how might you adjust your current practice with this in mind?

ACKNOWLEDGEMENTS

I would like to acknowledge that I am privileged to live, work, grow and raise my family on unceded Yaegl Lands, a place where my soul feels at home. I also acknowledge the ancestors of my Mother and Grandmother's lands from the Yuin Nation, somewhere that was once lost but now is found. I pay my deepest respects to the Elders of the past who have cared for and protected Country, the Elders of today who continue to nurture and share knowledge to grow the Elders of a thriving tomorrow.—Candace Angelo.

I would like to acknowledge my Elders who have come before me and have provided me a path and guidance to continue in my journey. I acknowledge the Bigambul people who are my traditional ancestors from the Goondawindii area and I would like to acknowledge and give my appreciation to Kalkadoon country, Mount Isa where I grew up and which has pathed my future today.—Madeline Ford.

The authors and editor would like to acknowledge Professor Rhonda Wilson, Wiradjuri woman, Professor of Nursing and Head of Indigenous Portfolio, School of Nursing and Midwifery University of Newcastle, for sharing her professional and cultural knowledge and wisdom, and her editorial advice in review of this chapter.

We would also like to acknowledge Boe Rambaldini, Bundjalung Elder and Associate Professor at Macquarie University and Poche Centre for Indigenous Health, University of Sydney, for reviewing the chapter and contributing his lived experience comment.

Useful websites

Australian Indigenous Health Infonet https://healthinfonet.ecu.edu.au/

The Centre of Best Practice in Aboriginal and Torres Strait Islander Suicide Prevention. Best practice screening and assessment: https://cbpatsisp.com.au/clearing-house/best-practice-screening-assessment/

WellMob healing our way: Social, emotional and cultural wellbeing online resources for Aboriginal and Torres Strait Islander People, https://Wellmob.org.au

Yarnsafe headspace resources https://headspace.org.au/yarn-safe/

References

Australian Bureau of Statistics (ABS) 2018. Estimates of Aboriginal and Torres Strait Islander Australians, June 2016. Cat. no. 3238.0.55.001. ABS, Canberra.

Australian Bureau of Statistics (ABS) 2019. National Aboriginal and Torres Strait Islander Health Survey. Online. Available: www.indigenoushpf.gov.au/measures/3-10-access-mental-health-services.

Australian Institute of Health and Welfare (AIHW) 2019. Rural and remote health 2019. AIHW, Canberra.

Beks H, Healey C, Schlicht K 2018. 'When you're it': A qualitative study exploring the rural nurse experience of managing acute mental health presentations. Rural and Remote Health 18(3):4616.

Berry S, Crowe TP 2009. A review of engagement of Indigenous Australians within mental health and substance abuse services. e-Journal for the Advancement of Mental Health 8(1):1–12.

Best O 2021. The cultural safety journey: An Aboriginal Australian nursing and midwifery context. In: Best O & Fredricks B (eds) Yatdjuligin. 3rd edn. Cambridge University Press, Melbourne.

Brand E, Bond C, Shannon C 2016. Indigenous in the city. Urban Indigenous populations in local and global contexts. UQ Poche Centre for Indigenous Health. Online. Available: https://poche.centre.uq.edu.au/files/609/Indigenous-in-the-city%281%29.pdf.

Burke D, Burke A, Huber J 2015. Psychogeriatric SOS (services-on-screen) – a unique e-health model of psychogeriatric rural and remote outreach. International Psychogeriatrics 27(11):1751–4.

Byrne L, Happell B, Reid-Searl K 2017. Acknowledging rural disadvantage in mental health: Views of peer workers. Perspectives in Psychiatric Care 53(4):259–65.

Chapman R, Smith T, Martin C 2014. Qualitative exploration of the perceived barriers and enablers to Aboriginal and Torres Strait Islander people accessing healthcare through one Victorian Emergency Department. Contemporary Nurse 48(1):48–58.

Commonwealth of Australia 2017. National Strategic Framework for Aboriginal and Torres Strait Islander Peoples' Mental Health and Social and Emotional Wellbeing. Department of the Prime Minister and Cabinet, Canberra.

Community Affairs References Committee 2018. Accessibility and quality of mental health services in rural and remote Australia. Commonwealth of Australia, Canberra. Online. Available: www.aph.gov.au/Parliamentary_Business/Committees/Senate/Community_Affairs/MentalHealthServices/Report.

Cox LG, Taua C 2013. Sociocultural considerations and nursing practice. In: Crisp J, Taylor C, Douglas C et al (eds) Fundamentals of Nursing. 4th edn. Elsevier Australia, Sydney.

Dorney K, Murphy M 2020. Recommendations for the medical work-up of first episode psychosis, including specific relevance to Indigenous Australians: A narrative review. Early Intervention in Psychiatry 2020:1–16.

Dudgeon P, Millroy H, Walker R (eds) 2014. Working together: Aboriginal and Torres Strait Islander mental health and wellbeing. 2nd edn. Commonwealth of Australia, Canberra. Online.

Available: www.telethonkids.org.au/globalassets/media/documents/aboriginal-health/working-together-second-edition/working-together-aboriginal-and-wellbeing-2014.pdf.

Gynther B. Charlson F, Obrecht K et al 2019. The epidemiology of psychosis in Indigenous Populations in Cape York and the Torres Strait. eClinicalMedicine. Online. Available: DOI: https://doi.org/10.1016/j.eclinm.2019.04.009.

Haswell M, Wargent R, Hunter E 2018. Indigenous adult mental health outcomes project in the Cairns Network, far North Queensland. University of Queensland, Queensland.

Hepworth J, Askew D, Foley W et al 2015. How an urban Aboriginal and Torres Strait Islander primary health care service improved access to mental health care. Int J Equity Health 14:51.

Hinton R, Bradley P, Trauer T et al 2014. Strengthening acute inpatient mental health care for Indigenous clients. Advances in Mental Health 12(2):125–35.

Inder K, Holliday E, Handley Tet al 2017. Depression and risk of unintentional injury in rural communities – a longitudinal analysis of the Australian rural mental health study. International Journal of Environmental Research and Public Health 14(9):1080.

Innes K, Morphet J, O'Brien A et al 2014. Caring for the mental illness patient in emergency departments – an exploration of the issues from a healthcare provider perspective. Journal of Clinical Nursing 23(13–14):2003–11.

Judkins S, Fatovich D, Ballenden N et al 2019. Mental health patients in emergency departments are suffering: the national failure and shame of the current system. A report on the Australasian College for Emergency Medicine's Mental Health in the Emergency Department Summit. Australasian Psychiatry: Bulletin of the Royal Australian and New Zealand College of Psychiatrists 27(6):615–17.

Kosiak M 2021. Midwifery practices and Aboriginal and Torres Strait Islander women: Urban and regional perspectives. In: Best O, Fredricks B (eds) Yatdjuligin. 3rd edn. Cambridge University Press, Melbourne.

Lim K, McDermott K, Read D 2020. Interpersonal violence and violent re-injury in the Northern Territory. The Australian Journal of Rural Health 28(1):67–73.

McGough S, Wynaden D, Gower S et al 2022. There is no health without cultural safety: Why cultural safety matters, Contemporary Nurse, Jan 25:1–10.

Memmott P, Long S, Bell M et al 2004. Between places: Indigenous mobility in remote and rural Australia. For the Australian Housing and Urban Research Institute, Queensland Research Centre. AHURI Positioning Paper No 81. Online. Available: www.ahuri.edu.au/sites/default/files/migration/documents/AHURI_Positioning_Paper_No81_Between_places_Indigenous_mobility_in_remote_and_rural_Australia.pdf.

Molloy L, Guha M, Scott M et al 2021. Mental health nursing practice and Aboriginal and Torres Strait Islander people: An integrative review. Contemporary Nurse 57(1–2):140–56.

Nasir BF, Toombs MR, Kondalsamy-Chennakesavan S et al. Common mental disorders among Indigenous people living in regional, remote and metropolitan Australia: A cross-sectional study. BMJ Open 2018;8:e020196.

Page IS, Leitch E, Gossip K et al 2022. Modelling mental health service needs of Aboriginal and Torres Strait Islander peoples: A review of existing evidence and expert consensus. Australian and New Zealand Journal of Public Health. https://doi.org/10.1111/1753–6405.13202.

Parker R, Milroy H 2014. Mental illness in Aboriginal and Torres Strait Islander Peoples.

Priest N, Paradies Y, Stewart P et al 2011. Racism and health among urban Aboriginal young people. BMC Public Health 11:568.

Ramsay N 2021. Remote area nursing practice. In: Best O, Fredricks B (eds) Yatdjuligin. 3rd edn. Cambridge University Press, Melbourne.

Ranzijn R, McConnochie K Nolan, W 2009. Psychology and Indigenous Australians: Foundations of cultural competence. Palgrave Macmillan, South Yarra.

Roberts R, Lockett H, Bagnall C et al 2018. Improving the physical health of people living with mental illness in Australia and New Zealand. Aust J Rural Health 26(5):354–62.

Ros K 1996. Population Issues, Indigenous Australians, AIHW Occasional Paper, ABS cat. no. 4708.0, ABS, Canberra.

Rouen C, Clough A, West C 2019. Non-fatal deliberate self-harm in three remote indigenous communities in Far North Queensland, Australia. Crisis: The Journal of Crisis Intervention and Suicide Prevention, 40(6):422–8.

Sayers J, Hunt G, Cleary M et al 2016. Brokering community engagement: Proactive strategies for supporting Indigenous Australians with mental health problems. Issues in Mental Health Nursing 37(12):912–17.

Sheldon M 2010. Reviewing psychiatric assessment in remote Aboriginal communities. In: Purdie N, Dudgeon P, Walker R, (eds). Working together: Aboriginal and Torres Strait Islander mental health and wellbeing principles and practice. Commonwealth of Australia, Canberra.

Sherwood J 2021. Historical and current perspectives on the health of Aboriginal and Torres Strait Islander peoples. In: Best O, Fredricks B (eds) Yatdjuligin. 3rd edn. Cambridge University Press, Melbourne.

Smith J 2016. Australia's rural, remote and indigenous health, 3rd edn. Elsevier Australia, Sydney.

Sutarsa N, Banfield M, Passioura J et al 2021. Spatial inequities of mental health nurses in rural and remote Australia. International Journal of Mental Health Nursing 30(1):167–76.

Vallmuur K, Pollard C 2017. Injury hospitalisations in public acute hospitals in Queensland: A five year snapshot 2011/12 – 2015/16. Metro North Hospital and Health Service.

van Spijker BA, Salinas-Perez JA, Mendoza J et al 2019. Service availability and capacity in rural mental health in Australia: Analysing gaps using an Integrated Mental Health Atlas. Australian & New Zealand Journal of Psychiatry 53(10):1000–12.

Wakerman J, Humphreys J 2019. 'Better health in the bush': Why we urgently need a national rural and remote health strategy. Medical Journal of Australia 210(5):202–203.e1.

Ward R 2021. Cultural understandings of Aboriginal suicide from a social and emotional wellbeing perspective. In: Best O, Fredricks B (eds) Yatdjuligin. 3rd edn. Cambridge University Press, Melbourne.

West R, Armao JE, Creedy DK et al 2021. Measuring effectiveness of cultural safety education in First Peoples health in university and health service settings. Contemporary Nurse 57(5):356–69.

Westerman T 2004. Engagement of Indigenous clients in mental health services: What role do cultural differences play? Guest editorial. Australian e-Journal for the Advancement of Mental Health AeJAMH 3(3):88–93.

Wilson RL, Waqanaviti K 2021. Navigating First Nations social and emotional wellbeing in mainstream mental health services. In: Best O, Fredricks B (eds) Yatdjuligin. 3rd edn. Cambridge University Press, Melbourne.

Wright M 2014. Reframing Aboriginal family caregiving. In: Dudgeon P, Milroy H, Walker R (eds) Working together: Aboriginal and Torres Strait Islander mental health and wellbeing principles and practice, 2nd edn. Commonwealth of Australia, Canberra.

Zubrick SR, Shepherd CCJ, Dudgeon P et al 2014. Social determinants of social and emotional wellbeing. In: Dudgeon P, Milroy H, Walker R (eds) Working together: Aboriginal and Torres Strait Islander mental health and wellbeing principles and practice, 2nd edn. Commonwealth of Australia, Canberra.

CHAPTER 3.2
Assessing and responding to people with co-occurring mental health and substance use concerns

Anthony O'Brien and Samantha Jane Clark

KEY POINTS

- Mental health and substance use concerns frequently co-occur and are common in people presenting to emergency care settings.
- Substance use may not be the presenting problem to emergency care, but will become apparent with comprehensive assessment, including carefully attending to the person's history.
- Responding to the person presenting with substance use and mental health concerns begins with forming a relationship of trust and respect.
- Physical health concerns need to be assessed and managed alongside substance use and mental health concerns.

LEARNING OUTCOMES

This chapter will assist you to:

- develop an understanding of concerns related to substance use and co-occurring mental health concerns
- apply principles of person-centred care to people presenting with substance use and mental health concerns
- develop therapeutic relationships with people who experience substance use and mental health concerns
- undertake comprehensive assessments with people who experience substance use and mental health concerns
- respond empathically and effectively to people presenting with substance use and mental health concerns
- use recognised frameworks of assessment and intervention when caring for people with substance use and mental health concerns.

Lived experience comment
by Helena Roennfeldt

LISTENING WITH OPENNESS AND CURIOSITY

Our histories often set the stage for emotional and relational intensity and instability – the connection between trauma and addiction is unquestionable. Emotions are a necessary part of how we experience life, and even painful emotions reflect something meaningful. Seeing substance use as self-medication reveals addictive behaviour as attempts to diminish acute feelings of anxiety, shame, loss and loneliness. While such self-medication can make sense as an attempt to soothe our intense emotional pain, using substances as an ongoing strategy can become a habit that evolves into a harmful spiral leading to loss of self-control, increasing our shame and ultimately resulting in greater withdrawal from life and social disconnection. It may be helpful to ask what does (or did) the alcohol or substance do for you? Be curious and invite the person to notice their own experience without judgement. Responding to someone struggling with substance use becomes a careful balance to avoid undue blame and restore personal autonomy. Significantly, hope and peer support can be a lifeline, and these social and emotional supports can restore a desire and build a willingness and capacity to tolerate dysphoria and distress.

Stigma surrounding people who use alcohol and drugs is very prevalent. As healthcare professionals, one of the ways that we can begin challenging this stigma is by becoming more conscious of the language we use. Throughout this chapter we will refer to substance use, rather than substance misuse – for the person who uses substances is often using the substance exactly as they intend to use them; the 'misuse' is our interpretation of what is occurring and can begin the process of stigmatisation.

INTRODUCTION

Substance use is a common health problem, with major impacts on individuals' health and wellbeing. Substances that are commonly used include prescription medication, cannabis, amphetamines, opioids and hallucinogens (Australian Institute of Health and Welfare (AIHW) 2017). While the use of some substances is socially validated and normalised, people who use drugs such as alcohol and opioids can experience a range of health problems ranging from dependence to physical illness and non-accidental injury. In addition, people who use substances experience higher rates of comorbid mental illness, especially anxiety and depression, and high rates of intentional self-harm and suicide (Moller et al 2013). Health problems associated with substance use frequently lead to people presenting for healthcare in primary and secondary care settings, often in crisis. Presentations to emergency departments (EDs) are common and these presentations sometimes involve suicidality or self-harm (Owens et al 2017). Although the substance use might not be the presenting problem, it may have contributed to the presentation and will have implications for further care. At the same time, physical health problems, such as injury, pain, toxidromes and dehydration, need to be addressed. Establishing priorities for care is an important nursing skill.

This chapter provides an overview of two prevalent substance use concerns – alcohol and opioid use – and their co-occurrence with mental health concerns. Two scenarios are presented. In the first scenario, Maria, who for several years has been taking oxycodone prescribed for pain, presents to the ED with gastrointestinal symptoms. Maria has a complex mental health history. The second scenario outlines the case of Neil, who also has a complex mental health history and has had many previous presentations to the ED. On this occasion he is intoxicated with alcohol after being found lying in the middle of the road, and is unable to explain how he came to be there. The scenarios are intended to capture some of the issues faced by nurses in caring for people with co-existing mental health and substance use concerns in the context of an emergency care setting, where there are also physical health problems. The chapter explores issues associated with assessment, emphasising the need for a holistic approach, including mental and physical health. The case scenarios are followed by an outline of the knowledge skills and attitudes that nurses need to respond to people with co-occurring substance use and mental health concerns. Nursing interventions needed for this population are also outlined.

ALCOHOL AND OTHER DRUG USE

In every practice setting nurses and other health professionals will encounter people who have substance use concerns. Substances may be legal or illegal, prescribed or non-prescribed (over-the-counter), and may be acquired through social networks or from health practitioners. In many cases, individuals use more than one substance; for example, alcohol together with cannabis (or 'synthetic' cannabis); stimulants such as amphetamines together with sedatives, or alcohol together with prescription opioids. Use of substances such as alcohol and tobacco are socially validated in our society and for many people are an integral component of their psychological and social functioning (Boyle et al 2021). Alcohol is the most commonly used recreational substance in Australia. It is a leading cause of death and disability, causing 5.1% of deaths, with 17% of adults consuming levels associated with long-term harm (Callinan & Livingston 2018). Another prevalent substance use problem in Australia is opioid use. Synthetic opioids are very effective in the management of some pain conditions, but can lead to overuse and addiction in vulnerable individuals. Prescriptions of opioids have increased markedly in the last two decades (Gisev et al 2018), with a consequent rise in recreational use and dependence (Kovitwanichkanont & Day 2018).

Alcohol and other substances are sometimes used as 'self-medication' for people who are struggling with difficult life problems, who have previous experience of trauma, are experiencing interpersonal conflict, or who find that substances provide relief from common mental health conditions, such as low mood or anxiety (Turner et al 2018). The immediate benefits, however, can eventually be overtaken by dependence on substances, while the original problems remain unresolved. People will often begin to use increasing amounts of substances, or multiple substances, to achieve a tolerable emotional state. It is not surprising, therefore, that people with substance use concerns commonly present to EDs (Smith et al 2015), in some cases involuntarily (Hughes et al 2018). It is important for nurses and other health professionals to be aware of how common substance use is and how it interacts with a person's mental health and wellbeing. A range of skills are required – in forming therapeutic relationships, empathetically inquiring about substance use and mental health, assessment of withdrawal and the physical impacts of intoxication, and supporting consumers in their recovery strategies (McKechnie 2020).

PREVALENCE OF CO-OCCURRING MENTAL HEALTH AND SUBSTANCE USE CONCERNS

Although rates of alcohol use have fallen in recent years, alcohol remains the most commonly used substance in Australia. Over 40% of Australians drink alcohol at a risky level at least once in a year, with the proportion of males significantly higher than that of females (AIHW 2021). Consumption of alcohol has reduced in younger age groups, but increased in older age groups. In addition to the physical harms arising from alcohol use, it is associated with high rates of anxiety and depression (Teesson et al 2010).

Although not as common as alcohol use, approximately 300 000 Australians are prescribed opioids each year, with almost half these prescriptions initiated by general practitioners (GPs), usually for pain (Lalic et al 2019). While many individuals are prescribed opioids for cancer pain, some are prescribed opioids for other forms of pain and are at risk of becoming opioid-dependent. Rates of mental illness are high among opioid users (Jones & McCance-Katz 2019), suggesting that services need to respond holistically to address both mental health and substance use.

Commonly, substance use co-occurs with significant mental health concerns, such as anxiety or depression. A recent systematic review of comorbid mental illness in people attending substance use services, found prevalence rates of between 47% and 100%, with rates of depression as high as 85% and anxiety up to 75% (Kingston et al 2017). Indigenous adolescents (Snijder et al 2020) and males (Harris et al 2015) have been shown to be at high risk of developing substance use disorders.

While substance use may contribute to the development of mental health concerns, for some people, substance use may be a consequence of adverse life events. People with co-occurring substance use and mental health concerns are more likely to have experienced adverse events in childhood, which may contribute to the development of both mental health and physical health concerns in adulthood (Wu et al 2010). People may also use substances to manage feelings of distress or symptoms of mental illness, such as voices (auditory hallucinations). While such 'self-medication' may meet immediate needs to reduce feelings of distress, over the longer term it can lead to dependence on substances, in addition to the associated physical health concerns.

CONSUMER EXPERIENCE OF SUBSTANCE USE

Recovery from substance use is described as a personal journey that involves reflection, commitment to change and a re-examination of personal values (McConnell & Snoek 2018). Consumers often begin their recovery after a long period of struggling with the effects of substances on their lives, including impairment in relationships, physical health issues, suicidality and legal issues. For many, the recovery pathway includes relapse, re-engagement in recovery and a long process of rebuilding their lives. Nurses caring for people with substance use concerns can help by ensuring they take a non-judgmental attitude, by listening, validating the person's experiences, and supporting consumers in their recovery journey. In the context of an emergency care setting, clinicians may feel frustrated when a person has presented many times and seems unable or unwilling to change. It is important, however, to demonstrate empathy, convey a sense of hope and communicate a belief that the person can take steps towards recovery. Reflecting on feelings of frustration and the impact they might have on practice is essential. (To read three consumers' narratives of their recovery journeys, see McKechnie 2020.)

ASSESSMENT OF THE PERSON WITH A CO-OCCURRING SUBSTANCE USE AND MENTAL HEALTH PROBLEM

Assessment of the person presenting with a co-occurring alcohol and other drug and mental health problems follows the same triage process used for all consumers presenting to emergency care (Australian College of Emergency Medicine 1997). Safety is the primary initial consideration, which means investigating the presenting problem and any acute physical health issue. For example, in the case of a person presenting with acute pain or injury, the severity and history of the pain or injury needs to be established and relevant investigations commenced. This initial interaction with the person is an opportunity to establish rapport and trust, which are invaluable as a basis for assessing substance use or mental health concerns. Baseline observations are important and provide an opportunity to assess whether the person is currently intoxicated or experiencing withdrawal symptoms. Behavioural changes, such as confusion, drowsiness and irritability, require a supportive response with clear communication that avoids complex language. Emergency care settings can be disorientating and frightening, so questions and explanations about what is happening may need to be repeated. In situations where initial triage suggests that a mental health issue is the primary presenting problem, Broadbent and colleagues (2010) suggest a secondary mental health triage process, which then leads to comprehensive mental health assessment, including assessment of alcohol and drug concerns. Assessment of substance use and mental health concerns will then usually proceed in tandem.

Stages of change and motivational interviewing

Awareness of the stages of change can be useful in the assessment process (Smith 2020). These stages reflect increasing recognition of substance use concerns, commitment to change and therapeutic work aimed at addressing the problem. The five stages are outlined in Table 3.2.1.

People may feel self-conscious about discussing substance use, so it is important that the initial stage of assessment is conversational, rather than a series of questions, which may feel overwhelming and lead to the person disengaging. What the person wants more than anything is to feel understood and supported.

Use of the OARS framework (open-ended questions, affirmations, reflective listening, summarising) (Table 3.2.2) can assist in applying the motivational interviewing model in clinical practice, enhance communication and build rapport between clinician and the person (Day et al 2017).

Standardised instruments and screening tools

Although not complete assessment tools, standardised instruments and screening tools can be a useful adjunct to assessment of the person with substance use concerns. For example, the Alcohol Use Disorders Identification Test (AUDIT) is a brief, widely validated alcohol

TABLE 3.2.1 Stages of change

Stage	Characteristics	Supportive actions
Pre-contemplation	Person is unaware that their behaviour is problematic and is leading to negative consequences. They may feel unable to change and be unaware of strategies and supports	Establish rapport and provide information about the effects of substance use. Suggest the possibility of change and express optimism
Contemplation	Person recognises the need to change, but feels ambivalent May be able to identify how life would be different without substance use	Work with the person's expressions of contemplation to reinforce the benefits of change. Work at the person's pace
Preparation	Person makes some steps towards change, such as contacting support services, or discussing their substance use with a family member or employer	Provide information and resources about support services. Encourage the person to make contact and make an appointment
Action	Person engages in a process of change and connects with support services	Reinforce the work the person is doing with their therapist or support service. Review progress made and next steps
Maintenance	At this stage sustained change has been achieved but may still be fragile. Plans are in place to deal promptly with any risk of relapse	Support the person in continuing their engagement with therapy and support services. Review skills gained and successful strategies

Adapted from Miller & Rollnick 2012.

TABLE 3.2.2 The OARS Framework

OARS: Putting motivational interviewing into practice		
Method	Description	Example
Open-ended questions	Using questions that invite discussion rather than a single word response	'Tell me about some of the strategies you've used to manage stress in your life'
Affirmations	Similar to validation, affirmations involve positive recognition of strengths and achievements	'It must have been hard to make the decision to seek help. That's something to feel proud of.'
Reflective listening	Paying attention to what the person is saying and responding in ways that recognise their concerns and experiences	'So you've reached out for support from your family and feel judged by them?'
Summarising	Providing brief summaries of points covered and issues addressed and seeking confirmation of those summaries	'It sounds like issues have been building for some time, but have become worse in the last few weeks. Does that sound right?'

Stewart & Fox 2011.

use assessment instrument of just 10 items, which can be completed either by the person as a self-report or administered by a clinician (Babor et al 2001). Ratings on the AUDIT scale give an indication of the severity of alcohol use. The Severity of Dependence Scale (SDS) (Martin et al 2006) is a brief, five-item instrument than is used for screening for a range of substance use issues and can be used in assessing people with opioid use. Discussion of the results of a standardised screening or assessment tool can provide a basis for further exploration of significant findings.

ASSESSMENT OF SUICIDALITY

Co-occurring mental illness and substance use and the distress related to crisis events means that suicidal thinking is common in this population (Yap et al 2019). Assessment of the use of substances and their effects on mental state and functioning includes a review of mood, thinking and social functioning. Nurses need to be alert for references to suicidality and thoughts of self-harm. People who are intoxicated or experiencing dysphoric states may express feelings of hopelessness and even suicidal thoughts while under the influence of substances. Withdrawal symptoms can also contribute to suicidal thoughts. Such expressions should be empathically validated and the person should be reassured that they will be kept safe. Suicidal thoughts may abate once intoxication or withdrawal symptoms diminish, and until this occurs, the person will need to be cared for with the appropriate level of observation. Exploration of suicidal thoughts can occur when the person's cognitions are not clouded by substances. This should include discussion of the intensity of suicidal thoughts, whether the person has specific plans, and what protective factors are present.

ASSESSMENT AND MANAGEMENT OF WITHDRAWAL

Drugs which can cause dependence, such as alcohol, benzodiazepines and opioids, can cause withdrawal symptoms if the person stops using the drug or significantly reduces the dose. While withdrawal syndromes share common features, there are also some features, such as the timing of the onset of symptoms, that are specific to individual substances. The signs and symptoms of alcohol and opioid withdrawal can vary in severity from very mild to severe. These are summarised in Box 3.2.1. Withdrawal might be apparent in the person's presentation (e.g. agitation and tremor), or the possibility of withdrawal might arise from the clinical history (long-term substance use and recent reduction or cessation).

In addition, there are standardised instruments that can be used to monitor patients in withdrawal. For alcohol withdrawal the Clinical Institute Withdrawal Assessment of Alcohol Scale – Revised (CIWA-Ar) (Reoux & Miller 2000) is a brief instrument that can be utilised in nursing practice, while for opioids the Clinical Opioid Withdrawal Scale (COWS) (Canamo & Tronco 2019) can be used. For benzodiazepine withdrawal the Clinical Institute Withdrawal Assessment for Benzodiazepines (CIWA-B) (Busto et al 1989) is recommended.

The use of standardised scales has the advantage of greater reliability of assessment and identifies changes in the person's presentation over time. Depending on the assessment findings, the person might be prescribed substitute medication to reduce withdrawal symptoms (or the risk of withdrawal symptoms). Medication will be prescribed on a reducing

Box 3.2.1 Identification of alcohol or opioid withdrawal

1. Cessation of or reduction in use that has been heavy or prolonged
2. Administration of an opioid antagonist drug such as naloxone (opioids only)
3. Onset of two or more of the following within hours or days of cessation or reduction:
   - Insomnia (trouble sleeping)
   - Autonomic symptoms (e.g. sweating or tachycardia)
   - Hand tremors (known as 'the shakes')
   - Nausea and/or vomiting
   - Psychomotor agitation (motor restlessness)
   - Anxiety
   - Perceptual disturbances (auditory, tactile, or visual type) and/or hallucinations
   - Seizures (tonic-clonic type, characterised by rhythmic, jerking movements, especially of the limbs).
4. The signs or symptoms in point 3 cause clinically significant distress or impairment in social, occupational, or other important areas of functioning.
5. The signs or symptoms are not attributable to another medical condition or mental disorder.

Adapted from McKechnie 2020.

basis, with the aim of ceasing administration once withdrawal is complete (Agnoli et al 2021). During the withdrawal process, consumers will need supportive care in relation to reorientation, psychological support, hydration, nutritional support, management of anxiety and safety when mobilising. Following detoxification, consumers should be offered the opportunity for rehabilitation to further support their recovery.

SCENARIO 3.2.1

Maria

Maria is a 35-year-old woman brought to the emergency department by a close friend late on Friday evening complaining of abdominal cramping, muscle aches, diarrhoea and nausea. Maria reports that she has been experiencing these symptoms for the past 24 hours and that the severity of her symptoms has been increasing. Maria is prescribed citalopram 20 mg daily; oxycodone controlled-release 20 mg tds (three times per day); temazepam 20 mg nocte (at night); paracetamol 665 mg tds and naproxen 500 mg bd (twice per day) as required. Maria had a motor vehicle accident in 2012; following this she was prescribed oxycodone to manage her pain. Maria also suffers from central sleep apnoea, fibromyalgia, lower back pain, PTSD from childhood trauma, depression and anxiety. Maria lives alone and has a small close circle of friends. She works part-time as a librarian, but has been off work on sick leave for the past four weeks.

Maria's GP for over 20 years has recently retired and she has been allocated to a new GP within the practice. Her new GP has recently reduced her oxycodone dose from 100 mg tds (40:20:40) to 60 mg tds (20:20:20). Maria has recently been experiencing sleep disturbance and she has been utilising temazepam 20 mg at night, which she has had on an as-required basis for previous insomnia. Maria has also been referred to the local alcohol and drug service by her new GP. She states that she feels ashamed and expresses concern that she will be perceived as an 'addict', as her treatment and prescribing will be taken over by this team and she is to be registered on the opioid treatment program.

You introduce yourself to Maria and explain that you will be taking some basic observations, monitoring her pain and other symptoms. Maria is very tearful, her eyes are downcast and she is very apologetic, stating that she is 'wasting your time', that this 'is all my own fault' and she can see that 'you're all very busy'.

RED FLAGS

- Exacerbation of symptoms of depression and anxiety, including tearfulness, poor eye contact, expressed feelings of shame, concern about time-wasting and self-blame.
- Statements indicating risk that she may self-discharge.
- Recent change in treatment team – particularly loss of a trusted GP with whom there was a long-term relationship.
- Recent change in long-term opioid prescription.
- Reduction in prescribed opioid dose with signs of opioid withdrawal evident.
- Experience of stigma and self-description as an addict.
- Diagnoses of PTSD, depression and anxiety.
- While there may be obvious opioid withdrawal, it is important that the mood disorder is given equal attention.
- Statements of low self-worth may be associated with suicidal ideation.
- Sleep disturbance.
- No work for 4 weeks.

PROTECTIVE FACTORS

- Works part-time. Maria's employment may be a source of social support and will probably provide a sense of meaning and purpose in her life.
- Supportive friends. A close friend has brought Maria to the ED. Friends can be enlisted in the consumer's care plan and can be an invaluable source of support.
- Previous engagement with her GP suggests that Maria accepts support from health professionals.

KNOWLEDGE

- Maria is presenting with gastrointestinal symptoms and these need to be assessed to exclude any new illness or an acute condition, such as bowel obstruction, appendicitis or ectopic pregnancy. Baseline observations should be taken, including vital signs and ECG.
- Maria's clinical symptoms and history of reduction in opioid dose suggest she may be experiencing opioid withdrawal. The COWS (see Useful websites) could be used to help with assessment. Observations of opioid withdrawal signs and symptoms should be made frequently in the initial period.
- Naloxone is used to treat opioid overdose; however, if Maria is already withdrawing naloxone would not be used as it is an opioid antagonist and would increase her withdrawal symptoms.
- Signs of depression and anxiety can present as complaints about physical health. Maria's presentation is complex as she has acute physical symptoms which may be explained by withdrawal, as re-emergence of mental health concerns, or as acute physical health

issues. Once her acute symptoms are safely managed, Maria will be better able to engage in assessment of her mood and thinking.

- Maria's comments that she is 'wasting your time', and that this 'is all my own fault', could suggest that she is feeling that she is not worthy of help. This may indicate that her mood is low and could be an indication that she may have suicidal thoughts. Once her acute symptoms have abated this possibility should be explored with her. In the meantime, Maria should be nursed in a high visibility area so that visual observation can be maintained. Regular recording of vital signs provides an opportunity to engage and monitor Maria's condition, relate empathically to Maria and help her to feel safe.
- It is important to be aware of other professionals in the hospital who can provide services (i.e. acute care teams, psychiatric liaison services etc.) and to ensure appropriate referral and collaboration in care provision.

ATTITUDES

- Be aware of and reflect on one's own feelings when working with people who have mental health and substance use concerns, including any feelings of frustration, disregard and/or hopelessness. Such feelings impact on practice and can affect the person's experience of being in hospital, help-seeking and recovery. Nurses may feel frustrated at Maria's level of complexity and challenged in responding simultaneously to her physical and mental health needs. Engage in clinical supervision if any negative feelings are triggered by working with someone with a mental health and/or substance use disorder.
- Reflect on the consumer's personal circumstances and history and how experiences of trauma and adversity may have contributed to use of substances as a way of coping. This can help with the development of empathy and supports interactions that are more therapeutic.
- Consider the stigma associated with receiving treatment from an alcohol and drug service and becoming registered onto an opioid treatment program; or the shame associated with presenting to the ED with substance-related concerns. Adopt a non-judgemental approach, taking care to suspend one's personal views of substance use and mental health concerns, in order to support the person to feel that they are able to be honest about their situation.
- Listen attentively and avoid dismissing or diminishing the person's expressed beliefs on how they are feeling.
- Reflect on issues of cultural identity and how differences between nurse and consumer might impact on the therapeutic relationship.

MENTAL HEALTH SKILLS

- On initial presentation, Maria is acutely distressed and in pain. Communication should focus on the immediate problems she is presenting with and should mirror the language Maria uses to communicate these problems. Medical and technical jargon should be avoided. Messages should be kept brief and the nurse should check Maria's understanding of information provided.
- Developing a relationship with the person based on warmth, empathy, genuineness and trust begins with treating the person with dignity and respect. In Maria's case, responding empathically to her presenting symptoms of pain and ensuring the pain is adequately managed are the first steps and will help her to feel that her attendance at the ED is valid and that her concerns will be taken seriously.
- Communication with a person with a substance use issue and mental health disorder is aimed initially at enabling the person to express what they are thinking and feeling.

Responding directly to Maria will promote communication. The OARS framework (see Table 3.2.2) can guide responses – from listening through to responding, and to offering summaries of what has been shared.

- Maria has made comments that suggest she may have suicidal thoughts. As rapport and trust are developed, and as her acute distress reduces, Maria can be sensitively invited to disclose any further thoughts of self-harm. Initial general questions can be followed up by more specific questions about intent and means. Assessment of thoughts of self-harm needs to take into account the effect of withdrawal symptoms on Maria's mental state. With further exploration, the nurse can discuss how Maria can keep herself safe while in the ED; for example, by calling the nurse if she feels she might harm herself or leave the department before completion of her episode of care.
- Maria has expressed a sense of shame because her GP has referred her to a specialist AOD (alcohol and other drugs) service. Assuring Maria that she is not wasting your time and that you are there to help can reduce the sense of shame she has expressed. If Maria experiences her interactions within the emergency care setting as non-judgemental she may be more likely to be open to engaging in recovery strategies and engaging further with health services.
- Once Maria's distress is relieved and she is not in acute pain, a gentle inquiry about her level of motivation can help to identify supportive responses. Maria is obviously past the stage of precontemplation, so interactions can focus on how the specialist service will be able to help. It may help to link service supports to the goals Maria wants to achieve in her life. Supporting Maria to consider the benefits of specialist treatment will help to encourage her and may enhance her motivation to engage.

NURSING ACTIONS AND INTERVENTIONS

- Welcome Maria to the treatment setting and establish a supportive relationship.
- Provide and maintain a safe environment in the ED.
- Check vital signs as indicated and use this opportunity to develop rapport.
- Complete comprehensive assessment (this may need to be staged in relation to Maria's presenting symptoms).
- Encourage and record fluid intake and output.
- Assign the same members of staff to work with Maria – limiting new contacts prevents Maria from having to explain her story multiple times and increases the likelihood that she will share information that she may feel ashamed about.
- Ensure appropriate laboratory tests are ordered; check results and discuss with other health professionals as needed.
- Monitor psychological symptoms of withdrawal (emotional lability, hallucinations, delusions).
- Ensure prescription and timely administration of medication to manage withdrawal symptoms.
- Explain symptoms of opioid withdrawal and inquire about the effectiveness of medication provided.
- Encourage Maria to talk about her feelings when she is not upset and tearful (she will be more able to verbalise feelings when not distressed).
- Promote rest and sleep.
- Refer Maria to a psychiatric consultation liaison service or to acute care team; or to alcohol and drug consultation liaison.
- Communicate with the GP. Include a summary of the presentation and actions taken to support Maria's referral to the specialist service.
- Collaborate on care planning with mental health and AOD services.

RELEVANT TREATMENT MODALITIES AND CONSIDERATIONS

- Appropriate care and treatment following standard withdrawal protocol.
- Referral to a relevant AOD service to initiate supplemental prescribing to manage and alleviate opioid withdrawal. Longer term medication will help Maria manage her opioid dependence (medication-assisted treatment of opioid dependence). This may include methadone or buprenorphine prescribed by a specialist addiction service. If Maria did not wish to commence a longer-term medication regime then symptomatic medications can be used to manage specific aspects of opioid withdrawal such as antiemetics for nausea and vomiting and NSAIDs for muscle and joint pain.
- Group or individual psychological therapy for people with substance use and mental health concerns might involve:
  - psychological strategies, such as working with Maria's personal belief system, clarifying values, setting realistic goals
  - brief intervention using motivational strategies
  - motivational interviewing techniques, which can help to enhance commitment to change
  - exploring strengths used in previous times of adversity
  - supporting connections between recovery and achievement of life goals.
- Community-based NGOs and consumer support organisations can help: services such as Narcotics Anonymous, where people with lived experience of addiction support each other to work towards recovery.
- People may feel reluctant to reach out to family, friends and other existing support networks. However, these connections help people to stay safe and recover.

SCENARIO 3.2.2

Neil

Neil is a 36-year-old man brought to the emergency department by ambulance. A community member called the ambulance after Neil was found lying in the middle of the road, and it was unclear whether or not he had been struck by a vehicle. Neil could neither confirm nor deny if he had been involved in an accident or answer how/why he was in the middle of the road. The police attended the scene, but were unable to ascertain any further details due to his level of alcohol intoxication and the lack of witnesses.

Neil has a diagnosis of borderline personality disorder (BPD), which is preceded by a long history of childhood sexual abuse from a youth worker, physical violence from his previous partners and trauma. He receives daily visits from a multidisciplinary community mental health team, who are working with him to improve his daily livings skills, help him to reduce his alcohol use and increase his coping skills. Neil's relationship with his 40-year-old partner has ended and he is now in temporary crisis accommodation. He has no contact with his family and only moved to the area 2 months ago following prison release.

Current medication is a multivitamin 1 tablet daily, thiamine 100 mg twice daily, folic acid 5 mg and olanzapine 5 mg. Neil takes all of his medication together in the morning, as this is the only time of day that he can remember to take it.

Neil regularly presents to the ED and today is the eighteenth time that he has attended the department in the past 4 weeks. He has previously presented with suicidal ideation and self-harm when intoxicated. During previous visits he has stated that he drinks 'three to four goon bags' daily (each 'goon bag' is 2L cask wine).

You introduce yourself to Neil and explain that you will be taking some basic observations. Neil is acutely intoxicated with alcohol. His speech is slurred and he smells strongly of alcohol. He is shouting very loudly that he is in pain and is 'dying', and can be heard throughout the department. Neil's observations show a fever and tachycardia.

RED FLAGS

- Alcohol intoxication.
- Known long-term high levels of alcohol consumption.
- Possible onset of alcohol withdrawal, including fever and tachycardia.
- Potential for severe alcohol withdrawal symptoms, including seizures.
- Inability to articulate what has occurred, or if any injury was sustained.
- Multiple presentations to the ED over the last 4 weeks.
- Recent relationship breakdown.
- No secure accommodation.
- Limited support network.
- Self-harm and suicide risk.
- Diagnoses of borderline personality disorder and substance use disorder.
- History of trauma.

PROTECTIVE FACTORS

- Active community mental health team involved in care.
- Seeks healthcare when in crisis.

KNOWLEDGE

- Alcohol withdrawal syndrome is triggered by the cessation of alcohol or reduction in level of consumption after prolonged periods of high consumption. Neil's current level of consumption, as described in recent presentations, is extremely high (8 L per day), suggesting withdrawal symptoms will develop quickly.
- Treatment of withdrawal should follow a standard protocol in terms of observation, pharmacological management, hydration and nutritional status.
  - Use of standardised withdrawal scale, such as the CIWA-Ar (see Useful websites) to monitor symptoms.
  - Standard pharmacological treatment for alcohol withdrawal is a tapering regimen of benzodiazepines. Most services will have a withdrawal protocol that will determine prescribing. If agitation persists, the dose may need to be increased from the standard protocol. An anti-emetic may be needed for nausea until withdrawal is controlled.
  - Intravenous fluids and nutritional support, especially B group vitamins.
- If it is not adequately treated, alcohol withdrawal progresses over 1–3 days, with worsening symptoms, and then abates. There is a possibility of seizures if withdrawal is not managed with appropriate medication.
- Wernicke's encephalopathy can develop when the person is rehydrated with intravenous fluids, causing a sudden fall in vitamin B levels. The classic triad for Wernicke's is confusion, ophthalmoplegia, and gait ataxia. Immediate intravenous B vitamin replacement is critical.
- Consumers can be confused when withdrawing, and confusion can fluctuate, so close observation is needed. The person will need assistance with mobilising and personal hygiene.

- Psychological safety is as important as physical safety during the withdrawal process.
- Familiarity with psychological strategies such motivational interviewing can be useful.

ATTITUDES

- Be aware of attributing all of Neil's behaviour to intoxication. Although intoxicated, there are multiple other physical and psychological issues that can manifest with similar symptomatology.
- Guard against the tendency to blame Neil for developing a substance use disorder.
- Consider the stigma associated with receiving treatment for alcohol withdrawal and from the social connotations of being perceived as an alcoholic. Reflect on your own attitudes regarding alcohol use. Self-awareness regarding one's own feelings when caring for people in withdrawal from persistent high levels of alcohol consumption is important.
- Be aware of any feelings of hopelessness that may arise when confronted with the severity and complexity of Neil's substance use and mental health concerns. Reflect on his personal history and how experiences of trauma and adversity may have led to his use of alcohol as a way of coping. Avoiding acknowledgement of a history of adversity and trauma can lead to the person feeling invalidated.
- Adopting a purely medicalised approach that does not engage with the consumer as a person is depersonalising. Active listening and responding with empathy and affirmations when someone comments on painful or difficult aspects of their lives can help to create a sense of safety and care.
- Reflect on issues of cultural identity and how differences between nurse and consumer might impact on the therapeutic relationship.

MENTAL HEALTH SKILLS

- Establish a rapport with Neil based on a non-judgemental approach. Develop your understanding of how to interact with someone who has multiple vulnerabilities and who may have difficulty trusting others. Genuine warmth and expressing empathy help to establish trust.
- Use focused communication skills while Neil is experiencing withdrawal symptoms, so that communication is clear; use simple language and repeat messages frequently, or as required.
- Regularly assess Neil's mental state, including thoughts, perceptions, orientation, attention, memory, cognition, mood and judgement. In particular, monitor Neil's thoughts or intentions for suicide and assess the risk of suicide or self-harm. In your assessment, take account of the context of withdrawal.
- Respond to any episodes of irritability without personalising the behaviour. This means responding calmly to the anxiety or fear Neil may be experiencing in the hyper-aroused state. Make careful judgements, based on symptoms, about when extra medication may be needed.
- Once the withdrawal syndrome begins to resolve, the focus can shift to assisting Neil to mobilise his strengths and resources towards recovery. Communicating messages of hope and confidence that Neil can make and sustain positive changes, focusing on recovery at his own pace, may help.
- Utilise psychological strategies to help Neil manage the anxiety he is experiencing (e.g. mindfulness) and motivational strategies to enhance motivation to change.
- Seek professional clinical supervision for yourself if you are working with people who present with a mental health or substance use issue that triggers concerns or any negative feelings.

NURSING ACTIONS AND INTERVENTIONS

- Introduce yourself and explain all actions and interventions, even if the person is intoxicated or does not appear to be listening.

- Provide a safe, low-stimulus environment during withdrawal to reduce exacerbation of symptoms.
- Provide nutritional support and monitor fluid intake and output.
- Monitor vital signs, including blood pressure, pulse and temperature.
- Review Neil's withdrawal status using a standardised instrument such as CIWA-Ar (see Useful websites), and document results.
- Monitor effects of medication given for withdrawal symptoms.
- Provide repeated assurances of safety and that symptoms will pass in time.
- Promote and monitor rest and sleep. Assist Neil with personal care as necessary while maintaining his sense of independence and dignity.
- Support and encourage Neil's referral to alcohol treatment services that will also address historic trauma experiences. Make a referral in collaboration with Neil and engage him in setting realistic initial goals, such as keeping his first appointment.
- Refer Neil to a psychiatric consultation liaison service or to alcohol and drug consultation liaison. If possible, have someone from the alcohol service meet Neil in hospital for warm handover.
- Communicate with the GP and mental health or alcohol treating team and ensure documentation is thorough and shared with all team members.

RELEVANT TREATMENT MODALITIES AND CONSIDERATIONS

- Motivational approaches can be integrated into routine care when working with Neil.
- Motivational interviewing skills can support people to consider or utilise strategies for change (see Table 3.2.1).
- The OARS framework (see Table 3.2.2) provides a helpful guide to positive communication with Neil.
- Once withdrawal symptoms abate, guide Neil towards commitment to further support from a specialist treatment service.
- Explore how unresolved issues of trauma might be impacting on recovery. Neil has a significant trauma history and might benefit from therapeutic work in relation to his trauma. This can be supportively explored with Neil without focusing on the details of traumatic events, which might be triggering for him.
- Refer Neil to a social worker to address housing issues.
- Communicate with a specialist mental health service with a summary of presentation.

> ### Reflection
>
> 1. How can you incorporate knowledge of substance use and mental health into your care of people presenting to an emergency care setting?
> 2. What strategies could you use to support people to manage their substance use?
> 3. What specific issues do you need to consider when assessing suicidality in someone who also has significant substance use concerns?
> 4. How could you use motivational interviewing skills to help someone contemplate a change in their pattern of substance use?

SUMMARY

Alcohol and substance use are prevalent issues in our society and commonly co-occur with mental health concerns, such as anxiety, depression and stress-related conditions. They can be used to 'self-medicate' feelings of anxiety and depression, or other distressing mental states. While overall alcohol use is decreasing in Australia, non-medical use of opioid analgesics is increasing. Presentations to emergency care services, including emergency departments, are common in this population, often precipitated by physical health issues, as demonstrated in Maria's scenario. In other situations, such as Neil's scenario, the person may present in circumstances that are unexplained, or with alcohol-related injuries.

All people presenting with co-occurring substance use and mental health concerns require timely and careful triage – with care and treatment focused on the areas of greatest immediate risk. Given the high rates of co-occurring substance use and mental health concerns, it should always be considered whether a person may be intoxicated or withdrawing from substances.

Responding to people experiencing these co-occurring concerns begins with taking a non-judgemental approach and establishing a relationship based on trust – which is facilitated by empathic inquiry, listening and validation. Nursing assessment requires knowledge of alcohol and other drug and mental health concerns, and how these problems interact. This includes knowledge of withdrawal syndromes and the physical health effects of co-occurring mental health and alcohol and drug concerns, as well as the mental health impacts of alcohol and/or substance use. Withdrawal can be assessed using standardised scales, and people should be provided with supportive care and an appropriate benzodiazepine regimen to avoid escalation of withdrawal symptoms.

During a presentation to an emergency care setting, people are at their most vulnerable, particularly when presenting with multiple physical and mental health concerns. Nurses engage in care that requires physical closeness, and are ideally placed through this role to establish a therapeutic rapport that can support, assist and encourage the person to engage or re-engage with the recovery journey. This requires both empathetic care and use of effective clinical tools and strategies that have been found to be effective and supportive. There are a number of frameworks to guide nursing practice, including motivational interviewing for enhancing the person's readiness to change, and the OARS framework for effective communication.

People who experience co-occurring substance use and mental health concerns often have complex lives, experiences of trauma and significant adversity. They may also carry multiple diagnoses that reflect a range of physical and mental health concerns. Person-centred care means attending to the individual as a person, with a focus on the issues they are experiencing, while still being mindful of the complexities associated with all conditions.

Medication has a role to play in managing acute distress and withdrawal, and it should be initiated with the intention to replace pharmacological support as the mainstay with psychological and social strategies. Friends, family and other personal supports play a critical role in supporting a person with co-occurring substance use and mental health disorders to build the life they want. The role of the nurse in the emergency care setting is to keep the consumer safe while they are vulnerable, and to instil hope that with ongoing support they can sustain their recovery.

Useful websites

ADIS – Alcohol and drug information service for consumers, carers and health professionals (Queensland): adis.health.qld.gov.au/

ADIS New South Wales: yourroom.health.nsw.gov.au/getting-help/Pages/adis.aspx

Alcohol and Drug Support Line (Western Australia): www.mhc.wa.gov.au/alcoholanddrugsupportline

CIWA-Ar. Clinical Institute Withdrawal Assessment of Alcohol Scale - Revised: insight.qld.edu.au/shop/clinical-institute-withdrawal-assessment-of-alcohol-scale-revised-ciwa-ar-insight-2019

CIWA-B Clinical Institute Withdrawal Assessment for Benzodiazepines: insight.qld.edu.au/shop/clinical-institute-withdrawal-assessment-scale-benzodiazepines-ciwa-b-insight-2019

COWS. Clinical Opioid Withdrawal Scale: nida.nih.gov/sites/default/files/ClinicalOpiateWithdrawalScale.pdf

Head to Health: www.headtohealth.gov.au

Healthdirect Drugs and Alcohol: www.healthdirect.gov.au/drugs-and-alcohol

Insight. Education training and workforce development: https://insight.qld.edu.au

Mission Australia. www.missionaustralia.com.au/what-we-do/mental-health-alcohol-other-drugs

Motivational interviewing – explained. A YouTube talk through motivational interviewing, including the four basic OARS skills. www.healthnavigator.org.nz/videos/m/motivational-interviewing-for-clinicians/motivational-interviewing-explained/

Narcanon Australia: www.narconon.org/

National MATOD guidelines. National guidelines for medication-assisted treatment of opioid dependence: www.health.gov.au/resources/publications/national-guidelines-for-medication-assisted-treatment-of-opioid-dependence

The Alcohol and Drug Foundation - Alcohol and Drug Foundation: adf.org.au

References

Agnoli A, Xing G, Tancredi DJ et al 2021. Association of dose tapering with overdose or mental health crisis among patients prescribed long-term opioids. JAMA 326(5):411–19.

Australian College of Emergency Medicine 1997. The Australian national triage scale: a user manual. Australian Government Publishing Service, Commonwealth Department of Health and Family Services (DoH&FS), Melbourne.

Australian Institute of Health and Welfare (AIHW) 2021. Alcohol, tobacco and other drugs in Australia. Online. Available: www.aihw.gov.au/reports/alcohol/alcohol-tobacco-other-drugs-australia/contents/drug-types/alcohol#consumption.

Australian Institute of Health and Welfare (AIHW) 2017. 2016 National drug strategy household survey – detailed report. AIHW, Canberra.

Babor TF, Higgins-Biddle JC, Saunders JB et al 2001. AUDIT: The alcohol use disorders identification test: Guidelines for use in primary health care. World Health Organization, Geneva, Switzerland.

Boyle HK, Gunn RL, López G et al 2021. Qualitative examination of simultaneous alcohol and cannabis use reasons, evaluations, and patterns among heavy drinking young adults. Psychology of Addictive Behaviors 35(6):638–49.

Broadbent M, Creaton A, Moxham L et al 2010. Review of triage reform: the case for clients with a mental illness in Australian emergency departments. Journal of Clinical Nursing 19(5–6):712–15.

Busto UE, Sykora K, Sellers EM 1989. A clinical scale to assess benzodiazepine withdrawal. Journal of Clinical Psychopharmacology 9(6):412–16.

Callinan S, Livingston M 2018. Drinking trends by age and over time among baby boomers and older drinkers. Foundation for Alcohol Research and Education, Canberra.

Canamo LJ, Tronco NB 2019. Clinical opioid withdrawal scale (COWS): Implementation and outcomes. Critical Care Nursing Quarterly 42(3):222–6.

Day P, Gould J, Hazelby G 2017. The use of motivational interviewing in community nursing. Journal of Community Nursing 31(3):59–63.

Gisev N, Pearson SA, Dobbins T et al 2018. Combating escalating harms associated with pharmaceutical opioid use in Australia: The POPPY II study protocol. BMJ Open 8(12):e025840.

Harris MG, Diminic S, Reavley N et al 2015. Males' mental health disadvantage: an estimation of gender-specific changes in service utilisation for mental and substance use disorders in Australia. Australian and New Zealand Journal of Psychiatry 49(9):821–32.

Hughes JA, Sheehan M, Evans J 2018. Treatment and outcomes of patients presenting to an adult emergency department involuntarily with substance misuse. International Journal of Mental Health Nursing, 27(2):593–9.

Jones CM, McCance-Katz EF 2019. Co-occurring substance use and mental disorders among adults with opioid use disorder. Drug and Alcohol Dependence 197:78–82.

Kingston RE, Marel C, Mills KL 2017. A systematic review of the prevalence of comorbid mental health disorders in people presenting for substance use treatment in Australia. Drug and Alcohol Review 36(4):527–39.

Kovitwanichkanont T, Day CA 2018. Prescription opioid misuse and public health approach in Australia. Substance Use and Misuse 53(2):200–5.

Lalic S, Ilomäki J, Bell JS et al 2019. Prevalence and incidence of prescription opioid analgesic use in Australia. British Journal of Clinical Pharmacology 85(1):202–15.

Martin G, Copeland J, Gates P et al 2006. The Severity of Dependence Scale (SDS) in an adolescent population of cannabis users: Reliability, validity and diagnostic cut-off. Drug and Alcohol Dependence 83(1):90–3.

McConnell D, Snoek A 2018. The importance of self-narration in recovery from addiction. Philosophy, Psychiatry and Psychology 25(3):31–44.

McKechnie M 2020. Substance use and co-occurring mental health disorders. In: Foster K, Marks P, O'Brien AJ et al (eds). Mental health in nursing: Theory and practice for clinical settings. Elsevier Australia, Sydney.

Miller WR, Rollnick S 2012. Motivational interviewing: Preparing people for change, 3rd edn. Guilford Press, New York.

Moller CI, Tait RJ, Byrne DG 2013. Self-harm, substance use and psychological distress in the Australian general population. Addiction 108(1):211–20.

Owens PL, Fingar KR, Heslin KC et al 2017. Emergency department visits related to suicidal ideation, 2006–2013. UMBC School of Public Policy Collection. Online. Available: https://mdsoar.org/bitstream/handle/11603/22067/sb220-Suicidal-Ideation-ED-Visits.pdf?sequence=1.

Reoux J, Miller K 2000. Routine hospital detoxification practice compared to symptom triggered management with an objective withdrawal scale (CIWA-Ar). Journal of Addiction 9:135–44.

Smith M 2020. The Transtheoretical model, stages of change and motivational interviewing. In: Smith M, Cavaiola A (eds) A comprehensive guide to addiction theory and counseling techniques. Routledge.

Smith MW, Stocks C, Santora PB 2015. Hospital readmission rates and emergency department visits for mental health and substance abuse conditions. Community Mental Health Journal 51(2):190–7.

Snijder M, Stapinski L, Lees B et al 2020. Preventing substance use among Indigenous adolescents in the USA, Canada, Australia and New Zealand: A systematic review of the literature. Prevention Science 21(1):65–85.

Stewart EE, Fox CH 2011. Encouraging patients to change unhealthy behaviors with motivational interviewing. Family Practice Management 18(3):21.

Teesson M, Hall W, Slade T et al 2010. Prevalence and correlates of DSM-IV alcohol abuse and dependence in Australia: Findings of the 2007. National Survey of Mental Health and Wellbeing. Addiction 105(12):2085–94.

Turner S, Mota N, Bolton J et al 2018. Self-medication with alcohol or drugs for mood and anxiety disorders: A narrative review of the epidemiological literature. Depression and Anxiety 35(9):851–60.

Wu NS, Schairer LC, Dellor E et al 2010. Childhood trauma and health outcomes in adults with comorbid substance abuse and mental health disorders. Addictive Behaviors 35(1):68–71.

Yap M, Tuson M, Whyatt D et al 2020. Anxiety and alcohol in the working-age population are driving a rise in mental health-related emergency department presentations: 15-year trends in emergency department presentations in Western Australia. Emergency Medicine Australasia 32(1):80–7.

CHAPTER 3.3

Assessing and responding to children and young people experiencing mental health concerns

Bridget Mulvey and Carla Trudgett

KEY POINTS

- The emergency department is often the entry point for young people seeking mental health support, treatment or access to services.
- Nurses and other health professionals require mental health knowledge and take a non-judgemental approach to young people presenting with mental health issues, to ensure a good experience and promote future help-seeking.
- Engaging the young person is important and can take time; see the young person alone, with their parents (if they agree), and also see the parents without the young person present.
- It is important to gather collateral information; this may involve liaison with agencies such as Child and Adolescent Mental Health Services (CAMHS)/ Department of Communities and Justice (DCJ)/the young person's school (with permission) to inform the treatment plan.

LEARNING OUTCOMES

This chapter will assist you to:

- develop awareness of the complex nature of adolescent mental health presentations and identify the knowledge and skills required to conduct a thorough assessment
- understand the role of the nurse working in the emergency department in relation to children and young people who present with mental health issues
- develop awareness of risks to assess for and interventions to implement when triaging young people presenting for mental health
- understand the impacts of stigma in mental health and the implications this can have on a person's willingness to seek or engage with treatment.

KEY POINTS—cont'd

- Most young people seen in the ED are discharged home with community follow-up. In situations where this cannot be coordinated, there is a mental illness that requires inpatient treatment, or the risks to self or others are considered too high, the young person may be admitted to a mental health unit.

Lived experience comment
by Helena Roennfeldt

I WAS NEVER THE SAME AGAIN

During the formative period of adolescence, being received into mental health care marks the crossing of a line, which can hold immense impact. Entry into mental health services as a young person interrupts our lives. It can feel like we are not the same person we thought we were; that we are not as capable as we had been earlier, and we don't fit in with our friends because they haven't had that experience. At the encounter with crisis services, there is potential for increased emotional and relational vulnerability. Having our experiences labelled can help, cause harm and everything in between. Labels can validate and invalidate emotional pain and distress. This has particular relevance for young people who have experienced trauma and abuse, to avoid the perception of locating the problem within individuals. It can feel like it discredits the impact and pathologises our response to trauma. The experience of crisis involves emotional experiences of overwhelm and powerlessness, uncomfortable bodily sensations, a need for connection and to be seen and heard. At this time of vulnerability, we desire openness to hear our personal experience, recognition of distress and a relational response.

INTRODUCTION

Emergency departments (ED) are often the entry point for children and young people presenting with mental health concerns, whether for an acute episode or due to an issue in accessing services elsewhere (e.g. primary care) – in fact, a large portion of paediatric ED presentations are related to mental health concerns. Children and young people present with varied and complex problems, including suicidal ideation and deliberate self-harm, depression and anxiety, eating disorders, behavioural disturbance (more common in children than adolescents), and less commonly, for psychosis or an elevated mood (Say et al 2021).

Almost 14% of Australian children and adolescents (4–17 years old) have been diagnosed with a mental health disorder – most commonly, attention deficit hyperactivity disorder (ADHD) (in 8.2% of all children and adolescents), anxiety disorders (6.9%), major depressive disorder (2.8%) and conduct disorder (2.1%). Boys are more commonly affected than girls (17% compared with 11%), and children living with one parent, those living with families with poor family functioning and those living in lower socio-economic areas more likely to experience mental health concerns (AIHW 2020). Many adult mental health problems begin in adolescence – 50% by age 15 and nearly 75% by age 18 – so presentations to health services for mental health concerns provide a valuable opportunity for early identification and intervention (Radez et al 2021).

Studies have shown that young people are generally hesitant to seek support for mental health problems, related to a number of barriers – including individual factors such as mental health literacy (i.e. recognising a problem and knowing where to seek help for it); social factors (stigma and embarrassment); concerns around confidentiality and about trusting a stranger; systemic factors (financial cost, waiting times); logistical barriers and perceived effectiveness of health professionals (Radez et al 2021). So, when they do present, it is imperative that they experience objective, non-judgemental, empathetic, evidence-based care that supports them with their presenting complaint and promotes future help-seeking. Young people are often brought to the ED by their parents or schools with injuries from self-harm or concerns about their safety. This can be an opportunity to assess their mental health status and risk, and refer them to mental health services where appropriate.

SELF-HARM AND YOUNG PEOPLE

Suicide and self-harm cause significant morbidity and mortality in adolescents worldwide. In Australia, suicide was the most common cause of death in 15–17-year-olds in 2016 and 11% of children and adolescents report self-harm at some point in their lives (AIHW 2022; Perera et al 2018). Recent Australian studies have identified that presentations to EDs of children and young people experiencing self-harm, suicidal ideation and behaviour, and intentional poisoning, has dramatically increased in 10–19-year-olds since 2010 (Hissock et al 2018; Perera et al 2018). In New South Wales in 2020, 79% of mental health presentations to EDs for 0–17-year-olds was for deliberate self-harm (MH-TRACE 2021).

Self-harm relates to intentional self-injury or poisoning that occurs without suicidal intent. It is generally an expression of personal distress aimed at achieving relief from overwhelming thoughts or feelings, and/or a way of managing distress associated with a range of issues – for example, abuse, bullying or trauma. In some instances, self-harm can be propagated in a friend group or cohort, or via social media when 'self-harm behaviour is modelled, normalized, and reinforced in media depictions' (Khasawneh et al 2020). Young people who experience cyberbullying are at greater risk of self-harm and suicidal behaviours than non-victims (John et al 2018). Some young people use self-harm to regulate their emotions when they are feeling distressed, and may present with superficial injuries in the context of more pervasive suicidal ideation. Other mental health conditions, such as anxiety, depression or psychosis, may also contribute to self-harm behaviour, and it is helpful for this to be identified as part of any assessment of a person who engages in self-harm (Hungerford et al 2018).

It is important for nurses and other health professionals to treat people who self-harm with respect and take a non-judgemental approach. People may feel shame regarding self-harming behaviours and fear of discrimination and stigma associated with self-harm behaviours can contribute to their reluctance to seek mental health support and treatment (Ramjan & Clark 2020). Medical risk is paramount, so young people who present with injuries related to self-harm should have their wounds reviewed, cleaned, treated and dressed, in the same way that they would be if sustained in any other way.

SUICIDE AND YOUNG PEOPLE

In Australia in 2017, suicide accounted for 2% of deaths among males and 1.2% of deaths among females aged 0–14 years. This increased to 36.4% of deaths among males and 32.9% of deaths among females aged 15–19 years, and 38.5% of deaths among males and 30.6% deaths among females aged 20–24 years (ABS 2018). Particularly vulnerable groups at risk include LGBTIQ+ youth (Rivers et al 2018) and Aboriginal and Torres Strait Islander youth (Dickson et al 2019; Westerman & Sheridan 2020).

Young people who have attempted suicide will be brought to EDs and will be initially managed by medical teams. It is essential that all nurses working in ED develop skills that enable them to comfortably address the complex issues surrounding suicide ideation or a suicide attempt with the person and their family in an empathic manner and to provide reassurance that the person's safety is priority (Foster et al 2020). The psychological and physical trauma experienced by a young person who has attempted suicide may be difficult for everyone to come to terms with, including the resulting fear and grief expressed by their parents/carers. Developing an understanding of these issues is important in order to be able to support everyone involved, and self-care for nurses and health professionals is also important.

PSYCHOSIS AND YOUNG PEOPLE

Psychosis usually emerges in late adolescence, i.e. people over 18 years of age, but a small number of young people experience their first episode of psychosis in mid-adolescence. Adolescents and young people experience the same symptoms as anyone with a psychotic illness; however, it is not uncommon for younger adolescents to present with a more limited range of symptoms. Symptoms of psychosis include thought disorder, hallucinations, delusional thinking, poor concentration, lack of energy/motivation and emotional blunting. There is a period of deterioration leading up to psychosis, known as the prodromal stage, which includes symptoms similar to depression, and can be misdiagnosed. If the prodromal phase of psychosis is identified early, this will have long-term benefits for the person, so it is important that problems are accurately identified as early as possible in order to offset the impacts that may occur with untreated psychosis (Ramjan & Clark 2020).

BEHAVIOURAL DISTURBANCE AND YOUNG PEOPLE

Behavioural issues that emerge in childhood or adolescence can be complex and difficult to resolve. These might include challenging and disruptive behaviours, such as:
- physical or verbal aggression
- defiance and non-compliance with reasonable requests
- disruption of the environment
- inappropriate vocalisations
- activities that irritate or aggravate others.

Disruptive behavioural problems might be diagnosed as attention deficit hyperactivity disorder (ADHD), oppositional defiant disorder (ODD) and conduct disorder (CD) (Ogundele 2018). These include behaviours such as oppositional behaviour, angry/irritable mood, inattention, intimidating and threatening behaviour, aggression and impulsivity (Perotta &

Fabiano 2021). Generally, early intervention is the most effective approach and naturally this requires early identification and close monitoring of behaviours of concern.

The causes of behavioural issues in children and adolescents are multifaceted. In some instances, difficult behaviour is a response to neglect, exposure to domestic violence, or physical, emotional or sexual abuse. Trauma has a significant impact on a young person's capacity to manage their behaviour. Children flourish in consistent, reliable, safe and predictable environments – and parents who are able to teach their children emotional regulation skills provide a language for emotions and help them manage the ups and downs of life. When parents are unable to support the child to develop these skills, for whatever reason, children can experience greater difficulty regulating their behaviour (Ramjan & Clark 2020).

TECHNOLOGY AND YOUNG PEOPLE

Children and young people, who are digital natives, are spending more and more time online or connected to devices – for entertainment, communication, education and socialisation (Crone & Konijn 2018). Device use became even more significant when there were lockdowns and school closures, during the first years of the COVID-19 pandemic, when digital technologies were being used to support learning from home (Graham & Sahlberg 2021). More than four out of five children, and nine out of ten Australian teenagers has a screen-based device (with an average of 3.3 devices owned by each child), and nearly all teenagers own a smartphone (Roy Morgan 2016). Digital media and technologies impact negatively on young people's physical activity, attention span and capacity for creative play. They also impact on learning – creating distraction, reducing focus on school work and lack of interest in learning. Children often lack the ability to self-regulate and control screen time, particularly when they need to manage online work – they can go to school tired and not ready to learn due to the use of technology after bedtime which interferes with sleep (Graham & Sahlberg 2021; Carter et al 2016). There are some benefits to the social connectedness that technology and social media affords, and there are also risks. Cyberbullying is a real risk and can be the source of emotional disturbances and substance use; it can lead to self-harm and thoughts of suicide in children and young people (Kids Helpline 2019; Graham & Sahlberg 2020). With the rise of connectivity, there has also been a rise in the use of social media. Fear of missing out (FOMO) means young people feel the need to be continually connected with what others are doing, which has significant effects on their mental wellbeing (Stephen & Edmonds 2018). Similarly, problem gaming, particularly for boys, may be a symptom of factors such as being lonely or feeling anxious or depressed (see Box 3.3.1 for warning signs). And while there is debate about whether it should be classified as a disorder, the amount of time a young person spends gaming can have significant negative effects on their daily life (including relationships, school or work, health and wellbeing) (Orlando 2019; Ramjan & Clark 2020).

Regardless of the reason for presentation, in the paediatric ED setting a triage nurse will conduct an initial assessment in order to identify the need for and coordinate the medical and mental health assessments. Many EDs nationally include a mental health clinical nurse consultant (CNC) or clinical nurse specialist (CNS), who will then conduct a mental health assessment for children or young people flagged as requiring mental health review. However,

Box 3.3.1 Warning signs of internet gaming disorder

- Tolerance – the need to play increasing amounts to get the same level of enjoyment
- Withdrawal – negative emotions if play is reduced or stopped
- Salience – video gaming dominating the person's thoughts
- Mood modification – using video games to modify mood, either to relax or to become excited
- Conflict – conflict about gaming both within the person and with other people
- Relapse – repeated failures to cut back or stop gaming, despite the desire to do so.

Paulus et al 2018.

it is important that all nurses and other health professionals working in paediatric emergency settings develop knowledge and skills in understanding common mental health presentations and supporting the mental health of children and young people, in order to provide holistic person-centred care. The two scenarios presented below demonstrate the knowledge, attitudes, mental health skills and nursing interventions required, and also demonstrate the role of the mental health clinical nurse consultant in the paediatric ED setting.

SCENARIO 3.3.1

Lily

'Lily' is a 14-year-old girl who presents to the Children's emergency department in an ambulance under a mental health schedule. Lily's father called the ambulance on direction from the community adolescent mental health services (CAMHS) team after she failed to attend the third consecutive appointment with her case manager and psychologist. Lily has experienced a 6-month decline in behaviour and mental state. She is refusing to attend school, isolating in her room, gaming until late at night, has poor food and fluid intake with a 5 kg weight loss and poor attendance to hygiene. Lily has become increasingly withdrawn from her parents and when she does interact with them she is hostile and abusive, telling them to 'fuck off' and saying she hates them. On the weekend her mother noticed cuts and scars on her arms and legs.

Background from CAMHS notes

Lily is a single child who lives with her mother Kate and stepfather Paul. She is in Year 8 at a local all-girls high school. Kate was diagnosed with schizophrenia in her teens and, according to the CAMHS notes, has experienced psychotic episodes on and off for much of Lily's childhood, at times requiring hospital admission. Lily had a supportive primary school and a good group of friends; however, she left many of these connections when she moved on to high school. Shortly after Lily started Year 8 her parents and school teachers noticed she became irritable and anxious; she started missing days of school and isolated in her room at home gaming until late at night. The school counsellor suggested to her parents that they arrange to have an assessment at their local CAMHS service, which they did. Lily attended a few appointments initially, where she talked about hating high school and her mother.

The CAMHS assessment noted that Lily described symptoms of depression, which included withdrawal, reversed sleep cycle, irritability, and thoughts of self-harming. After the initial assessment, Lily was not consistent in attending appointments, and treatment for depression was not commenced. Over recent weeks, Lily stopped going to school completely. Kate contacted the CAMHS clinician after noticing wounds on Lily's arms and legs, and also advised them that Lily was not eating properly and appeared to have lost weight. The CAMHS clinician asked her to call an ambulance to bring Lily to the ED for assessment.

Background from parents
Kate and Paul are in attendance; Kate has English as a second language, and she provides an account as best as she can, but you notice that Paul is answering for her a lot of the time. Lily's parents, Kate and Aryan, separated when she was a baby, and Kate and Paul have been together since Lily was 5. Paul is a high school teacher. They report that Lily has not coped with the transition to high school, that she has been in conflict with peers and teachers because she's 'so cranky' and as a result has stopped going to school. At times, it appears that Kate doesn't follow the conversation, but offers to arrange an interpreter are refused by Paul. Lily's parents seem worried, but are not very forthcoming with information about Kate's illness or any other stressors that may have contributed to Lily's decline in mental health.

Triage assessment
Lily is superficial in engagement. When asked why she thinks she has been brought to the ED she minimises the account that has been given by the ambulance officer, stating she hates her parents and they are punishing her for telling them what she thinks of them. Lily's affect appears flat. She is malodorous and her clothes are dirty and dishevelled. She is very thin and pale with hair unkempt and hanging in her face. She has visible scars on her arms and injuries that look recent, with dried blood. Lily explains that when she hurts herself it makes her feel better, and particularly when she is feeling really angry, she says, 'It stops me bashing my mum'. She has no current suicidal or self-harm thoughts or intentions, and is willing to stay to speak to a mental health clinician.

Lily is categorised as a '3' (ATS – Australasian triage scale), and the medical registrar and mental health clinical nurse consultant (CNC) are contacted to see her. The medical registrar is advised that Lily has had minimal nutritional intake over the past week.

Mental health CNC assessment
When asked why she has stopped going to school, Lily replies, 'Because there's no point and I can't concentrate anyway'. She says the teachers are trying to make her 'join the groups' at school and that they 'have a plan to make her conform'. Lily will not elaborate on this. She says she isn't eating because her parents aren't giving her the right food. She denies restricting her food intake with the intention of losing weight and she denies body image concerns, but she does minimise the weight loss. Lily is spending most days sleeping and nights gaming; she tells the CNC she enjoys this and just wants to be left alone. The CNC asks Lily about her mood, asks her if she feels sad or tearful; Lily responds, 'Not really', then says that she has lost touch with her old friends and she doesn't care about the girls in her year at school. She has stopped playing netball and swimming, which she used to enjoy, but says she can't be bothered with sport any more.

The CNC explains that there are some unusual questions she needs to ask as part of the mental health assessment (this is important to normalise the process for Lily and gain her trust). She then asks Lily if she has experienced anything unusual, such as hearing voices outside her head or getting messages from the TV or laptop. Lily reports she has heard voices when she is in her room gaming at night, and says this has happened on a few occasions over the past few weeks. Lily denies any illicit drug use.

Continued

The CNC asks about the cuts on Lily's arms. Lily explains that she does this when she is angry. When asked if she has thoughts to end her life, Lily replies she does not want to be here and sees no hope for the future; however, she does not have any plans to kill herself. The CNC then asks Lily if there is anything else she would like to tell her or that she feels is important for her to know – such as whether she has experienced or witnessed anything traumatic in her life. Lily does not respond at all to this question.

Medical assessment

Lily is medically assessed with possible malnutrition considered; she is medically cleared, but it is noted her BMI is 16. The mental health CNC, with the psychiatrist on call, discuss their concerns with Lily and her parents – particularly, that it has been difficult for her parents to keep Lily engaged with community services and that she is presenting with risk factors to herself and that without intervention and treatment it is likely that her mental health will continue to decline. They recommend Lily be admitted to the mental health unit for a period of observation, to clarify exactly what is going on for her, and to develop a plan to support Lily to reintegrate back to school. Lily's parents agree with the plan. Lily is non-committal, but says she will be happy to get away from them. As there is no bed available in the mental health unit, Lily spends the night in the ED, nursed on Therapeutic Supervision Level 1 (TSL 1) (see Box 3.3.2).

⚑ RED FLAGS

- Lily is dismissive of/minimises the severity of her current situation.
- Lily's parents seem unable to influence her or ensure she will receive treatment in the community.
- Family history of psychotic illness.
- Symptoms could be explained by depression, prodromal or first episode psychosis and need to be explored and clarified.
- Experience of trauma or disruption to attachment in childhood in relation to her mother's illness needs to be investigated, including whether there is any ongoing trauma or issues at home.
- Interruptions to education and social development need to be addressed.
- Low weight and poor nutritional intake. Level of malnutrition and its impact on mood need to be assessed, as does any potential refeeding risks.

Box 3.3.2 Therapeutic supervision level (TSL)

- Hospitals will have their own local policies and guidelines regarding the use of therapeutic supervision levels or 'care levels'.
- Typically TSL 1 refers to 1:1 nursing or 'specialling', where the nurse will be either at arm's length (specified) or in line of sight of the patient at all times.
- TSL 2 requires the patient is sighted every 10–15 minutes and TSL 3 – every 30 minutes.
- The ED nurse needs to be aware of the role of the 'special nurse', which should include a friendly, caring and compassionate approach, rather than one that is simply observing or monitoring the young person, which can feel awkward or intimidating for the young person.
- Be mindful that TSLs can feel like an intrusive intervention and ensure support for the person by ensuring dignity is maintained.

PROTECTIVE FACTORS

- Lily is a likeable girl; she did engage with the CNC, and was cooperative and willing to stay in the ED for the assessment, and also responded positively to the suggestion of an admission to the mental health unit.
- Lily has an open case file with the local CAMHS team, who will remain connected and provide follow-up care.
- Lily's parents have sought help and followed advice from CAMHS and the mental health clinicians in the ED.
- Lily has had friends and consistent relationships in the past.

KNOWLEDGE

- Screening for acute risk will determine the level of urgency with which the young person should be seen (what triage category to apply) and identify the need for the triage nurse to coordinate the interventions required, such as a mental health assessment. This will include medical risk, whether the young person has engaged in deliberate self-harm (do they have wounds that need attention?), or taken any medications or other drugs. Such questions should be asked in a discreet and non-judgemental manner, and it may be necessary to separate the young person from their parents to ensure an honest response.
- Questions about immediate risk to self through intent to self-harm or suicidal ideation are important. The nurse needs to ascertain the person's willingness to remain in the waiting room, or identify whether they are at risk for leaving without being seen, in which case, a more urgent response and a Therapeutic Supervision Level (TSL) may be required.
- Collecting additional collateral information is important. Background information can help streamline the assessment process and provide accurate clinical details and history. Reviewing previous assessments or discharge summaries can be helpful. Meeting with parents/carers separately may enable them to provide information they don't necessarily want to share in front of their child.
- Once a picture of the presenting problem has been identified, e.g. that Lily has cut herself and her wounds will need attention, and that she has not been eating, the next steps of treatment can be prioritised.
- For adolescents, the issue of confidentiality is particularly important. It is important to spend some time explaining that the conversation is private, but that certain issues, such as risk of (or actual) harm to self or others, will need to be shared with other members of the team. Advise the young person that if any element of what is discussed is to be raised with other members of the team, you will discuss it with them first.

ATTITUDES

- It is important to consider and reflect on our own values and bias regarding mental health as this can impact on the type of treatment experience and care a young person will have.
- If a young person is seeking (or needing) mental health intervention, particularly for the first time, their current experience is likely to directly impact on their level of willingness to engage or re-present for care in future. Experiencing practitioners who demonstrate a judgmental or stigmatising approach can increase risk, as the person may disengage from any future contact with health services and this can impact on social and emotional wellbeing, illness and future mental health.

MENTAL HEALTH SKILLS

Developing rapport and engagement is essential to enable the young person to feel comfortable and safe enough to tell their story and of conducting an accurate mental health assessment. Consider:

- it can take time for a young person to feel safe enough to talk openly

- approaching the young person with unconditional positive regard and using non-judgemental inclusive language
- normalising the young person's experience in the context of the situation/stressors they are experiencing
- outlining the parameters for confidentiality to put their mind at ease and allowing for forthcoming and honest responses
- using language that the young person can understand.

Using a curious tone and non-judgemental approach, conduct a risk assessment, including:

- asking whether Lily is experiencing current thoughts or plans to hurt herself
- asking about self-harm such as cutting/burning, taking tablets or ingesting substances or foreign bodies
- identifying whether Lily is willing to remain in the department to see a mental health clinician.

Consider and respond to issues that might contribute to increasing risk:

- Extended delays that may occur in the ED may contribute to someone becoming agitated or wanting to leave.
- Observe for signs of increasing distress or agitation. If the person appears to be escalating, de-escalation strategies may assist. This may involve simply providing information about why there is a delay or it may require reassurance, for example if the person is experiencing symptomatology such as anxiety or paranoia.

NURSING ACTIONS AND INTERVENTIONS

Triage assessment:

- Introduce yourself and get a brief description of the presentation. Ensure privacy when discussing sensitive issues.
- Conduct a risk assessment – this should be done in triage before the mental health assessment takes place, to identify whether immediate medical attention is required.
- Conduct initial physical assessment:
  - Seek permission to clean and dress Lily's cuts
  - Take a set of observations and weigh Lily.
- Lily is identified as Category 3 due to identified risk (medical and mental health) and mental health CNC (or local equivalent) is contacted.

Mental health clinical nurse consultant (MHCNC):

- Gather collateral information about Lily's mental state from her parents, the CAMHS team (verbal and, if possible, access notes on electronic medical record (EMR)), and any other relevant agencies that are involved, to help inform the assessment and development of the treatment plan. If possible, this should be done prior to seeing the patient so that pertinent questions are asked and the person is not asked to repeat elements of their story that should already be known.
- Introduce yourself and explain the CNC role with mental health, engaging in light conversation initially to help establish rapport and trust.
- Discuss confidentially (your conversation will remain confidential between you and relevant staff members, other than anything that is disclosed relating to risks to herself or others, where additional notifications may need to be made) and explain what the assessment will involve.
- Conduct a mental health assessment, which includes:
  - asking Lily for her understanding of why she is in the ED
  - screening for eating disorder
  - screening for psychotic phenomena
  - screening for current risk to self or others
  - screening for previous or current trauma

- mental state examination and impression
- developing plan in collaboration with the person and their family.

RELEVANT TREATMENT MODALITIES AND CONSIDERATIONS

- Immediate risk and long-term risk should be considered when planning treatment. In this case, the decision to admit Lily to a mental health unit was made due to Lily's clinical risk of harm to herself, combined with her previous lack of engagement with CAMHS and some uncertainty about her parents' ability to support her and access treatment.
- An admission to a mental health unit can provide:
  - containment of risk
  - a period of observation for diagnostic clarification
  - an opportunity to gather more information regarding any potential issues, such as child protection or domestic violence concerns
  - the opportunity to engage with Lily's parents and identify information or supports they may need to ensure Lily gets back to school and maintains contact with CAMHS post discharge
  - the opportunity to engage with Lily's school to establish a return to school plan and ensure support and understanding of the issues by teachers and relevant staff.
- Treatment should include a trauma-informed approach and should reflect the evidence base.
- The *Mental Health Act* 2007 (NSW) may need to be considered if treatment is refused.

SCENARIO 3.3.2

Mark

Mark is a 13-year-old boy who presented to his local emergency department via ambulance with police escort. Police had completed the relevant documentation under the state's Mental Health Act to enable Mark to be legally transported to hospital for a mental health assessment. Mark's parents report they called the police when he suddenly became very angry after being told it was time to get off his gaming device. Mark shouted and swore at them, threw things around the house and grabbed a knife from the kitchen. Mark's parents feared for their safety and also for the safety of Mark's younger siblings. They called police for support as they were unable to calm him down, despite multiple attempts.

History from paramedics and police
Police reported Mark was very agitated and upset when they arrived at the house, but that he followed all their directions and calmed down somewhat shortly after their arrival. Mark admitted to taking a knife from the kitchen, but stated that he did not intend to harm himself or anyone else. Mark's parents were very distressed as they had not seen Mark behave in this way before. Mark has no known mental health history or previous contact with police.

Triage assessment
On arrival in ED, Mark was teary and gave limited eye contact. He was able to engage in some conversation with the nursing staff, however, remained guarded and made relatively brief responses. When asked, he informed the triage nurse he was not feeling suicidal or experiencing thoughts of hurting himself or others. Mark was given a triage category of 3 (ATS – Australasian triage scale).

Medical assessment
The ED doctor completed a physical assessment of Mark and obtained brief details about what had occurred in the lead-up to him arriving at the hospital. There were no concerns

Continued

for Mark's physical health. The doctor completed a HEEADSSS Assessment (Klein 2014) as an age-appropriate psychological assessment to ascertain Mark's current mental state. This can be an effective framework to screen a full range of psychosocial issues that may impact on a young person's health and wellbeing – it includes asking about a young person's Home, Education and employment, Eating, Activities, Drugs, Sexuality, Suicide/depression and Safety. See Box 3.3.3 for Mark's HEEADSSS assessment.

Mental health CNC assessment

Mark reported he became angry quite suddenly after his parents removed his PlayStation™. He was upset about having police at his house and worried about what that might mean for his future. He denied any current issues or stressors that may have contributed to the night's events.

Mark is functioning well in Year 8 and has been attending school without incident, completing his schoolwork and has a stable group of friends. He has never had an angry outburst at school or been given a suspension or expulsion. There is no history of physical fights or any previous contact with a mental health professional or school counsellor.

Mark denied any significant issues with his mood, rating his mood on average over the last two weeks as 7/10 (10 being a great mood, 0 being a terrible mood). He didn't feel like he worries excessively or over-thinks things, and reported no issues with his sleep. He acknowledged that he does tend to stay up late at night playing video games and that perhaps this has been getting later.

Mark said he became frustrated tonight as his parents would not listen to him and he wanted to finish the current level in a game he was playing as he had been working towards achieving it for some time. Mark plays online with his friends and said he became distressed as his parents turned it off abruptly and he was not able to save his level or say goodbye to his friends. He expressed some embarrassment about this during the assessment.

Mark described feeling guilty and was remorseful about his actions. He was worried about seeing his parents. Mark said he had grabbed the knife impulsively, but did not know why. He felt frustrated at the fact that no one was listening to him. He emphatically denied any intent to harm himself or anyone else with it and continued to re-state this throughout the assessment. There have never been any previous episodes of thoughts of self-harm or harm to others.

Mark denied having difficulties managing anger or frustration, although reported that sometimes 'things can escalate quickly'. He acknowledged he has had other occasions where he has become angry or not followed his parents' directions, but that it has never been as bad as tonight.

Collateral information from parents

Mark's parents attend the ED shortly after Mark's arrival. They were upset and anxious over tonight's events and worried about what is happening for Mark.

They provided Mark's developmental history, with no issues noted during pregnancy or after birth. They described Mark as having met all developmental milestones on time or early.

Mark was described as an easy-going kid with a wide circle of friends, who was above-average at school and enjoyed playing a few sports. They had not noticed any particular changes in Mark's mood or behaviour and could not identify any significant changes in routine or current stressors for either Mark or the family.

As Mark got older, they noted him beginning to push parental boundaries at home, but thought this was probably typical teenage behaviour. Mark had been spending longer time periods gaming with peers. His parents became increasingly concerned about the amount of time he spent on devices and felt it was becoming increasingly difficult to set limits around his game use, particularly as he was wanting to stay up later and later. They reported that tonight's episode was out of character and was a sudden and acute change in Mark's behaviour.

They noted that Mark's maternal grandmother had a history of depression and his paternal uncle experienced anxiety.

RED FLAGS

- Mark's level of anger rapidly escalated to a point where he felt out of control.
- Mark's impulsivity in grabbing a knife could have resulted in serious injury to Mark or a member of his family.
- The amount of time Mark spends on video games is increasing and his response to limit-setting around this was uncharacteristic. Is Mark developing (or at risk of developing) a video game addiction or obsession?
- Mark's parents were not able to calm him down using their usual parenting methods.

PROTECTIVE FACTORS

- Mark has been polite and cooperative in ED and able to engage with multiple health professionals.
- There was no evidence of ongoing behavioural disturbance on or after his arrival to the ED.

BOX 3.3.3 Mark's HEEADSSS assessment

H – Home Mark lives with both parents and his younger 10-year-old sister and 8-year-old brother. He has lived in the same home his entire life.

E – Education and Employment Mark attends a local high school; he is in Year 8 and is doing very well academically. There are no issues with discipline or attendance.

E – Eating Mark describes a healthy appetite, enjoys sports and is physically fit. There are no current concerns about his weight or development.

A – Activities Mark plays in two team sports and describes close friends and also other friends from a nearby neighbourhood school, teams and family. He enjoys gaming and does this online with his friends.

D – Drugs Mark denies any substance use. He has not tried smoking, vaping or alcohol.

S – Sexuality Mark is not in a current relationship, nor sexually active. He identifies as heterosexual.

S – Suicide/depression Mark denies any suicidal or self-harm thoughts currently. He says he has never intentionally hurt himself. Mark does not voice any concerns about low mood.

S – Safety Mark feels safe in hospital, but is a bit concerned about tonight's events and police attending his house, but otherwise is settled and cooperative. He denies any past traumatic experiences.

Klein 2014.

- Mark has a close, supportive family, who are help-seeking and willing to engage in care.
- He is a high achieving student with good friends and social supports.
- No trauma history.
- Mark has communicated remorse for his actions and a desire to prevent it from occurring again.

KNOWLEDGE

- Adolescence is a time of dynamic maturation and rapid brain development. A cascade of neurobiological changes occur – there is rapid growth, major physiological changes and hormonal fluctuations, as well as changes in learning styles, emotional reactivity and behaviour. It is a time that is associated with increased reactivity to emotional and social cues as well as impulsive behaviour (Casey et al 2019).
- It is more common for young people to experience symptoms of mental disturbance than a clinically diagnosable mental disorder. Understanding adolescent development will help to differentiate between normal emotions and 'normative' adolescent behaviours with early signs of mental health problems. The duration of emotions and the concerns of the parents will help to support this assessment.
- It is not uncommon for adolescents to experience distressing and disruptive emotions, thoughts or behaviours, which are only diagnosed as a behavioural disorder when they are severe, persistent and adversely affect daily functioning.
- An acute behavioural disturbance is not necessarily a behavioural disorder, but may be an externalising way of expressing strong emotion. Behavioural disorders involve a pattern of disruptive behaviours in children that last for at least 6 months and cause problems in various settings, including school, at home and in social situations (Perrotta & Fabiano 2021).
- Adolescents may be difficult to engage as they often do not seek help and often do not see their behaviours as problematic. A range of barriers exist, including limited mental health knowledge, perceived social stigma, embarrassment, concerns over confidentiality, and not knowing who to trust (Radez et al 2021).

ATTITUDES

- Young people with challenging behaviours may be seen as 'naughty' by others; therefore it is essential to reflect on your own beliefs and values to ensure that these do not impact on the provision of safe, non-judgemental, and culturally sensitive healthcare.
- Likewise, health professionals' attitudes towards the parents' capacity to manage their child's behaviour and perceived lack of parenting boundaries and limits could potentially impact on the assessment process.

MENTAL HEALTH SKILLS

- It is important to build rapport with the young person and develop an environment of trust before undertaking a psychosocial assessment. Talking about topics not related to the reason for presentation (e.g. school, pets, interests, movies) can be an effective way to facilitate building rapport and improving engagement.
- Provide psychoeducation to Mark and his family about the impacts on health and mental health of excessive screen time, the importance of good sleep hygiene and the link between poor sleep and irritability and/or low mood. Discuss with Mark and his parents the need to structure in daily routine, socialisation and exercise, and the benefits of these on overall health and wellbeing. Nurses can support families with setting screen time guidelines and family media agreements to help young people 'stay safe', 'think first' (before posting), 'stay balanced' and 'communicate openly'. An example of an agreement

can be found on the Common Sense Media website (see Useful websites) (Ramjan & Clark 2020).
- Children and young people can be taught various strategies to help them recognise signs of building frustration and to then use coping skills to defuse anger or aggressive behaviour. These strategies include: learning alternative ways to manage and express feelings of anger, and relaxation strategies such as use of sensory modulation and stress management skills.

NURSING ACTIONS AND INTERVENTIONS

Factors to be considered prior to commencing assessment when someone arrives with a police escort.
- The place of assessment needs to provide privacy and a safe environment with access to emergency supports if required.
- Staff safety must be considered when someone first arrives in the ED with a history of aggression. Do police need to remain present? Is security required?

Structure of assessment
- Ideally, if it is safe, the nurse would see Mark alone – to assist with rapport building. Ensure a child-friendly approach, using age-appropriate language and explain confidentiality and any limitations around this.
- Engagement with family members is a priority – manage parental expectations by providing information and explaining assessment process. Ensure opportunities for them to ask questions.
- Observe the family as a unit – including interactions and communication style.
- Prior to discharge, ensure that Mark can sustain his current mood and behaviour in the presence of his parents. Observe how they interact, and how Mark is when they are present.

Safety planning
- Develop a plan with Mark and his parents to identify early warning signs, triggers, patterns of behaviour (e.g. time of day or particular feelings) and consequences of these behaviours.
- Discuss with family about what usually works and what does not. Develop strategies to prevent future escalation and reduce anxiety.
- Assist with the development of an agreement between Mark and his parents about appropriate limits for time spent on devices or gaming for the immediate future.

RELEVANT TREATMENT MODALITIES AND CONSIDERATIONS
- Immediate care planning is focused around risk assessment of Mark's safety and his current supports. In this case, Mark was not found to have any acute risks and he demonstrated calm and appropriate behaviour over time while in hospital. There was no evidence of him being at risk of harm to others.
- Provide the young person and their family with written resources regarding supports in the community, including a list of private psychologists, HeadSpace and 24-hour crisis support lines (phone, text and online). Speaking to the young person about when they can use crisis support lines and reassuring them that their contact will be anonymous may increase the likelihood that they will use them if they need to.
- Follow-up with the young person's general practitioner (GP) is aways a good idea. Send ED assessment notes to the GP with the parents' consent, with a view to them attending for a health check-up and consideration of a mental health care plan (MHCP), in order to obtain a referral for accessing some psychology support in the community.

- It may be appropriate to provide parents with parenting resources and courses for example, Tuning into Teens, or for younger children, Triple P Positive Parenting Program (see Useful websites).
- Discuss with the young person and their parents the potential for the development of an internet gaming disorder and the warning signs to watch out for (see Box 3.3.1). Recommend they discuss with the GP the possibility of a referral to a psychologist with expertise in this area to assist the family prevent the development of any problematic behaviours.

Reflection

1. Adolescence is often seen as a time of angst and risk. How might you work with young people to build on their strengths and promote their confidence and self-efficacy?
2. Parents often find episodes of acute behavioural disturbance confronting and unsettling. How might you reassure parents during these times to ensure they do not lose confidence in their parenting abilities?

Useful websites

Common Sense Media website: www.commonsensemedia.org/family-media-agreement
HeadSpace: www.headspace.com
Kids Helpline: kidshelpline.com.au
Tuning into Teens: www.resourcingparents.nsw.gov.au
Triple P Positive Parenting Program (for younger children) www.triplep-parenting.net.au/au-uken/triple-p/

References

Australian Bureau of Statistics (ABS) 2018. Causes of death, Australia 2017. Cat. no. 3303.0. ABS, Canberra.

Australian Institute of Health and Welfare (AIHW) 2022. Suicide and self-harm monitoring. Online. Available: www.aihw.gov.au/suicide-self-harm-monitoring/data/populations-age-groups/intentional-self-harm-hospitalisations-among-young.

Australian Institute of Health and Welfare (AIHW) 2020. Australia's children. Cat. no. CWS 69. AIHW, Canberra.

Carter B, Rees P, Hale L et al 2016. Association between portable screen-based media device access or use and sleep outcomes: A systematic review and meta-analysis. JAMA Pediatrics, 170(12):1202–8.

Casey BJ, Heller AS, Gee DG et al 2019. Development of the emotional brain. Neuroscience Letters 6:693:29–34.

Crone EA, Konijn EA 2018. Media use and brain development during adolescence. Nature Communications 9:588.

Dickson JM, Cruise K, McCall CA et al 2019. A systematic review of the antecedents and prevalence of suicide, self-harm and suicide ideation in Australian Aboriginal and Torres Strait Islander Youth. International Journal of Environmental Research and Public Health 16:3154.

Foster K, Marks P, O'Brien AJ et al 2020. Mental health in nursing: Theory and practice for clinical settings. 5th edn. Elsevier Australia, Sydney.

Graham A, Sahlberg P 2021. Growing up digital Australia: Phase 2 technical report. Gonski Institute for Education. UNSW, Sydney.

Hiscock H, Neely RJ, Lei S 2018. Paediatric mental and physical health presentations to emergency departments, Victoria, 2008–15. Medical Journal of Australia 208(8):343–8.

Hungerford C, Hodgson D, Bostick R et al 2018. Mental health care. 3rd edn. John Wiley, Milton.

John A, Glendenning AC, Marchant A et al 2018. Self-harm, suicidal behaviours, and cyberbullying in children and young people: Systematic review. Journal of Medical Internet Research 20(4):e129.

Khasawneh A, Madathil KC, Dixon E et al 2020. Examining the self-harm and suicide contagion effects of the blue whale challenge on YouTube and Twitter: Qualitative study. JMIR Mental Health 7(6):e15973.

Kids Helpline 2019. Insights 2019: Insights into Young people in Australia. Online. Available: www.yourtown.com.au/sites/default/files/document/KidsHelpline-Insights2019-Report-APPROVED.pdf.

Klein D, Goldenring A, Adelman WP 2014. HEEADSSS 3.0: The psychosocial interview for adolescents updated for a new century fuelled by media. Contemporary Pediatrics. Online. Available: www.trapeze.org.au/sites/default/files/2014_01_Klein_Goldenring_HEEADSSS3.0_Contemporary%20Pediatrics.pdf.

MH-TRACE 2021. Indicators of NSW Mental Health Service Demand and Care, June 2021. NSW Ministry of Health, Sydney.

Ogundele M 2018. Behavioural and emotional disorders in childhood: A brief overview for paediatricians. World Journal of Clinical Pediatrics 7(1):9–26.

Orlando J 2019. How to know if your child is addicted to video games and what to do about it. The Conversation. Online. Available: www.joanneorlando.com.au/articles/2019/7/9/how-to-know-if-your-child-is-addicted-to-video-games-and-what-to-do-about-it/.

Paulus F, Ohmann S, Von Gontard A et al 2018. Internet gaming disorder in children and adolescents: A systematic review. Developmental Medicine and Child Neurology 60(7):645–59.

Perera J, Wand T, Bein KJ et al 2018. Presentations to NSW emergency departments with self-harm, suicidal ideation, or intentional poisoning, 2010–2014. Medical Journal of Australia 208(8):348–53.

Perrotta G, Fabiano G 2021. Behavioural disorders in children and adolescents: Definition, clinical contexts, neurobiological profiles and clinical treatments. Open Journal of Pediatrics and Child Health 6(1): doi.org/10.17352/ojpch.000030.

Radez J, Reardon T, Creswell C et al 2021. Why do children and adolescents (not) seek and access professional help for their mental health problems? A systematic review of quantitative and qualitative studies. European Child and Adolescent Psychiatry 30(2):183–211.

Ramjan L, Clark, G 2020. Mental disorders of childhood and adolescence. In: Foster K, Marks P, O'Brien A et al (eds) Mental health in nursing: Theory and practice for clinical settings. Elsevier Australia, Sydney.

Ray Morgan 2016. Nine in 10 Aussie teens have a mobile (and most are already on their second or subsequent handset) 22 August. Online. Available: www.roymorgan.com/findings/6929-australian-teenagers-and-their-mobile-phones-june-2016-201608220922.

Rivers I, Gonzalez C, Nodin N et al 2018. LGBT people and suicidality in youth: A qualitative study of perceptions of risk and protective circumstances. Social Science and Medicine 212:1–8.

Say DF, Carison A, Hill A et al 2021. Mental health presentations to the paediatric emergency department. A retrospective study. Journal of Paediatrics and Child Health 57(5):684–95.

Stephen R, Edmonds R 2018. Briefing 53: Social media, young people and mental health. Centre for Mental Health, London.

Westerman T, Sheridan L 2020. Whole community suicide prevention forums for Aboriginal Australians. Australian Psychology 2020: doi.org/10.1111/ap.12470.

CHAPTER 3.4

Working with families of people experiencing mental illness or distress

Sophie Isobel

KEY POINTS

- Individual experiences of illness occur within a wider context of people's lives and can affect family members, who may also play supportive or caregiving roles.
- Families supporting a loved one in an emergency care setting often experience significant stress and worry. Many issues can be resolved through transparent and clear communication, validation of concerns and genuine recognition that families are interwoven with people's experiences of health and illness.
- Nurses are ideally placed to engage with families, support families and also advocate for families within treatment planning.
- Empathic and non-judgemental interactions with families can improve individual experiences, as well as efficacy of care in emergency settings.

LEARNING OUTCOMES

This chapter will assist you to:

- identify the importance of families in the delivery of care for people experiencing mental illness or distress
- consider how to engage with families in emergency settings using strengths-based approaches
- apply a systems lens to interactions with families that recognises the 'lived expertise' of both people accessing care and their families
- prioritise the delivery of family-inclusive care through compassionate caregiving and engagement, alongside collaborative care planning and information sharing.

Lived experience comment
by Helena Roennfeldt
....
NEED FOR PRIVACY

People in distress often experience the ED environment as overstimulating and chaotic. A lack of privacy also contributes to feeling vulnerable. Family members often accompany someone in a mental health crisis to the ED and can be a vital source of support during the long wait times. Family support can mitigate the emotional impact and embarrassment of being distressed in a busy ED environment during a mental health crisis. However, a lack of privacy amplifies the struggle for both the person in distress and families to articulate their experiences. We can feel judged that our ED presentation is inappropriate or less legitimate than physical health presentations. Kindness and compassion from nurses can lessen the impact of the chaotic and clinical ED environment. At the same time, acts of hospitality demonstrate that we are worthy of care and that our mental health crisis and suicidality are valid reasons for seeking support.

INTRODUCTION

Any experience of illness, including accessing care and treatment, occurs in a wider context of people's lives. Most people's lives include key relationships with people who are considered family. The construction of a 'family', and who is included, is determined by individuals and can often take diverse forms, including relationships determined by origin, birth or choice (Foster et al 2020).

In healthcare, family members may be referred to as 'carers', although not all family members will identify with this term. The person considered to be important in their care can also differ from individuals identified as 'next of kin', and may change over time. It is essential that nurses and other health professionals are comfortable in identifying family roles and relationships, and recognise the interplay of these relationships with experiences of health and illness, including in acute situations. Recognising the vital importance of relationships in the lives of people accessing care is essential to providing effective care and supporting wellbeing (e.g. Baker et al 2019; Nickel et al 2018; Victorian Government 2018).

Families are often present in the emergency department (ED), and will need to be actively engaged; this includes being provided with information and support. Including families in a person's care can be particularly complex in an emergency setting, due to the acuity of care and unpredictable aspects of the environment (Sagoo & Grytnes 2020). However, it is essential that care be delivered in ways that acknowledge the importance of families in the lives of people receiving care and also the importance of family roles (such as parent, sibling, carer or partner), held by people who may themselves experience mental illness or experience health/mental health impacts related to the 'caring' role. Family members of people who experience mental illness often provide vital informal caregiving (Foster et al 2020) that ensures safety, quality of life and access to treatment. Yet, as with any family or relationship, roles are likely multifaceted and caregiving pathways should not be assumed.

When beginning to work in ways that recognise the importance of families, conceptualising the family as a 'system' can be helpful, where separate parts of a larger system rely on each other for functioning. In a family system, all members are connected and the functioning or wellbeing of one person influences the others (Bowen 1978). This can lead to patterns of reciprocal functioning, where members can 'borrow' strength from each other during periods of need, as well as patterns of relating, where control and levels of functioning are developed and maintained between members. This might mean, for example, that one family member routinely takes a 'role' of being bossy or presents as highly capable, while another may take a 'role' of being more submissive or seemingly inept. Such patterns exist in all families, but can be amplified or altered when there is illness. Patterns of relating observed during healthcare interactions may be representative of longstanding ways that family systems cope. Experiences of illness with a family member are known to affect the whole family (Soklaridis et al 2019). Recognising families as systems where each member is affected by the others also highlights why providing care or treatment to one member of a family needs to incorporate other family members.

While healthcare delivery overall is increasingly inclusive of families, families of people who experience mental illness often report interactions with services that are not inclusive, sensitive, or collaborative, and encounters with healthcare professionals who do not share information, consult or support them (Schaffer 2020). Families can feel (and/or be) blamed for their loved ones' illness, leading to stigmatisation by services, exclusion from care or positioning as either 'burdened' or 'overinvolved'. Fear of blame can also make family members reluctant to engage with services. To add further complexity, many healthcare workers may feel that they lack the skills, knowledge and time to engage effectively and work collaboratively with family members (Shah-Anwar et al 2019).

THE NEEDS OF CHILDREN

When thinking about families, it is essential to also consider the needs of children. Children and young people can be overlooked when considering the impacts of mental illness on families and can also be overlooked when considering how to engage with families in healthcare delivery. Many children and young people who live in families where someone experiences mental illness provide psychological or physical care for their family member or may take on additional caregiving or other responsible roles. It should not be assumed that children in families are not aware of what is happening or do not require information about treatment of their family member. Children can experience a range of impacts from mental illness in the family, but with support and information, these effects can be buffered. Interactions with services provide a window of opportunity for health professionals to engage directly with children and to support families to identify and address the needs of children.

WORKING WITH FAMILIES IN EMERGENCY SETTINGS

Working with families in emergency settings brings unique challenges. EDs are often busy and crowded, staff are focused on prioritising care, and interactions are brief. Family members have reported feeling disrupted by the unfamiliar environment, having their concerns dismissed and feeling 'invisible' and powerless (Emmamally et al 2020a). Conversely, having positive interactions with nurses and other health professionals in these settings can improve experiences of care and overall pathways through services and treatment. Nurses are often the healthcare professionals who interact the most with families in EDs, and as such it is essential that they strive to have the necessary knowledge, confidence and skills to best support families. Even in brief interactions in high acuity settings, simple strategies can be used to ensure family members are recognised, heard and included, and that people's family roles are incorporated into care.

In EDs, people often prefer to have their family member with them when receiving medical or nursing interventions. Having family present can reduce worry and enhance engagement with care. However, when people are presenting for reasons associated with mental health and wellbeing, issues of confidentiality and privacy require consideration, at times leading to complexity when attempting to respect the individual's autonomy while also including family members in care. Transparent communication, discussion among the team and professional judgement are required. Including family members in care can be mutually beneficial, as family members can be very useful sources of information to inform treatment. For example, family members may identify changes in behaviour or mood or propose strategies that have been effective for the person in the past. Many families provide high levels of care to their family members that experience mental illness and to ensure ongoing support post discharge, need to be actively engaged in any treatment planning or delivery. While issues of confidentiality and privacy can be tricky, fears about compromising the autonomy of the individual should not thwart all contact with families. While, of course, there are exceptions; for example, when people specifically ask staff not to communicate with their family, these situations should not determine usual practice. While personal and specific information may at times not be able to be shared, general information-giving and engagement with all families remains essential.

In emergency settings, people may be accompanied by family members who themselves are experiencing distress, agitation or fear – regardless of the reason for presentation. On top of this, seeking treatment for a person with a mental illness can at times be frustrating and can lead to high levels of agitation directed at healthcare workers. Nurses are therefore often confronted by families who are experiencing sudden or unanticipated emotional disruption or crisis and require support themselves, while simultaneously playing crucial roles in providing support for their loved one.

SCENARIO 3.4.1

Sasha

Sasha is an 18-year-old young woman waiting in the sub-acute section of an emergency department in a regional hospital. Sasha was brought in by her family who were concerned after she stopped engaging in her daily treatment required for her physical health issues and subsequently expressed suicidal ideas, telling them there was 'no point'. Sasha reports a recent history of low mood and decreased enjoyment of usual activities. She describes exhaustion and loss of appetite. Sasha has a diagnosis of cystic fibrosis (CF) since age 6 months, and reports being tired of the daily treatment regimen required for her CF and feeling like a burden on her parents, who often disagree about her care.

Sasha has been in the department for 4 hours and is awaiting psychiatric review. She has been seen by the medical team and medically cleared, with a plan to refer her back to her specialist team in the community for ongoing monitoring and treatment of her CF, pending outcome of the psychiatric assessment. Sasha's parents, Kate and Jill, are also present and want to take Sasha home. Jill is Sasha's primary carer; she accompanies Sasha to her appointments and physical therapies and is also the primary carer of Sasha's brother, Jim, who is 6 years old, and is also present in the ED and appears occupied on an iPad. Kate has taken time off work today and has been increasingly expressing frustration at having to wait for the psychiatry team and worried at the potential for Sasha to be exposed to pathogens in the context of the ED environment. Kate has approached the nurses' station a number of times, becoming increasingly demanding in wanting to know when the doctor will arrive. Both Kate and Jill deny that Sasha has any mental health issues, are stating she is 'now fine' and will be safe to go home, and that they do not want Sasha admitted to a mental health unit. Kate has stated that if the doctor doesn't come in the next 20 minutes they will leave. Sasha presents as teary and withdrawn.

◤ RED FLAGS

- There are well-known reciprocal relationships between mental health and physical health. Sasha is experiencing a sustained physical health issue and an entwined mental health presentation. Sasha is in the role of child in the family unit, but is an adult in the healthcare environment. Issues of consent relating to involving family, and the level of engagement with family that Sasha desires, need to be discussed.
- Increasing agitation of a family member (Kate) requires consideration of what engagement, information, communication or de-escalation may be beneficial.
- Expressed intent to self-discharge before psychiatric review.
- Sasha's current presentation and recent actions are incongruent with the family's expressed perception that she is fine.
- There is a need to assess ongoing risk of harm through careful conversations with both Sasha and her family and the establishment of trust, engagement and a private space.
- The assumed gender of Sasha's parents may have an impact upon how some staff interact or engage with the family.

PROTECTIVE FACTORS

- Sasha's family are present, engaged, supportive and seemingly cohesive.
- Sasha's age may allow her access to specialised youth services for proactive community follow-up.
- Sasha has a team of engaged health professionals who manage her CF in the community who can provide sustained follow-up. Communication with this team will be important for transition of care.
- Sasha voiced her suicidal thoughts to her family, which suggests she is open to receiving help and feels safe to talk to them.
- Sasha came voluntarily to the ED.

KNOWLEDGE

- Be aware of the interplay between physical and mental health experiences and take time to both disentangle this relationship and recognise its inherent nature. People may present with physical symptoms of mental health origin, may present with mental health symptoms linked to physical changes, or may be experiencing both physical and mental health disruptions concurrently. It will be important to consider what impact Sasha's current mental state may be having on her physical health (including through decreased adherence to treatment), and also what the relationship is between her current physical health state and recent deterioration in mental state.

- Rarely are family relationships all positive or all negative – excluding in situations of abuse or violence. It is important to recognise that families can be protective and supportive at the same time as causing challenges or contributing to difficulties.
- Further conversations are required, both with Sasha on her own and with her family, particularly in relation to the expressed desire to leave prior to psychiatric assessment. While this is a choice Sasha can make, it may also mean the loss of a window of opportunity to provide crucial mental health support and services to her. It will also be necessary to ensure it is Sasha's choice to leave and not her parents. Nurses may be best placed to explore what Sasha thinks will be helpful.
- Expressed fear of admission to the mental health unit by Sasha's parents and comments that she is 'fine' despite the presenting circumstances, may relate to concerns around stigma, fear of blame or lack of understanding. Brief supportive enquiry may help identify concerns, and providing information and psychoeducation may help address these.
- Knowledge of the relevant Mental Health Act, including understanding of how the local Mental Health Act provides for families, helps ensure the delivery of safe, legal and humanising care. For example, most Acts explicitly state that, to the greatest extent practicable, family members should be involved in decisions about care and treatment. The Act may also guide communication with families, matters of consent and issues of confidentiality. Being knowledgeable about what is possible and necessary in relation to including families will aid in talking with consumers and family members.
- Knowledge of local policies related to confidentiality, privacy, next of kin, primary carers and nominated persons is critical. These may be helpful in determining who the treating team can and cannot communicate with and how to proceed when there are differing perspectives about how much information can be shared and with whom.
- Knowledge of child protection legislation is also important when working with families, both in the provision of care to children, who may be at risk of harm, but also in recognising the potential impacts of parental or family illness upon caregiving roles and child wellbeing, and for ensuring the safety of all children during opportunistic encounters with services.
- Presence of a child (brother Jim) on the unit requires consideration – including what explanation he has been given about the events leading up to the presentation, and whether Kate and Jill require support in explaining it to him in age-appropriate ways, alongside caution in undertaking assessments and conversations with him present, despite appearing distracted.

ATTITUDES

- It is essential that heteronormative assumptions about what a family should look like do not direct, impact or influence staff interactions or the provision of care. Self-reflection on biases or judgements about 'traditional' family structures or roles is required. To enact this may require keeping an open mind, clear communication and respectful questioning, using non-assumptive language and careful use of pronouns and titles. While directly clarifying roles and relationships may be important, and family members expect to be asked direct questions in emergency settings, such as 'What is your relationship to the person accessing care?', questions regarding people's sexual orientation or gender identity are not usually appropriate unless directly relevant to care, engagement or treatment.
- Attitudes about mental illness and families need to be actively reflected upon and challenged where necessary. This will include self-reflection about any assumptions related to blame or stigmatising attitudes. Clinical supervision may also be helpful with this.
- To enact cultural safety, nurses need awareness of their own experiences of culture, family and illness, with reflection on how this may lead to unconscious bias or assumptions

about other people's experiences. Reflective questions may include: 'Why am I reacting so strongly to this person?', 'What assumptions am I making about this family and why?' and 'How do my cultural beliefs alter how I perceive this person/family?'.

MENTAL HEALTH SKILLS

- All nurses, regardless of their speciality, require skills in assessment, engagement and care delivery for people who experience mental health challenges and their families. This requires knowledge of the interplay between physical and mental health, understanding of the varied ways mental illnesses can present and attention to the centrality of the therapeutic relationship in being able to ensure people are comfortable to answer questions honestly about their mental health.
- Family members often report that they are not included in assessments; however, collaborative and holistic assessments are likely to yield more clinically useful information to guide care. While nurses may fear that this process may take additional time, it can also lead to more streamlined care.
- EDs are high-load work environments where communication is central to safe and effective care. Effective communication requires introducing yourself, providing regular updates and transparent information, reassurance to both individuals and family members, validation of emotional responses, including frustration, minimising defensive or rushed responses and even in brief interactions, ensuring you are present, engaged and focused on what is being said.
- Conversations about risk need to be undertaken with confidence and competence.
- Compassion and empathy underpin all mental health care. This involves establishing a therapeutic relationship with people that makes them feel safe and supported, often through the use of active listening, appropriate eye contact and validating statements.
- Empathy is a core aspect of nursing and requires trying to see things from another perspective, avoiding judgement, and recognising and responding to emotion. For example, in EDs when talking to families, statements such as: 'I can see that you are upset; it is understandable that you would feel overwhelmed at the moment' or 'I notice that you seem frustrated. Can I suggest ...?' may be helpful.
- Often people wait for extended periods of time in EDs. Family members experience uncertainty and a lack of control associated with waiting (Sagoo & Grytnes 2020). Experiences of 'waiting' can be buffered when family members are actively informed about progress and their basic needs are attended to in empathic ways. While these actions can take extra time, they can also reduce the likelihood of incidents occurring or distress escalating.
- Respectful language and professional communication, both about and to people accessing care and their families, is important. In relation to mental health, it is important to check what words and labels people feel comfortable using and referring to a person by name rather than by their diagnosis.
- Family relationships and roles should be part of any assessment. This could involve questions such as: 'Who supports you and who do you support?' and 'Is there anything about your family that it would be helpful for me to know?'. Family resilience can be enhanced by supporting shared narratives of events, mapping existing resources, developing collaborative plans, engaging supports or services, and listening to both the positives and negatives of experiences.
- Nurses are well placed to identify subtle changes in the presentation of people accessing services or their family members, before agitation progresses to aggression. Skills of de-escalation involve recognising unmet needs that may be leading to agitation, expressing genuine concern, promoting dignity and autonomy, intervening early and remaining calm. Communication is the most important skill of de-escalation. The focus should be

on establishing rapport, answering questions, and finding agreements without making unreasonable concessions or appearing uncompromising. Many incidents in ED occur due to family members feeling ignored or excluded from care.

NURSING ACTIONS AND INTERVENTIONS

- Include family in processes of assessment by seeking information about the person's usual levels of health and functioning and any observed changes.
- Provide information and education about mental health, wellbeing and treatment to families, including pathways to carer support resources.
- Undertake collaborative care planning with families through engaging families in decisions about care, ensuring feasibility of treatment decisions and promoting dignity of choice.
- Provide supportive interventions to families; for example, ask family members about their wellbeing and needs, ensure everyone gets heard in consultations, observe family dynamics and provide family members with the information, hope and reassurance they need to be able to cope with the stress of the crisis.

RELEVANT TREATMENT MODALITIES AND CONSIDERATIONS

- Many interactions with families in emergency settings are brief and focused on the person presenting for care; however, these brief interactions can also be therapeutic.
- When care and treatment are viewed through a family-oriented lens, alongside any biological or pharmacological treatments, there is a need for family psychoeducation and support.
- Psychoeducation in this context encompasses the provision of holistic information about mental illness and treatment, which can enhance engagement with care and the family's ability to provide support.
- Strengths-based approaches are important when working with families – focus on what is working well in families and what can be further enhanced. This does not dismiss the 'problem' but focuses on using and accessing existing resources and capacities to support coping.
- Family systems approaches in practice require healthcare professionals to be conscious of how they may interact with the (family) 'system', and to recognise that often dynamics in families have been longstanding and have served some purpose. The nurse's role may be to ensure that individual voices get heard, that the healthcare team don't get 'caught up' in the family's anxiety, and to prompt families to notice their own ways of responding to stress. Taking a moment to step back from intense emotions, to consider 'what else may be going on here' can be helpful, as well as trying not to take sides with family members. Other examples of systems-oriented strategies include suggesting that you hear from one person in the family at a time while also promoting shared problem-solving, for example, by asking: 'What strategies have you tried as a family to manage so far?'
- One of the most useful interventions for families who support someone with mental illness may be to link them in to services run by and for people in similar situations. Local carer, sibling, children and relationship services often run groups, counselling services and provide resources that can support family members to access their own sustained supports to enable them to maintain their caring roles.

SUMMARY

Through reflection on underlying assumptions, fears, biases and expectations about encounters with families in the ED, it becomes easier for nurses to engage with families in genuine, compassionate and respectful ways. In an emergency situation, families are often experiencing significant stress and worry. Many issues and tensions can be resolved through transparent and clear communication, validation of concerns and genuine recognition that families are interwoven with people's experiences of health and illness.

At times, staff in emergency settings need to make decisions on behalf of families and individuals, as they may lack the capacity, knowledge or time to make the decision themselves, or may be too overwhelmed. In these circumstances, communication, transparency, professionalism and respect are also essential. Nurses are ideally placed to engage with and support families, but they may also be required to advocate for families within multidisciplinary team approaches to ensure that treatment is delivered in family-inclusive ways.

Engaging with families in the ED does not involve standardised steps, but instead requires consideration of each individual situation, with a focus on creating authentic connections with families, respect and empathy for families and clear communication. Families may bring different coping styles, communication styles and beliefs to the ED, which play out in differing responses to illness and treatment, indicating a need for ongoing vigilance to taking a non-judgmental stance and spending time ensuring cultural safety within the delivery of care (Emmamally et al 2020a).

Engagement with a person's family should be underpinned by understandings that prioritise authentic engagement and experiences of care, not just health outcomes, and that recognise the 'lived expertise' of both people accessing care and their families. This includes recognising the potential for non-traditional family structures and memberships, and providing equitable approaches to all families. Family members consistently report wanting compassionate and reassuring displays of care and opportunities to have their concerns heard, alongside the sharing of information about their loved one's condition and plans for treatment (Emmamally et al 2020b).

Nurses and other health professionals working in emergency settings need to ensure that they treat all people accessing care and their families with respect, that they consider the wider context of people's lives and how this intersects with care, that they take the time required to provide information in accessible formats and without jargon, that they value the expertise of family members and proactively engage in collaborative decision-making with the person accessing care and the people that person identifies as their family.

Reflection

1. What assumptions, beliefs or experiences impact upon how you perceive family members of people accessing care?
2. Can you recall a positive interaction you have had with family members of people accessing care, or as a family member of someone accessing care? What actions or words from yourself or others facilitated this interaction to go well?
3. What specific words might you use to open up conversations with people accessing care about their family?
4. If you observed concerning interactions among family members accompanying their loved one to an ED, what steps or actions could you take? In your local context, who would you access for further information if you were not sure how to proceed?

Useful websites

Australian Institute of Family Studies: aifs.gov.au/
Bouverie Centre Family Institute: www.bouverie.org.au/
Carers Australia: www.carersaustralia.com.au/
Mental Health Carers Australia: www.mentalhealthcarersaustralia.org.au/
National Children of Parents with a Mental Illness Initiative: www.copmi.net.au/
National Workforce for Child Mental Health: emergingminds.com.au/

References

Baker D, Burgat L, Stavely H 2019. We're in this together: Family inclusive practice in mental health services for young people. Orygen, Melbourne.

Bowen M 978 Family therapy in clinical practice. Jasonn Aronson, New York, NY.

Emmamally W, Erlingsson C, Brysiewicz P 2020a. Describing healthcare providers' perceptions of relational practice with families in the emergency department: A qualitative study. Curationis 43(1):1–7.

Emmamally W, Erlingsson C, Brysiewicz P 2020b. Families' perceptions of relational practice in the emergency department: A qualitative study. International Emergency Nursing 51:100877.

Foster K, Isobel S, Usher, K 2020. Working with families in mental health. In: Foster K, Marks P, O'Brien A et al. Mental health in nursing: Theory and practice for clinical settings. Elsevier Health Sciences, Sydney.

Nickel WK, Weinberger SE, Guze PA 2018. Principles for patient and family partnership in care: An American College of Physicians position paper. Annals of Internal Medicine 169(11): 796–9.

Sagoo SN, Grytnes R 2020. Involvement un-enabled? An ethnographic study of the challenges and potentials of involving relatives in the acute ambulatory clinical pathway. BMC Health Services Research 20(1):1–18.

Schaffer MA 2020. Family perspectives of healthcare for relatives living with a mental illness. Perspectives in Psychiatric Care. PMID: 33373064.

Shah-Anwar S, Gumley A, Hunter S 019 Mental health professionals' perspectives of family-focused practice across child and adult mental health settings: A qualitative synthesis. Child and Youth Services 40(4):383–404.

Soklaridis S, McCann M, Waller-Vintar J et al 2019. Where is the family voice? Examining the relational dimensions of the family-healthcare professional and its perceived impact on patient care outcomes in mental health and addictions. PLOS ONE 14(4):e0215071.

Victorian Government 2018. Working together with families and carers: Chief psychiatrist's guideline. Department of Health and Human Services, Melbourne. Online. Available: www2. health.vic.gov.au/about/key-staff/chief-psychiatrist/chief-psychiatrist-guidelines.

CHAPTER 3.5

Assessing and responding to an older person presenting with confusion, agitation and delirium

Scott Lamont and Sally Matthews

KEY POINTS

- Delirium is a consequence of physical changes relating to illness or related treatment, but the underlying cause is not always known.
- Delirium is highly prevalent in older persons within community, residential and acute care settings.
- Delirium is underdiagnosed, and often mistaken for a primary mental health disorder.
- If not recognised and treated promptly, delirium can lead to increased morbidity and mortality.

LEARNING OUTCOMES

This chapter will assist you to:
- understand the risk factors, signs and symptoms commonly associated with the development of delirium
- identify screening and assessment tools for delirium, and relevant referral processes for its optimum management
- initiate evidence-based interventions and a psychosocial care plan to reduce the severity and duration of delirium
- engage patients with delirium using person-centred principles
- recognise the key features in responding to and de-escalating agitation in the clinical environment.

Lived experience comment
by Helena Roennfeldt

GATHERING AND RESPECTING THE UNIQUE KNOWLEDGE OF FAMILIES

In an environment where problems and even solutions are individualised, it can be easy to dismiss the unique role of family. This includes, but is much more than, obtaining information from families. Family relationships have a role in fostering wellbeing across the whole life span. As family members, we can feel excluded and want someone also to acknowledge our needs and fears. Involving families and carers builds a trusting relationship with the treatment team, and strengthens the relationship between the person and their family. Listening and sharing information with families shows an appreciation for the family's unique knowledge about how best to support their older relatives, including their usual behaviour and warning signs that they are unwell. Families may also have a role in advocating for their relative's needs, relaying information, and rallying services and support together if needed. However, it is always important to respect the person's wishes and the family in the level of involvement they want.

INTRODUCTION

Presentations to emergency departments (ED) have been increasing globally, with older persons being disproportionately represented in these increases due to higher rates of illness in the ageing population. Transfers from residential aged care facilities (RACF) in Australia to EDs are common, with particular diagnostic and treatment challenges for this sub-group being noted (Hullick et al 2021). Older persons transferred from RACFs may present with impaired cognitive functioning, confusion and agitation, and assessment difficulties may ensue if the person is unable to provide an accurate medical history or details of current medications, both essential information for ED staff in the provision of timely, and safe, person-centred interventions and care. Consequently, presentations of people from RACFs to EDs often present a range of complexities not present in many other ED presentations.

Internationally, 'deficient information' is cited as a common complaint in relation to transfers between aged care and emergency care facilities. Deficient information from RACFs regarding the person's presentation and medical history can lead to delays in, or inappropriate care and iatrogenic harm (harm caused by treatment), all of which can compromise the quality of care and patient flow in EDs (Munene et al 2020). For these reasons, ED nurses should ensure they seek comprehensive clinical handovers from RACFs, often via paramedics, which includes the reason for the transfer, presenting symptoms and the person's medical history.

RESIDENTIAL AGED CARE TRANSFERS TO EMERGENCY DEPARTMENTS

Comprehensive handover and transfer of care information is often highlighted and takes on greater importance in older persons transferred to EDs from RACFs with delirium, which may not be recognised by referring facilities or the receiving healthcare specialists. Delirium is recognised as a serious medical condition and is characterised in the *Diagnostic and Statistical*

Manual of Mental Disorders (DSM-5) as the following: a disturbance in attention (reduced ability to focus or concentrate) and awareness (impaired orientation to the environment), which develops over a short period of time (usually hours to a few days), representing a change from the person's baseline attention and awareness, and which fluctuates in severity throughout the course of the day. Impaired cognition is also present, which may manifest as a disturbance in memory, language, perception or visuospatial ability (APA 2013). While some of these disturbances may be visibly evident, others may be subtle (see Table 3.5.1), and thus require careful consideration in all older persons transferred from RACFs.

It is important to note that delirium must be differentiated from dementia and depression, which are also common in older people, and are both risk factors for delirium. Although they may share some common features in clinical presentations, a comprehensive and collateral history will help differentiate between these conditions, as will knowledge of the different associated characteristics (see Table 3.5.2).

TABLE 3.5.1 Delirium subtypes: hypoactive, hyperactive and mixed

Hypoactive	Hyperactive	Mixed
Apathy, lethargy or psychomotor retardation may be present, and a person may appear drowsy or withdrawn	Restlessness, hypervigilance, or irritability may be present, and a person may present as agitated and combative, with disturbance of thinking, or hallucinations	A person may fluctuate and show signs of hypoactive and hyperactive symptoms throughout the day

Robinson-Reilly & Marks 2020.

TABLE 3.5.2 Differentiating delirium, dementia and depression

Features	Dementia	Delirium	Depression
Onset and duration	Slow deterioration over time – months to years	Sudden onset – hours or days	Mood change over 2 weeks, and may coincide with a life event or change such as death of a loved one
Course	Slow and progressive cognitive decline; non-reversible	Sudden, short and fluctuating; reversible underlying cause	Diurnal fluctuations – can be worse in the morning or evening; reversible with treatment
Signs and symptoms	Wandering, agitation, sleep disturbance, fluctuations in behaviour during the day, generally alert, depression may be present, difficulty with word recall	Restless and uneasy, with fluctuations in agitation, restlessness and hallucinations, impaired attention, mood changes from anger, tearful outbursts and fear, disorganised thinking	Withdrawn, apathetic, feelings of hopelessness and alert, though attention fluctuates with mood; appetite may be increased or diminished

DELIRIUM IN THE EMERGENCY DEPARTMENT

Despite its known high prevalence, delirium is unrecognised and underdiagnosed in up to 75% of older persons presenting to EDs when structured screening is not present (Émond et al 2017). This situation is not unique to EDs and is prevalent in other acute care specialties, with approximately 50% of cases going undetected (Boucher et al 2019). Research identifies that delirium is present in 8–17% of older persons in ED (Giroux et al 2018), and has a higher prevalence in those older persons experiencing cognitive disorders, and in those transferred from RACFs. Its prevalence in those transferred to ED from RACFs is posited to range between 9.6% and 89% (Émond et al 2018).

The dynamic and busy nature of the ED environment can make early detection of delirium challenging. Early detection of delirium is critical in treating its underlying cause, and providing early and targeted intervention and appropriate management strategies to prevent and mitigate against its severity and trajectory. Undetected delirium is associated with adverse health outcomes for older people, and consequences for health organisations. For example, delirium is associated with increased morbidity and mortality in older ED patients (Yadav et al 2020), which includes cognitive and functional decline, and occupational health and safety issues related to the person's confusion, irritability or agitation. Delirium is also associated with increased length of stay and re-admissions (Choutko-Joaquim et al 2019), and increased health costs throughout organisations, as a high percentage of undetected delirium in EDs also goes undetected in receiving specialty wards (Voyer et al 2017). Expert groups have recommended that all older persons presenting or transferred to EDs are assessed or screened for delirium, to assist with early detection and management (Pérez-Ros & Martínez-Arnau 2019).

RISK FACTORS FOR DELIRIUM

Prominent risk factors, which should flag the need for delirium screening in older persons in EDs, include, but are not limited to (Robinson-Reilly & Marks 2020):
- age 70 years or older
- diagnosis of dementia or depression
- chronic health conditions, or recent onset acute illness (e.g. infection)
- dehydration, malnutrition
- polypharmacy
- sensory impairment (e.g. eyesight or hearing)
- drug or alcohol withdrawal
- undergoing surgical procedures requiring a general anaesthetic (e.g. hip fracture).

While only one triggering factor is required to precipitate delirium, older persons in the ED, and in particular those transferred from RACFs, can often have several triggers present. Consequently, delirium screening is warranted.

DELIRIUM SCREENING

Increased screening and detection of delirium in older persons presenting to EDs allows for early interventions, care and treatment, to mitigate its trajectory and reduce morbidity and mortality. A plethora of screening instruments have been identified for delirium screening in

EDs, with varying degrees of validation, and complexities associated with their use (Carpenter et al 2021). Commonly used instruments for delirium screening in the ED include, but are not limited to, the Confusion Assessment Method (CAM), the 4AT, the Delirium Triage Scale (DTS), and the Delirium Rating Scale (DRS). The development of delirium pathways and enhancement of electronic health record systems have also been posited as supporting an increased screening uptake in EDs (Vardy et al 2020).

STRATEGIES FOR MANAGING DELIRIUM

The management of delirium requires a collaborative, multifaceted approach, which includes a range of measures that aim to identify and treat its underlying cause or combination of causes. A combination of diagnostic (e.g. bloods, urinalysis), environmental (e.g. reduce noise, clutter and stimulation, soft lighting, ensure sensory aids for any impairment), supportive (e.g. assistance with ADLs, reorientation, reassurance, presence and assistance of family members or carers), and pharmacological measures (treatment of underlying cause, distress/agitation), is usually indicated. It should be noted that pharmacological interventions for distress or agitation should be used with caution and as a last resort, as medications used in this context can cause complications, and may in fact worsen the delirium. Consequently, non-pharmacological interventions for distress and agitation are recommended (de-escalation, reassurance and distraction). However, if these approaches are unsuccessful, then medications should be dosed cautiously, and monitored carefully and frequently (Shenvi et al 2020).

The following scenario illustrates the need to consider the presence of delirium in an older person transferred from an RACF. Following this, key aspects related to assessment, management, and the provision of person-centred care will be highlighted.

SCENARIO 3.5.1

John

John is a 78-year old man who has been residing in a residential aged care facility for the previous three years. John is brought to the ED via ambulance, following an assault by a fellow resident of the RACF the previous evening, where he experienced bruising and swelling to his face, and a fall. John has had no previous altercations during his time in the RACF. The paramedics report that John's medical history includes type 2 diabetes, COPD, hypertension, hypercholesterolemia and mild cognitive impairment. Staff at the RACF gave the paramedics a medication pack, which includes the following medications prescribed for John: Metformin, tiotropium, amlodipine, rosuvastatin and omeprazole. Ventolin and Seretide inhalers are also handed over.

John is accompanied by his wife Rita, who visits John most days in the RACF. Rita states that John had been incontinent of urine for several days, and that this had been making him irritable. Rita feels the incontinence is 'getting John down', and he has 'not been him-self at times'. As the triage nurse, you note that John presents as lethargic and has difficulty focusing on your questions. John provides an incorrect day and month of the year when asked, and is reluctant to have his baseline vital signs taken, batting your hands away when attempting this. John appears fidgety and is looking around the assessment room. John is also becoming irritable when you repeat questions, and shouts at you to 'go away'.

RED FLAGS

- John has several chronic co-morbid health issues.
- John is prescribed more than five regular medicines (polypharmacy) for his health issues.
- Rita has indicated that there has been a recent change in John's behaviour.
- At interview, John presents with an altered level of consciousness, and has difficulty with attention, concentration and orientation.
- A potential for aggressive behaviour exists, as John is becoming irritable and has a low tolerance for assessment/questions.

PROTECTIVE FACTORS

- Critical information about John's medical and medication history has been provided by the RACF.
- The change in John's behaviour appears to be acute in nature and consistent with the incontinence, potentially indicating a reversible urinary tract infection.
- Rita has accompanied John to the ED and can assist in orientation and reassurance.
- John has no prior history of challenging behaviour or altercations with fellow residents in the RACF.

KNOWLEDGE

- Delirium is a serious medical condition, which has an acute onset and fluctuating course. It is predominantly characterised by disturbance of consciousness and cognition, but may also feature hallucinations and delusions.
- Identify the underlying cause of delirium and treat this, while providing other environmental and supportive measures. Note: Delirium can eventuate in the absence of an identifiable underlying cause; however, the delirium can still be diagnosed and manifesting symptoms can still be managed as investigations continue.
- Older persons are at greater risk of developing delirium due to the higher prevalence of severe and chronic illness, and polypharmacy in the older population, both of which are risk factors for delirium.
- A comprehensive collateral history (from RACFs and family) is essential for assessment, and in determining appropriate diagnostic investigations and interventions.
- Identify and familiarise yourself with your organisation's delirium pathway, and/or preferred screening tool.
- Familiarise yourself with escalation and referral processes to specialist services (e.g. geriatricians, consultation liaison psychiatry) within your organisation.

ATTITUDES

- Engage in a respectful person-centred manner. This requires empathy and patience, active listening, reassurance of safety and a calm demeanour.
- Be mindful of expectations regarding how a person behaves when they have a delirium.
- Be aware of your own emotional responses when someone shouts, is hostile, or is verbally abusive. Look beyond the behaviour, don't judge or personalise it, and consider the context in which it manifests.
- In the context of challenging behaviour, avoid taking control, and consider how you can assist a person to maintain, or regain, a safe space (care versus control is a helpful philosophy to have).
- Know when to ask for support.

MENTAL HEALTH SKILLS

- Developing a therapeutic alliance with John is essential in engaging him throughout the assessment process. This requires the use of empathy, active listening skills and validation.
- Effective communication skills are essential when assessing and caring for persons with cognitive impairment. The 'what' and the 'how' of communication are equally important. Be clear and concise (avoid medical jargon) about what is happening and what needs to happen. Use a soft tone of voice, as well as a considered rate and volume in your speech. Ask yourself: 'Am I too loud?', 'Am I loud enough?' or 'Do I sound threatening?'
- Congruent (harmonious) words and behaviour are required to instil a sense that you are 'present' with a person. If our words and behaviour do not match, we may appear inauthentic and untrustworthy.
- An enquiring mind and critical thinking skills are important when presented with challenging diagnostic dilemmas, or acute changes in a person's condition. Looking 'beyond' what is in front of us will often reveal important information, and aid assessment and care. For example, aggressive or violent behaviour is often a way of communicating that something is not right with someone. Looking beyond this behavioural manifestation will aid identifying what this is, and how you can help.
- Risk assessment skills underpin a collaborative and dynamic approach to ensuring safety for both consumers and nurses. Risk assessment should be undertaken in partnership with consumers and family/carers.
- De-escalation skills and reassurance are integral in assessing and managing persons with confusion, agitation, or irritability (see Lamont & Brunero 2021 for more information on de-escalation skills). Note: engage assistance from family members, carers or friends where possible.
- Use skills in redirecting and negotiating during challenging encounters, or when a person has difficulty engaging with assessment processes.

NURSING ACTIONS AND INTERVENTIONS

- Revisit and check John's vital signs. Have Rita sit with John to assist with these and explain/reiterate what you are doing every time.
- Perform other investigations, such as routine bloods, urinalysis (acute onset of symptoms consistent with a UTI), blood glucose level, pain assessment.
- Complete delirium screen and any other relevant screens as per your department's protocols.
- Assess current mental state and baseline mental state – include collateral information from Rita and the RACF. What is John usually like? What has changed?
- Assess for risks such as: falls, aggression, leaving the department, poor oral intake, skin integrity.
- Care planning: does John require any further nursing assessments/interventions based on his presentation and history? For example, food/fluid chart.
- Care management: consider where to locate John in the department to minimise noise and stimulus. Also, consider Rita's needs during this challenging time.

RELEVANT TREATMENT MODALITIES AND CONSIDERATIONS

- Treat the underlying cause of the delirium – have any of the investigations highlighted any abnormalities (e.g. infection)?
- Initiate relevant environmental (e.g. low noise/stimulus, sensory aids etc.) and supportive (fluid and electrolyte hydration, companion, reorientation etc.) measures.
- Use non-pharmacological interventions in the first instance, to manage any challenging behaviours occurring as a result of delirium (e.g. maintain a calm demeanour, offer reassurance and provide redirection).

- If antipsychotic or benzodiazepine medications are required, use cautiously (start low and go slow) and consistently with local protocols, pathways or guidance.
- Make referrals for specialist assessment/consultation as required (e.g. geriatrics, liaison psychiatry, drug and alcohol). For example, specialist consultation may be helpful when considering differential diagnoses such as dementia, depression or psychosis, when acute behavioural disturbance is prominent, or when substance use/misuse is indicated.

SUMMARY

Delirium is a serious medical condition which is associated with increased morbidity and mortality. Early diagnosis, treatment and care are essential in mitigating its deleterious effects, and optimising person-centred outcomes. Comprehensive transfer of care information from RACFs and relevant others is integral to assessment and planning processes. This chapter has highlighted delirium subtypes and differentiating factors from other common presentations in older adults; some of the common aetiological factors associated with delirium; screening for, and management of delirium. The clinical scenario presented within this chapter was then followed by red flags and protective factors associated with the clinical presentation, as well as specific knowledge, attitudes and skills relevant to providing person-centred care for John. The chapter concluded with guidance relating to nursing interventions, and evidence-based treatment options for John.

Reflection

1. What factors indicate the need to screen for delirium in older persons presenting to the ED?
2. What assessment and management strategies are important in providing person-centred care for older persons with a delirium in the ED?

Useful websites

Agency for Clinical Innovation: Care of Confused Hospitalised Older Persons (CHOPs) project: www.aci.health.nsw.gov.au/chops

Australasian Delirium Association: www.delirium.org.au/

Australian Commission on Safety and Quality in Health Care (ACSQHC): Caring for Cognitive Impairment: cognitivecare.gov.au/

Australian Government Department of Health: Delirium Care Pathways: www1.health.gov.au/internet/main/publishing.nsf/Content/Delirium-Care-Pathways

References

American Psychiatric Association (APA) 2013. Diagnostic and statistical manual of mental disorders: DSM-5, 5th edn. American Psychiatric Association, Washington DC.

Boucher V, Lamontagne ME, Nadeau A et al 2019. Unrecognized incident delirium in older emergency department patients. The Journal of Emergency Medicine 57(4):535–42.

Carpenter CR, Hammouda N, Linton EA et al 2021. Delirium prevention, detection, and treatment in emergency medicine settings: A geriatric emergency care applied research (GEAR) network scoping review and consensus statement. Academic Emergency Medicine 28(1):19–35.

Choutko-Joaquim S, Tacchini-Jacquier N, D'Alessio GP et al 2019. Associations between fraity and delirium among older patients admitted to an emergency department. Dementia and Geriatric Cognitive Disorders Extra 9(2):236–49.

Émond M, Boucher V, Carmichael PH et al 2018. Incidence of delirium in the Canadian emergency department and its consequences on hospital length of stay: A prospective observational multicentre cohort study. BMJ Open 8(3):e018190.

Émond M, Grenier D, Morin J et al 2017. Emergency department stay associated delirium in older patients. Canadian Geriatrics Journal 20(1):10.

Giroux M, Sirois MJ, Boucher V et al 2018. Frailty assessment to help predict patients at risk of delirium when consulting the emergency department. The Journal of Emergency Medicine 55(2):157–64.

Hullick CJ, Hall AE, Conway JF et al 2021. Reducing hospital transfers from aged care facilities: A large-scale stepped wedge evaluation. Journal of the American Geriatrics Society 69(1):201–9.

Lamont S, Brunero S 2021. Managing challenging behaviours, aggression and violence. In: Roberts L, Haines D (eds) Mental health and mental illness in a pre-hospital setting. Elsevier Australia, Sydney.

Munene A, Lang E, Ewa V et al 2020. Improving care for residents in long term care facilities experiencing an acute change in health status. BMC Health Services Research 20(1):1–10.

Pérez-Ros P, Martínez-Arnau FM 2019. Delirium assessment in older people in emergency departments: A literature review. Diseases 7(1):14.

Robinson-Reilly M, Marks P 2020. Mental disorders of older age. In: Foster K, Marks P, O'Brien A et al (eds) Mental health nursing: theory and practice for clinical settings, 5th edn. Elsevier Australia, Sydney.

Shenvi C, Kennedy M, Austin CA et al 2020. Managing delirium and agitation in the older emergency department patient: The ADEPT tool. Annals of Emergency Medicine 75(2): 136–45.

Vardy E, Collins N, Grover U et al 2020. Use of a digital delirium pathway and quality improvement to improve delirium detection in the emergency department and outcomes in an acute hospital. Age and Ageing 49(4):672–8.

Voyer P, Émond M, Boucher V et al 2017. RADAR: A rapid detection tool for signs of delirium (6th vital sign) in emergency departments, Canadian Journal of Emergency Nursing 40(2): 37–43.

Yadav K, Boucher V, Carmichael PH et al 2020. Serial Ottawa 3DY assessments to detect delirium in older emergency department community dwellers. Age and Ageing 49(1):130–4.

CHAPTER 3.6

Assessing and responding to someone who presents following intentional self-harm

Enara Larcombe and Paul McNamara

KEY POINTS

- Borderline personality disorder is often misunderstood and many people who have been given this diagnosis feel that it has stigmatised their care in the hospital and health system.
- Intentional self-harm is a complex phenomenon; it does not always indicate a wish to die.
- Nurses and other emergency care professionals are well placed to provide both physical and mental health care to the person who presents following intentional self-harm.

LEARNING OUTCOMES

This chapter will assist you to:

- improve your understanding of the diagnosis of borderline personality disorder and what this means for the person
- articulate the differences and similarities between a suicide attempt and non-suicidal self-harm
- describe examples of stigma that the person who self-harms experiences and consider how this might impact on practice
- identify nursing interventions and practices that are helpful to the person who self-harms
- describe the communication and interpersonal skills that can be deployed to support the person who intentionally self-harms/who has been diagnosed with borderline personality disorder.

Lived experience comment
by Helena Roennfeldt

STIGMA

Stigma is highly prevalent for people diagnosed with borderline personality disorder (BPD). This scenario chapter highlights the judgemental comments and attitudes that people with BPD may experience. The impact of this discriminatory treatment can leave people feeling shame and consequently may impact any future help-seeking. The voice of lived experience woven through the chapter offers powerful personal testimony of the experience of someone with BPD, including some of the reasons for self-injury. The reasons for self-injury are varied, reinforcing the importance of gently asking questions and not making assumptions. Similarly, the high prevalence of trauma enhances the need for trauma-informed approaches when providing care. This chapter also highlights the potential positive impact of kind and compassionate responses, which may be particularly impactful given the predominance of these negative experiences.

Autoethnography, with its origins in the post-structuralist paradigm, was first used as a research term by Hayano in 1979 to describe studies in which the researcher is a member of the group being studied (Luggins et al 2013). In this scenario chapter, the otherwise unreferenced sections in *italics* are informed by the lead author's lived experience of hospitalisation following intentional self-harm.

INTRODUCTION

From July 2008 to June 2019 there were an average of over 28 000 hospitalisations per year in Australia secondary to intentional self-harm (National Hospital Morbidity Database 2019). The true statistics around self-harm are unknown due to poor reporting systems and individual factors – including whether a person reports self-harm or just the resulting injury (Sveticic et al 2020). *This represents a significant onus on emergency services and departments as the first points of contact for those patients presenting with self-harm. This initial interaction can be a polarising experience for these individuals and be highly influential in terms of future help-seeking behaviours. Subsequently, there is a need for healthcare practitioners to have a thorough understanding of the needs of the consumer, both in terms of physiological and mental health, and to respond to self-harm presentations with safe and appropriate knowledge, professionalism and empathy.*

Intentional self-harm occurs with or without suicidal intent (Edmondson et al 2016; Hooley et al 2020). *The lived experience is that there is rarely any correlation between the objective lethality of injury and the intent. Clinicians should be wary of projecting their estimation of the objective of self-harm onto the people in their care – I have been close to death when aiming only to release intense emotions and have been sutured in ED and sent home when I wanted to die.* To further complicate matters, there is little consensus as to the definitions of self-harm and/or suicide, with terms such as 'intentional self-harm', 'deliberate self-harm', 'non-suicidal self-injury (NSSI)', 'suicide', 'completed suicide' and 'suicide attempt' being used in different contexts (American Psychiatric Association 2013). However, there is some consensus around the lived experience of self-harm; Box 3.6.1 identifies a range of 'truths' around self-harm for people who experience it.

Complex trauma and the diagnosis of borderline personality disorder (BPD) often coincide (Jowett et al 2020). People with a diagnosis of BPD are known to have experienced

Box 3.6.1 Self-harm truths from the lived experience perspective

A seminal study found that – from a lived experience point of view – the following statements can be true.

Self-harm:
- *is a form of communication*
- *provides a way of staying in control*
- *provides distraction from thinking*
- *can create feelings of euphoria*
- *is a release for anger*
- *expresses emotional pain*
- *can be a response to sexual abuse*
- *is a coping strategy*
- *helps a person maintain a sense of identity*
- *provides an escape from depression*
- *helps to deal with problems.*

Warm et al 2003, p. 76.

a significantly higher rate of childhood abuse than the general population, including sexual abuse, neglect and emotional abuse; they are up to 13 times more likely to report historical childhood abuse (Porter et al 2020). People who have experienced complex trauma are more likely than the general population to self-harm as a way to ventilate or regulate emotions (Bradley et al 2019). Emotional regulation or a desire to avoid emotions entirely has also been cited as a major factor in self-harm (Brereton & McGlinchey 2020). Alexithymia (i.e. difficulty identifying and communicating emotions) has been shown to be prevalent among people diagnosed with BPD and is also thought to play a considerable role in why some people self-harm (Sleuwaegen et al 2017). Dissociation of moderate–severe intensity is commonly experienced among people diagnosed with BPD (Jaeger et al 2017) and influences both the risk of engaging in self-harm behaviours and the severity of physical injuries as a result of the self-harm act (Dorahy et al 2019). *Dissociation is a separation of mental processes, a feeling of detachment from the world, like you aren't really present. Time, places, people and actions have very little significance – it's like you're floating and your senses have all been altered. Sometimes it feels like your mind is trying to protect you, but it can be a dangerous thing as you can easily act impulsively and perilously, with little knowledge of or regard for the consequences of your actions.*

People with the diagnosis of BPD access the emergency department (ED) for all sorts of reasons, including safety (Vandyk et al 2019). Research has found that there can be empathy failure from nurses towards people who present to the ED after intentional self-harm (Baker et al 2021; Rayner et al 2019). A recurrent theme in the literature is that people diagnosed with BPD experience stigma from health professionals (Vandyk et al 2019); some studies contend that nurses are the health professionals who have the poorest attitude towards this cohort (Dickens et al 2019). Consumers who present to the ED after repeated self-harm are sensitive to this empathy failure, and identify where improvements can be made (Meehan et al 2021). *My presentations to hospital have been varied. On some occasions I have walked into the emergency department with relatively serious injuries and little shame, then barely a week later reappeared with intense shame and higher distress, but with smaller wounds. Occasionally, I present not with injuries, but for my own safety, when I (or my treating team) feel that I cannot cope safely at home with the distress I am experiencing.*

Healthcare practitioners commonly misunderstand the intentions behind presentations for self-harm behaviour, believing it to be purely 'attention-seeking' or 'manipulative' (Day et al 2018). Language historically associated with self-harm and people with a diagnosis of BPD includes words such as 'difficult, manipulative, attention-seeking and self-destructive' (Vandyk et al 2019, p. 758). Unsympathetic judgements or remarks, even when said without malicious intent, can result in a reluctance to seek help or engage in continued support for self-injurious behaviour (Owens et al 2016).

Statements like 'Try harder next time', 'What a waste of time and resources', 'There are real emergencies', 'You did this to yourself', etc. are not only unhelpful, but are seriously damaging to a person's perception of the practitioner, the health industry and themselves. These words and phrases are hurtful and only serve to further stigmatise. In fact, they can perpetuate further self-harm and result in an increased risk of suicidal behaviour.

Diagnosis of borderline personality disorder carries stigma, but can also be a useful adjunct to insight and understanding for the individual, and facilitate more informed and evidence-based treatment for practitioners (Campbell et al 2020). Diagnosis of BPD need not be a barrier to therapeutic consumer–nurse relationships, and there are strategies that have been shown to help enhance the therapeutic rapport (Romeu-Labayen et al 2020). Responding with empathy, understanding or a sincere effort to understand, is much more conducive to a therapeutic relationship. Communicating harm minimisation strategies or suggesting alternatives to self-injurious behaviour may be helpful substitutes (Pengelly et al 2008).

Neutral statements, or where possible, positive and empowering words and phrases such as 'courageous for seeking help,' 'resilient' and 'self-aware', should be used instead.

Many people who self-harm recognise when their emotions, ideation or actions have reached crisis point and other resources have been exhausted (Vandyk et al 2019).

Personal experiences have shown serious physical and emotional consequences to occur as a result of these people in crisis not being seen as a matter of urgency. As a practitioner, it is imperative to fully engage with these individuals to prevent further harm. Asking individuals to rate their current level of distress provides a good indication as to how treatment needs to be prioritised.

Where possible, it is helpful for the person's individual needs to be accommodated (e.g. avoiding certain beds/bays or minimising waiting room times), as they may have the potential to provoke or escalate maladaptive coping mechanisms (Stanley et al 2019). Additionally, the association between impulsivity and self-harm should be considered (Lockwood et al 2017). It is a balancing act: constant supervision (nurse specials and security) and removal of personal belongings is associated with higher levels of resentment and dissatisfaction, and an increased risk of violence towards both self and others (Pengelly et al 2008).

People who present to ED after self-harm commonly experience guilt, shame, feelings of isolation, unworthiness, fear and failure (Owens et al 2016). Medical trauma from previous presentations (e.g. having self-inflicted lacerations repaired without local or parental analgesia) can significantly impact on the person's willingness to seek and accept external assistance (Hall 2017) and their ability to regulate emotions during this process. In certain circumstances and for some individuals, exposure to negative attitudes and unhelpful interactions from health practitioners can have such a significant impact as to induce or exacerbate violence, either towards the self or others, and can result in a person subsequently being unwilling or refusing to seek or accept help (Shaikh et al 2017).

People who self-harm should be invited and encouraged to actively participate in their own care and be empowered to make decisions regarding their ongoing needs (Ntshingila 2020).

While this can sometimes be difficult in an emergency environment, it is imperative to keep people updated on their care, on timelines, on procedures and referrals. Even the simple action of reassuring the person that their needs are still being considered can be effective in helping them regulate their emotions and adjust expectations.

Patients who experience positive interactions with health practitioners report higher levels of trust, an increase in help-seeking and greater participation in treatment; in contrast, patients with more negative interactions reported isolation, resistance to treatment and a reluctance to engage with services (Cully et al 2020). Early, positive intervention and support for patients presenting with self-harm have been found to reduce future self-harm presentations, and a decreased risk of suicide ideation and attempts (Cripps et al 2020).

Reflection

A helpful question for practitioners to ask themselves is: 'What is the person trying to communicate or regulate?' Gently asking this question may be appropriate in some circumstances. Be sure to reassure the person that they did the right thing by presenting to hospital/calling an ambulance, and that their needs are valid and they are deserving of care and treatment. Recognise and verbalise that the hospital or prehospital environment may be a trigger or a distressing environment for them.

The following scenario illustrates possible challenges for the person presenting to hospital after self-harm, and some considerations for the nurses providing care. The example is based on an amalgamation of actual events. Put yourself into the shoes of the nurse and reflect on how you would respond under similar circumstances. Following the scenario, key aspects related to assessment, management and the provision of person-centred care will be highlighted.

SCENARIO 3.6.1

Taylor

Taylor is a 20-year-old woman diagnosed with borderline personality disorder (BPD), who has presented to the emergency department via triage at 2300 hours. She presents alone with significant new lacerations to her left forearm, which she has covered with a clean towel. There are seven lacerations made with a razor blade, they range in depth from 5 mm to over 15 mm. Taylor explains that she has had a series of stressors over the past few days and has cut herself tonight to help 'release' these emotions. She was recorded as being calm and cooperative in her interactions with the triage nurse.

You have just come on shift and are receiving a bedside handover from your colleague on the earlier shift. In contrast to her earlier calm demeanor, during this handover Taylor is visibly distressed, wringing her hands, crying and refusing to make any eye contact. Your co-worker states, 'She's only here because she's cut herself up.' He does not offer any clinical information beyond Taylor's name and age, her mechanism of injury and the location of the injuries. No basic observations have been taken.

▤ RED FLAGS

- Taylor was calm and cooperative when she presented at triage, now she is distressed and not engaging. Consider what has changed for Taylor since she has been in hospital.
- Taylor is distressed. Consider whether she is at risk of further self-harm while in hospital, or of leaving the department against medical advice. Consider what steps can you take to decrease Taylor's risk.
- A colleague displays a negative attitude towards Taylor's presentation. Consider whether the negative counter-transference from your co-worker is contributing to Taylor's distress.

PROTECTIVE FACTORS

- Self-initiated, voluntary presentation – Taylor has demonstrated that she can identify when to seek help.
- At triage Taylor was able to verbalise emotions and identify stressors/triggers for self-harm.
- To date Taylor has been playing her part in harm minimisation by keeping the wounds clean and covered, and staying in hospital for wound review.

KNOWLEDGE

- Vital signs and vascular observations of the affected limb are required. The physical care of the person who self-harms should be no different to the care of someone who sustained the same sort of injuries in an accident.
- Assessment and ongoing monitoring of Taylor's mental state in the ED is important – especially to monitor and document changes. Any increase in distress should be considered a sign that extra support may be required.
- An awareness of and willingness to practise trauma-informed care (TIC) is required. As described by (Isobel et al 2021), elements of TIC include:
  - being aware of trauma
  - collaborating in care
  - building trust
  - creating safety
  - offering a diversity of treatment options, with a decreased focus on medications
  - staff practising with consistency and continuity.
- Taylor presented to hospital of her own volition. However, under some circumstances, people presenting with self-harm may need to be treated under the Mental Health Act, e.g. if the person remains actively suicidal, is showing signs of mental health problems, lacks capacity for decision-making, and is refusing to remain in hospital as a voluntary patient. An awareness of the legal requirements of providing treatment under the Act relevant to the jurisdiction, as well as knowledge of local policies and procedures is essential. Regardless, the person should be treated in a non-threatening, non-judgemental way, where decisions around treatment are discussed in an open and honest manner.
- How and when to refer to the mental health team/consultation liaison psychiatry service. This should be routine part of practice when a person presents with intentional self-harm. Knowledge of local policies and practices is essential.

ATTITUDES

- Empathy not sympathy: Unlike sympathy, which can be disempowering and minimising of a person's suffering, empathy is a compassionate recognition and validation of suffering. In her landmark paper, Wiseman describes empathy as 'a skill which is crucial to the helping relationship' (1996, p 1164). An empathetic approach enables a person-to-person connection, and can include acknowledging that, while you don't fully understand self-harm, you would like to know more and gain insight into the person's experience, so as to assist if you can.
- Professional curiosity: *There is literally no other way to explain this. Clinicians always have something to learn from patients and particularly so from people who engage in self-harm behaviours. It gives clinicians the opportunity to reflect on their own knowledge of why people self-harm, of emotion regulation, and the ability for people with BPD to define and describe their own emotions. People with BPD may also have the experience of being deemed a 'frequent flyer', and while this often has negative connotations, it also means that they are in a unique position to be able to offer a new perspective on the continuity of mental health care and attitudes within the health service.*
- Reflective practice. Take time to consider the person's lived experience and be informed by the principles of trauma-informed care (as above). Be mindful that some people who have experienced trauma are very sensitive to feelings of neglect or rejection. Your communication skills, collaborative approach and warmth are the best antidotes to this.
- Whether they are self-inflicted or not, wounds need to be repaired. Most nurses will attempt to live-up to nursing's reputation of providing kind and compassionate care. See Box 3.6.2 for tips from someone with lived experience of both BPD and intentional self-harm to assist you to do so.

MENTAL HEALTH SKILLS

- Use active listening. To ensure that you are accurately understanding the content of the person's narrative, check occasionally by rephrasing or asking follow-up questions, e.g. 'When you say "I just want it to end", are you talking about wanting the intrusive negative thoughts to end, or are you saying you want your life to end?'
- The personal competencies of self-awareness and self-management, and the social competencies of social awareness and relationship management are known as emotional intelligence (Hurley & Linsley 2012). These skills are helpful in all nursing settings, especially when working with people who have been diagnosed with BPD. Reflecting on your practice with a trusted colleague (aka clinical supervision) may assist in developing confidence with emotional intelligence.
- 'Therapeutic use of self' is an essential mental health nursing skill used to assist the people in our care towards recovery (Wyder et al 2017). This is the opportunity to use your communication skills, your empathy, your warmth, your clinical skills, your communication skills and your personality in the service of someone in need. Mental health nurses working in this way are humble enough to know that we cannot impose change onto someone else, but we are confident in our ability to create a space where the person can make changes when they are ready.
- Recognise and manage transference (the patient's unconscious bias about the clinician) and counter-transference (the clinician's unconscious bias about the patient). This emotionally intelligent approach to care is important; without it there is a risk of empathy failure and/or escalation of harmful behaviours.
- Attend to the changing needs and nuances of establishing and maintaining a therapeutic relationship. As articulated in trauma-informed care, this will include building trust, collaborative care planning, and consistent practice.

Box 3.6.2 Tips for care of person with borderline personality disorder and intentional self-harm

Instead of telling me that I am a 'waste of time and resources,'

Try: 'I am so proud of you for seeking help.'

Instead of saying, 'You did this to yourself,'

Try: 'You appear to be in so much pain.'

Instead of telling me to 'try harder next time,'

Try: 'How can we help you?'

Instead of calling me 'attention-seeking,'

Try: 'I recognise that you are coping in the best way you know how.'

Instead of guilt-tripping me by saying 'there are real emergencies,'

Try: 'Your feelings and your injuries are real and valid.'

Instead of saying 'you are ruining your body,'

Try: 'You are resilient.'

Instead of asking me, 'Why are you doing this?'

Try: 'I don't understand why you hurt yourself, but I'd like to know why you are in distress, and I want to help you.'

Instead of telling me I am 'not worth the time' (of mental health services),

Try: 'Would it be useful to involve the crisis team? Would you like me to ask them to see you now?'

Please treat me with respect, care and be honest with me. Positive interactions with clinicians influence my help-seeking actions in the future, and significantly affect my future self-injurious behaviours. If you can't maintain a positive attitude towards me, please try to remain neutral. I am placing a lot of trust in you by asking you for help.

- Basic skills in mental state assessment, i.e. looking, listening and asking. Looking at the person's behaviours, listening to the content and meaning of the person's speech, and asking about their concerns and needs.
- Understanding the uses and limitations of the Mental Health Act as a means to decrease risks. The Mental Health Act may be useful as a short-term tool to prevent discharge against medical advice in someone who meets criteria (i.e. has a mental illness, is at risk to self/others, lacks decision-making capacity, and unreasonably refuses treatment). However, the Mental Health Act is not a long-term solution to addressing underlying problems or preventing future self-harm.

NURSING ACTIONS AND INTERVENTIONS

- Introduce yourself, ideally using your first name. *Likewise, use my name. We are both humans. If you like my tattoos, tell me. Ask me what music I'm listening to. Forming a rapport without volunteering too much information about yourself is relatively easy if you can show interest in me beyond my wounds or diagnosis.*
- Maintain the person's dignity and privacy at all times. *If you afford this to every other patient, I deserve it too.*

- Undertake a risk assessment – including risk of further harm to self or to others. *You'll need to ask me; I'll need to trust you with the answer.*
- Evaluate the safety of the person in a busy environment. *Consider the risk of me leaving if I am placed in a 'busy' waiting room with any number of triggers. This doesn't mean I expect to be seen straight away, but offering a quiet space to wait can help me.*
- Provide adequate information about treatment and procedures and gain consent. *Don't assume anything, including the extent of the treatment I am seeking. Just because I have presented to hospital does not mean I want stitches, etc. Sometimes I have presented just for my own safety. Keep me informed about my care. Please acknowledge tedious processes and long waits.*
- Remain positive and recovery-oriented. *Recognise positives without being condescending. Saying, 'I'm really glad you presented tonight' is a lot more helpful than 'You've done a good job this time'.*
- Encourage people with BPD to identify triggers and maladaptive behaviours and enable choices that lead to the mitigation of these. *Give options (does the person want to sit on the bed or on a chair?) If possible, allow them to make a choice in which area to be seen and where they feel safest (this can help minimise trauma).*
- While still following local policy and procedure, consider the necessity of security specials and other actions that may be viewed negatively by the person or by others. *Unless the person is an acute risk to themselves or they are under the Mental Health Act, do not remove belongings, do not request they turn their phone off, do not use a scanning wand – it's embarrassing and feels like a violation. It also elicits trauma responses and can disrupt emotion regulation and distraction techniques currently being used.*
- Offer a standard of care equivalent to that of any other patient. *Treatment as usual please. If it's a wound that would normally be sutured, please suture my wound too. Please don't punish me for causing the wound – I will notice it. I will be offended by it.*
- Patient advocacy should remain a priority for nurses working with people who have self-harmed. *Nurses are often the strongest advocate for patients regarding the provision of adequate analgesia. There was an occasion when I cut into a tendon and was refused paracetamol, let alone offered anything stronger. It REALLY hurt! Please don't let the fact that I caused the wound cloud your common sense or change your usual practice – of course I don't want long-lasting pain. Would you offer me analgesia if my wound was caused by an accident? If the answer is 'yes', you should offer me analgesia for self-harm too.*
- Local procedures may necessitate the use of mental health outcome measures, which should be undertaken in a safe and efficient manner. *I understand that you will need to assess my mental state, risk and safety, but I would be grateful if you could do so without reading off a formal checklist (even if you must document using one). It's much more helpful to me if you integrate your questions into a conversation. You will probably realise that I will catch onto you quickly and volunteer the information anyway.*
- Be aware of your language and the content of your conversations with colleagues, during handover. *Language is powerful. Use facts, communicate my needs and desires to the treating team and address my need to be included in clinical decisions where appropriate.*
- Be conscious of your language and judgement in your documentation. *It is relatively easy for me to access my own medical information (especially with MyHealthRecord) and it can cause me significant emotional distress should you use language that portrays me negatively, including making assumptions about me or my history.*
- Maintain a clinical focus and be alert to any other concurrent mental or physical health issues that may be occurring, and the risk of serious complications. *Be aware of my other potential health concerns, including further self-harm that I may not be disclosing.*

- Consider the potential for deterioration both mentally and physically, and encourage the person to communicate any concerns. *Take my observations. Sit with me. Reassure me. Trust me, I've probably been in this position before and if I tell you that I'm not okay, then I'm definitely not okay.*

RELEVANT TREATMENT MODALITIES AND CONSIDERATIONS

- Be kind.
- A person-centered and holistic approach to all physical and mental health treatments is required.
- Engage the mental health team as early as is practical, not just to refer the person for assessment or admission, but for support and to advise the clinical team as well. The mental health team may be able to facilitate access to evidence-based outpatient treatment specific to the person's needs, e.g.:
  - Dialectic behaviour therapy (DBT) was developed specifically to treat people who experience BPD. Therapy can be delivered individually or in a group program. It includes strategies relating to acceptance and change, mindfulness, distress tolerance, emotional regulation and enhancing interpersonal effectiveness.
  - Cognitive behaviour therapy (CBT) is a psychological therapy which focuses on recognising and addressing thoughts and behaviours that are unhelpful and ineffective at managing the symptoms which are impacting on their life.
  - Eye movement desensitisation and reprocessing (EMDR) is a psychotherapy which targets traumatic memories and distressing life experiences, helping to alleviate the person's distress and develop insights into the impact of trauma on their life experiences.
  - Acceptance and commitment therapy (ACT) uses experiential exercises to help people change their relationship with painful thoughts and feelings, and to take actions that are guided by their own personal values in order to create a life that is meaningful to them.

SUMMARY

There are many instances where the health system has failed to provide compassionate, effective care to people diagnosed with borderline personality disorder who present to hospital following intentional self-harm. This empathy failure is evident in the literature and reflected in the voices of lived experience. The focus for all health professionals should not be on what mistakes have been made in the past, but on how we can 'do better' in future.

The person who presents to hospital following self-harm is not necessarily suicidal. They may be suicidal, but we know that self-harm can serve a number of purposes: it may provide relief, release, distraction, a form of communication, and may prevent distress from escalating. People present to hospital for safety because their needs are not being adequately met at home/in the community. The hospital becomes – temporarily – the safest place for the person to receive support.

The clinical skills honed by emergency clinicians caring for accident survivors can be equally useful to the person who has self-harmed. Wounds need evaluation, cleaning, care, repair and maintenance, no matter the aetiology. Similarly, clinicians can be therapeutic by using the communication and interpersonal skills they have already developed and used with other patients in the emergency setting. When these skills are deployed with patience, persistence and intent to assist a person who is experiencing distress, positive outcomes can be generated.

A trauma-informed approach provides a framework for clinicians to contextualise their understanding and work in partnership with the person who has presented with self-harm.

Being understanding of, and respectful about, the person's experience of trauma, positioned not as 'What is wrong with you?', but as 'What has happened to you?', enables reflection on the clinical approach that will be most helpful. Collaborating with the person about the plan and delivery of care moves hospital clinicians from a paternal 'doing to' approach, to an interpersonal 'working with' model of care. This is likely to be much more satisfactory for the consumer and the clinician.

General hospital clinicians can borrow the mental health meaning of recovery when working with people diagnosed with BPD who self-harm. That is, 'recovery' can be considered a direction in which a person is travelling, rather than as a point at which they have arrived. In this context, a person who self-harms less frequently this year than they did last year can be considered to be working towards (or being in) recovery – depending on the person's own definition of what recovery means to them. We should be encouraged and encouraging about that sort of progress; sometimes the person experiencing distress relies on others to hold hope for them on their behalf.

Caring for people who experience BPD and intentional self-harm is an aspect of nursing that enables and encourages us to stretch our skill set. Yes, it can be challenging at times, but when we draw on principles and practices that enable and support the person who is in distress, it can also be a very rewarding aspect of our work. In this chapter, we have used examples from the lead author's lived experience to add clarity and nuance to the academic content. It is our hope that this approach has provided clinicians with a deeper understanding of the issues, that it has highlighted the power and importance of your words, attitudes and actions, and provided the opportunity to reflect on how to help.

To succinctly summarise, the best first step for anyone providing care for a person diagnosed with borderline personality disorder who self-harms, is this: be kind.

Reflection

1. In the text above, there are 11 reasons for self-harm identified by people who have self-harmed. Reflecting on that list, how many myths about self-harm that you have been told/heard can you identify?
2. What interpersonal skills and personality traits do you have that allow 'therapeutic use of self' when providing care to the person diagnosed with borderline personality disorder who intentionally self-harms?

References

American Psychiatric Association (APA) 2013. Diagnostic and statistical manual of mental disorders (DSM-5), 5th edn. APA, Arlington VA.

Baker D, Blyth D, Stedman T et al 2021. Case manager perceptions of emergency department use by patients with non-fatal suicidal behaviour. International Journal of Mental Health Nursing 30:487–94.

Bradley A, Karatzias T, Coyle, E 2019. Derealization and self-harm strategies are used to regulate disgust, fear, and sadness in adult survivors of childhood sexual abuse. Clinical Psychology and Psychotherapy 26(1):94–104.

Brereton A, McGlinchey E 2020. Self-harm, emotion regulation and experiential avoidance: A systematic review. Archives of Suicide Research 24(sup1):1–24.

Campbell, K, Clarke K-A, Massey D et al 2020. Borderline personality disorder: To diagnose or not to diagnose? That is the question. International Journal of Mental Health Nursing 29: 972–81.

Cripps RL, Hayes JF, Pitman AL et al 2020. Characteristics and risk of repeat suicidal ideation and self-harm in patients who present to emergency departments with suicidal ideation or self-harm: A prospective cohort study. Journal of Affective Disorders 273:358–63.

Cully G, Leahy D, Shiely F et al 2020. Patients' experiences of engagement with healthcare services following a high-risk self-harm presentation to a hospital emergency department: A mixed methods study. Archives of Suicide Research 1–21.

Day NJS, Hunt A, Cortis-Jones L et al 2018. Clinician attitudes towards borderline personality disorder: A 15-year comparison. Personality and Mental Health 12:309–20.

Dickens GL, Lamont E, Mullen J et al 2019. Mixed-methods evaluation of an educational intervention to change mental health nurses' attitudes to people diagnosed with borderline personality disorder. Journal of Clinical Nursing 28(13–14):2613–23.

Dorahy MJ, Carrell JM, Thompson N 2019. Assessing the validity of the quartile risk model of dissociation for predicting deliberate self-harm. Journal of Trauma & Dissociation 20(5):548–63.

Edmondson AJ, Brennan CA, House AO 2016. Non-suicidal reasons for self-harm: A systematic review of self-reported accounts. Journal of Affective Disorders 191:109–17.

Hall MF 2017. Managing the psychological impact of medical trauma: A guide for mental health and health care professionals. Springer, New York.

Hooley JM, Fox KR, Boccagno C 2020. Nonsuicidal self-injury: diagnostic challenges and current perspectives. Neuropsychiatric Disease and Treatment 16:101–12.

Hurley J, Linsley P 2012. Emotional intelligence in health and social care. Radcliffe, London.

Isobel S, Wilson A, Gill K et al 2021. 'What would a trauma-informed mental health service look like?' Perspectives of people who access services. International Journal of Mental Health Nursing 30: 495–505.

Jaeger S, Steinert T, Uhlmann C et al 2017. Dissociation in patients with borderline personality disorder in acute inpatient care – A latent profile analysis. Comprehensive Psychiatry 78:67–75.

Jowett S, Karatzias T, Albert I 2020. Multiple and interpersonal trauma are risk factors for both post-traumatic stress disorder and borderline personality disorder: A systematic review on the traumatic backgrounds and clinical characteristics of comorbid post-traumatic stress disorder/borderline personality disorder groups versus single-disorder groups. Psychology and Psychotherapy: Theory, Research and Practice 93(3):621–38.

Lockwood, J, Daley D, Townsend E et al 2017. Impulsivity and self-harm in adolescence: a systematic review. European Child and Adolescent Psychiatry 26(4):387–402.

Luggins J, Kearns RA, Adams PJ 2013. Using autoethnography to reclaim the 'place of healing' in mental health care. Social Science and Medicine 91:105–9.

Meehan T, Baker D, Blyth D et al 2021. Repeat presentations to the emergency department for non-fatal suicidal behaviour: Perceptions of patients. International Journal of Mental Health Nursing 30:200–7.

National Hospital Morbidity Database 2019. Table NHMD S2: Intentional self-harm hospitalisations by age and sex (2008–2009 to 2018–2019). Online. Available: www.aihw.gov.au/suicide-self-harm-monitoring/data/data-downloads.

Ntshingila N 2020. Mental health nurses' experiences of implementing a model to facilitate self-empowerment in women living with borderline personality disorder in South Africa. Nursing and Health Sciences 22:769–76.

Owens C, Hansford L, Sharkey S et al 2016. Needs and fears of young people presenting at accident and emergency department following an act of self-harm: Secondary analysis of qualitative data. The British Journal of Psychiatry: The Journal of Mental Science 208(3): 286–91.

Pengelly N, Ford B, Blenkiron P et al 2008. Harm minimisation after repeated self-harm: development of a trust handbook. Psychiatric Bulletin 32(2):60–3.

Porter C, Palmier-Claus J, Branitsky A et al 2020. Childhood adversity and borderline personality disorder: A meta-analysis. Acta Psychiatrica Scandinavica 141(1):6–20.

Rayner G, Blackburn J, Edward K-l et al 2019. Emergency department nurses' attitudes towards patients who self-harm: A meta-analysis. International Journal of Mental Health Nursing 28: 40–53.

Romeu-Labayen M, Rigol Cuadra MA, Galbany-Estragués P et al 2020. Borderline personality disorder in a community setting: service users' experiences of the therapeutic relationship with mental health nurses. International Journal of Mental Health Nursing 29: 868–77.

Shaikh U, Qamar I, Jafry F et al 2017. Patients with borderline personality disorder in emergency departments. Front Psychiatry 8:136.

Sleuwaegen E, Houben M, Claes L et al 2017. The relationship between non-suicidal self-injury and alexithymia in borderline personality disorder: 'Actions instead of words'. Comprehensive Psychiatry 77:80–8.

Stanley IH, Hom MA, Boffa JW et al 2019. PTSD from a suicide attempt: An empirical investigation among suicide attempt survivors. Journal of Clinical Psychology 75(10):1879–95.

Sveticic J, Stapelberg NCJ, Turner K 2020. Suicidal and self-harm presentations to emergency departments: The challenges of identification through diagnostic codes and presenting complaints. Health Information Management 49(1):38–46.

Vandyk A, Bentz A, Bissonette S et al 2019. Why go to the emergency department? Perspectives from persons with borderline personality disorder. International Journal of Mental Health Nursing 28:757–65.

Warm A, Murray C, Fox J 2003. Why do people self-harm? Psychology, Health and Medicine 8(1):71–9.

Wiseman T 1996. A concept analysis of empathy. Journal of Advanced Nursing 23:1162–7.

Wyder M, Ehrlich C, Crompton D et al 2017. Nurses experiences of delivering care in acute inpatient mental health settings: A narrative synthesis of the literature. International Journal of Mental Health Nursing 26:527–40.

CHAPTER 3.7

Assessing and responding to someone who presents with suicidal behaviour

Justin Chia and Tim Wand

KEY POINTS

- Suicidal behaviours include thinking about, planning or attempting to take one's own life by suicide.
- Therapeutic engagement from a person-centred, strengths-based perspective is essential and will maximise the potential of being able to verbally de-escalate someone who is distressed and agitated.
- If verbal de-escalation is unsuccessful, physical restraint or sedation with medication may be required and must be done in a safe manner, complying with all local policy and legislative requirements.
- Physical health comorbidities must be considered.

LEARNING OUTCOMES

This chapter will assist you to:

- identify protective factors in a situation where they may not be immediately obvious
- understand considerations when engaging in physical restraint or administering sedative medication
- understand the importance of considering physical health comorbidities in the care of people who present with mental health issues.

Lived experience comment
by Helena Roennfeldt
....
DO NOT SKIRT AROUND ASKING ABOUT SUICIDE

After self-injury or a suicide attempt, we want our emotional pain to be recognised and taken seriously. Honest discussions about self-injury and suicide are often welcomed. Talking about suicide does not increase suicide risk, possibly due to the act of asking, conveying compassion and validation of distress and suffering. An open, authentic conversation creates a safe space for dialogue to explore experiences, understandings and an appreciation for the individual nature and complexities of suicide. These conversations may give new insight into and exploration of meanings for suicide and suicidal behaviour. The opportunity to talk with someone who neither lectures nor judges suicidal thinking and behaviour can be a positive and deeply connective experience. Centring personal narratives of suicide rather than relying exclusively on assessment tools can allow an emotional space for processing and ultimately understanding experiences that may be silenced or misunderstood. Promoting these conversations and experiences can support freedom from the silence and shame surrounding self-injury and suicide.

INTRODUCTION

Suicide is a devastating event that leaves long-lasting impacts on the person's family, friends and community. There is no one cause of suicide and the reasons people take their own life vary and are complex, with influences including a range of social (e.g. unemployment, relationship breakdown, parental discord), economic (e.g. recessions, depressions) and environmental factors (Hill et al 2021; Jorm 2020).

While thoughts of suicide may be common (Slade et al (2009) reported 13% of Australians aged 16–85 have had thoughts of taking their own life at some point), making plans to take one's own life (suicidal ideation/thoughts) and suicide attempt are less so (4% and 3% respectively), and completed suicide remains a relatively rare occurrence. That said, suicide is the leading cause of death for Australians aged 15–44 years of age, the leading cause of death among Australians aged under 25 years of age and the second highest cause of death in people who are aged 45–65 years (ABS 2019; AIHW 2021). Suicide was the second leading cause of maternal death in Australia in 2017 (AIHW, Pointer 2019) and men aged 85+ years have been identified as having the highest suicide rate of any age group in Australia (ABS 2019).

Both intentional self-harm and suicide constitute a significant burden of disease on the population, ranking as the third leading cause of premature death in Australia in 2015 (AIWH, Pointer 2019). This is particularly true for young Aboriginal and Torres Strait Islander people, who experience intentional self-harm, suicide and suicidal thinking at a significantly higher rate than their non-Indigenous peers, with this higher prevalence correlating to the Aboriginal and Torres Strait Islander population's disproportionately poor experience of the social determinants of health (Dickson et al 2019; Gibson et al 2021) and the significant barriers to accessing culturally appropriate mental health support in general and culturally appropriate support for suicidality in particular (Dickson et al 2019; Soole et al 2014; Stapelberg 2020).

Emergency care settings such as ambulance and emergency departments (EDs) are often the first point of contact for people experiencing suicidal behaviours (Perera et al 2018). Between 2010 and 2019, rates of presentations to Australian EDs for suicidal behaviours were reported to have increased significantly (and are greater relative to the general increase in presentations and increased mental health presentations) (Alarcon et al 2015; Perera et al 2018; Stapelberg et al 2020; Tran et al 2020). Similarly, increased suicidal presentations reflect increased deaths by suicide, which rose from 10.5 deaths per 100 000 population in 2010 to 12.9 per 100 000 in 2019 (ABS 2020; Stapelberg et al 2020). During this 10-year period, there was also a consistently disproportionate number of suicides by males relative to females, although the rate for females has increased proportionally higher than for males (ABS 2020). For Aboriginal and Torres Strait Islander people, the rate of increase remained approximately 13%, but the absolute numbers remain nearly double the overall population figures, with an increase from 21.3 deaths per 100 000 to 24.6 deaths per 100 000 in the same timeframe (ABS 2020).

Self-harm behaviour needs to be considered as distinct from suicidal thinking and behaviour. While people might engage in self-harm behaviours such as cutting, burning or pharmacological overdose with the intention of ending their life, self-harm may also be utilised for a variety of other non-lethal reasons, such as coping with distress (see Chapter 3.6). Importantly though, there is a correlation between self-harm behaviour as coping and self-harm behaviour with suicidal intent, with statistical estimates indicating that around 1 in 25 people who engage in self-harm behaviour will go on to die from suicide in the 10 years from their initial index presentation (Carroll et al 2014).

While there are numerous factors and circumstances which combine to result in suicide, and while not all individuals who die by suicide experience a mental illness, statistically it has been estimated that those with a diagnosed mental disorder are around eight to nine times more likely to die from suicide than individuals without a diagnosis (Too et al 2019). People who are diagnosed with borderline personality disorder are among those most associated with statistical risk of suicide (Chesney et al 2014). Suicidal thinking can increase, particularly during an episode of depression, but also in the manic phase of bipolar disorder, so it is important to enquire about suicidality with all people who experience mental illness (Clark & Temmhoff 2021). Other risk factors include gender (males are consistently more likely to die by suicide than females), those living in a rural area (Kennedy et al 2020), and alcohol consumption, which is known to be 'one of the most significant proximal risk factors for suicidal behaviour' (Borges et al 2017).

In spite of the statistics discussed above, it is important to remember that statistically derived risk factors cannot be directly applied to any given individual consumer presenting to an ED. There is strong recognition of the limited utility, and even harms, associated with the practice of stratifying an individual consumer's level of risk in order to allocate care (Carter & Spittal 2018; Ryan et al 2015; Wand 2015). What is suggested instead is a focus on therapeutic engagement and an individualised assessment of each consumer's situation, including modifiable risk factors and strengths.

While assessment is important in nursing, the word carries a fairly procedural connotation and it is important to remember that effective assessment requires effective therapeutic engagement. This serves not only to provide the consumer with a therapeutic experience, but also maximises the quality of data gathered by the clinician (Shea 2017). Moreover, holistic person-centred engagement is central to the practice of nursing (Santangelo et al 2018), with some suggesting ED nursing teams may benefit from an increased focus on non-judgemental, therapeutic engagement (Rayner et al 2019). The importance of therapeutic engagement in the ED setting is underscored by previous research, indicating that consumers presenting to the ED frequently express a preference to leave the ED feeling assisted rather than simply assessed (Wand et al 2016). The importance of therapeutic engagement can also be viewed through the lens of a person's neurobiological fear response, with an emphasis on what could simply be called a pleasant bedside manner being required to overcome this fear response and thereby effectively assist the consumer (Parnas & Isobel 2017).

While it is important for EDs to have access to additional specialist resources on-hand to provide timely care, and to support ED staff, the knowledge and skills of ED nursing and medical staff also need to expand to address this clinical need.

The following scenario illustrates the importance of appreciating that the majority of people with mental health challenges have experienced some form of trauma or adversity, particularly in early childhood, and this is common in people who frequently attend the ED. This perspective also recognises that people who have experienced trauma are more likely to experience distress and re-traumatisation as a result of encountering the healthcare system (Reeves 2015) and, as outlined above, may be at greater risk of suicidal behaviours and completed suicide.

SCENARIO 3.7.1

Rachel

Rachel is a 27-year-old woman who has been brought in by ambulance to the ED having called a telephone counselling crisis line saying she was having thoughts of killing herself by taking an overdose of her prescribed medication. The crisis line worker then called emergency services.

Rachel is well known to the ED, the toxicology service at the hospital, and the local mental health service. She carries a diagnosis of complex PTSD secondary to childhood trauma, and a history of long-standing suicidal ideation, difficulty managing her emotions, and frequent episodes of both intentional self-harm and serious suicidal behaviour. She has previously taken large overdoses requiring intubation and ICU admission. While Rachel has her care coordinated by the local community mental health service, she frequently presents to the ED under similar circumstances, and frequently accesses the local mental health acute care team after-hours. Rachel also has significant medical comorbidities. These include morbid obesity (weight of 147 kg and BMI of 57), type 2 diabetes mellitus, obstructive sleep apnoea, sinus tachycardia, and chronic knee and back pain.

On arrival in ED Rachel is lying on the ambulance stretcher screaming and swearing at staff, saying 'Let me out of here!' She is agitated and thrashing her arms and legs against the seatbelt restraints on the stretcher. Rachel has been transported under the Mental Health Act by the ambulance due to her reluctance to attend hospital and the suicidal thoughts she has continued to voice to the paramedics.

RED FLAGS

- Be mindful of the risk of causing further psychological harm through re-traumatisation.
- Recall that intentional self-harm and suicidal ideation can be two distinct experiences for a person, and it is important consider both possibilities, using a gentle exploration of their stated intentions. The possibility of suicidal ideation should never be overlooked simply because the person has a history of using self-harm as a coping behaviour.
- Characteristics of the ED physical environment (multiple entry/exit points, other vulnerable healthcare consumers in close proximity, an abundance of medical equipment hanging from walls and ceilings, etc) may increase the challenge in managing Rachel's risk of further self-harm, harm to others or absconding.
- High BMI, respiratory comorbidities and cardiac comorbidities should all be considered when weighing up risks and benefits of acute sedation.

PROTECTIVE FACTORS

- Rachel chose to call for assistance today rather than acting on her suicidal thoughts. (There have previously been times where she has acted on similar thoughts without calling for assistance, so this is a positive).
- Rachel has previously found strategies that have been helpful in managing her acute distress and suicidal ideation.
- Rachel is well known to the community mental health team.

KNOWLEDGE

1. General principles of trauma-informed care.
   - Emphasis on therapeutic engagement and verbal de-escalation skills to respond to Rachel's agitation and distress, prior to considering any need for sedation.
   - Provide a psychologically and physically safe environment for Rachel, being mindful that EDs can be noisy, busy places. Is there a suitable place in the department that is lower stimulus and clinically appropriate to care for Rachel? Will a lower stimulus space be likely to assist Rachel to de-escalate, or will she require a high (possibly resuscitation bay) level of care due to her heightened level of distress?
2. Therapeutic engagement and verbal de-escalation may not be entirely effective and sedation may need to be considered. Risks of engaging in further restrictive practices and complications of sedation should be weighed against the benefits of keeping Rachel in hospital for further review and risks associated with her leaving the ED without waiting for psychiatry review. Risks associated with sedating Rachel include:
   - inducing further psychological harm due to restrictive practices if required
   - obesity-related increase risk of respiratory, airway or other complications related to physical health comorbidities
   - common side-effects of medications used for acute sedation
   - an understanding of the medications used for acute sedation of consumers presenting with behavioural disturbances is required.
     - For example, NSW Guidelines for Management of Patients with Acute Severe Behavioural Disturbance for Adults < 65 years old (NSW Ministry of Health 2015) recommend first offering oral sedation of diazepam 5–20 mg PO (orally) or lorazepam 1–2 mg PO and/or olanzapine 5–10 mg PO. If the person is not accepting of oral sedation, if oral sedation has not been effective after 45 minutes or if behaviour escalates, move to parenteral sedation – first dose droperidol 5–10 mg IM (intramuscular – by injection). If not settled in 15 minutes, then second dose: further droperidol 10 mg IM/IV (IV – intravenous). The maximum dose of droperidol is 20 mg per event.

3. Systems issues which apply to the care and treatment of consumers with mental health issues in the ED.
   - In case of physical restraint and/or chemical sedation, consideration of obligations under local policy, health department policy, and local legislation in terms of documentation are required.
   - The legal requirements for review of consumers involuntarily detained in the ED under the Mental Health Act of your state or jurisdiction, and how this applies in your local setting also need to be considered. For example, are there provisions for senior ED medical officers to review and discharge someone who has been initially detained under the Mental Health Act where they consider psychiatry consultation is not required? This may be the preferred option if the person is not deemed to be acutely suicidal and a risk to themselves, and is adamant they want to leave and will require significant physical restraint and sedation in order to ensure they stay.
   - Consider the ED's capacity to provide safe, clinically appropriate care given the resources on hand at any given time.
     - How readily accessible are psychiatry staff (e.g. on-site, on call, or video-link accessible only)?
     - How does Rachel's acuity and need for care fit with the competing workload and acuity demands of other healthcare consumers in the department?

ATTITUDES

- Ensure a calm, non-judgemental, empathetic, validating approach with all healthcare consumers, regardless of their presenting issues.
- Consider potential for a past trauma history, including possible trauma Rachel may have experienced in the hospital environment when accessing healthcare previously.
- Pay attention to medical comorbidities that require consideration in the emergency/acute setting, remembering that a consumer's physical health condition frequently impacts on their mental health.
- In allocating limited ED resources, remember that Rachel's presentation may be the psychological equivalent of a serious medical emergency and her care should be prioritised as such.

MENTAL HEALTH SKILLS

- Engaging in a person-centred approach, with a focus on therapeutic engagement, which forms the basis for verbal de-escalation skills, is essential. This may minimise any potential for causing further psychological harm and requires that empathy and validation are conveyed to start building therapeutic rapport. It also involves conveying a genuine interest in hearing what Rachel has to say in an effort to understand what her experiences mean for her, while being mindful of your non-verbal communication (posture, gestures, eye contact; facial expression; rate, pitch, tone of your voice). These skills also positively affect bedside manner, facilitating an environment that is both physically and psychologically safe; and enables a person's neurologically-based fear response to be calmed, thereby maximising engagement and promoting recovery (Parnas & Isobel 2017).
- Use of verbal de-escalation skills to calm the consumer and reduce their level of arousal/agitation/distress.
- Using therapeutic engagement discussed above, gently encourage Rachel to elaborate on her suicidal thinking.
  - Did she feel so distressed she actually had a desire to end her life?
  - Were her earlier statements made while acutely distressed and more an expression of her distress at the time, as opposed to an actual wish to die?
  - Does she currently still feel like she wants to die?

- o If she appears ambivalent, gently explore strengths, including helping Rachel identify ways in which she has safely managed her suicidal thinking in the past.
- o It is important to recognise that for many consumers, cutting or other intentional self-harm behaviour may be a coping mechanism for them to manage their suicidal thoughts, and is actually done with the intention of avoiding taking action to end their lives.
- In the event that physical restraint and administration of parenteral sedation are required, it is important to have the knowledge and skills to do this in a safe manner.
- Consider the use of a solutions-focused approach. Given Rachel frequently presents to ED, this might involve reminding Rachel of strategies she has discussed as helpful on previous presentations to ED.

NURSING ACTIONS AND INTERVENTIONS

- Use verbal de-escalation strategies and a calm and empathetic approach in an effort to calm Rachel.
- Therapeutic engagement from a strengths-based point of view.
- Assess risks related to both Rachel's mental state and her physical health issues.
- Identify whether Rachel may be intoxicated.
- Ensure physical restraint in a safe manner.
- Administer oral or parenteral medication as required.
- Ask Rachel to identify the triggers for her current situation.
- Collaborative care planning with Rachel, the community mental health team and other relevant supports.

RELEVANT TREATMENT MODALITIES AND CONSIDERATIONS

- Once calmed, a solution focused-brief therapy (SFBT) approach may be useful to collaboratively identify a positive outcome for Rachel.
  SFBT:
  - o is a strengths-based approach, which empowers the consumer by inviting them to explore their own resources and past successes as solutions to achieve their identified future hopes and goals (Franklin 2015; Franklin et al 2016)
  - o assumes the consumer is their own expert as to what is helpful for them
  - o draws attention to those occasions in the past where individuals have successfully coped with a challenging or stressful situation, and assists them in articulating, to the clinician and themselves, how they achieved that
  - o assists the individual to build a positive picture of what their life will look like without their current problems, and the ways their current life is even a bit like that preferred future.
- A consistent, coordinated approach across all service delivery locations and teams involved in Rachel's care is also important, as there are a multitude of services she accesses concurrently.
  - o This could take the form of an inter-service agreement document briefly outlining her background history, a consistent approach to be taken by all teams/clinicians, and specific strategies to use in each setting.
  - o Examples of possible agreed upon aims or general principles for the plan could be to:
    - support Rachel to develop safe ways of coping with stress, as opposed to her current ones which put her at significant risk of harm
    - support Rachel's recovery within the community
    - facilitate psychotherapy within the community to support recovery
    - reduce hospital and ED presentations and admissions
    - provide a consistent and coordinated approach between services if admission is required

- allocate a lead clinician who is readily accessible for consultation by other clinicians to discuss Rachel's care.
  - ○ Examples of a treatment strategy specific to the ED context might be to provide:
    - prompt review by an ED medical officer (senior medical officer only) with a specialist mental health nurse on arrival to the ED
    - early liaison with the lead clinician on every presentation to ED during lead clinician's operating hours
    - a reminder to staff of the importance of using a calm, empathetic, validating approach when engaging with Rachel.

SUMMARY

Presentations to ED for suicidal thoughts, suicide attempt, or intentional self-harm behaviour are fairly common, with many mental health consumers who present also having a background history of previous traumatic experiences.

Therapeutic engagement from a person-centred, strengths-based perspective is essential and will maximise the potential of being able to verbally de-escalate someone who is distressed and agitated. It should be recognised, however, that verbal de-escalation may not always be possible, and sedation with medication or physical restraint is sometimes necessary.

In prioritising ED resources, care should be taken in recognising that presentations of this nature may be the psychological equivalent of a serious medical emergency, and prioritised as such.

It is important to remember that people presenting with suicidal behaviours may be experiencing a range of emotions and thoughts, encompassing everything from despair and hopelessness to anger and agitation, to shame or embarrassment, or even calm acceptance that they require assistance.

It is also important to remember that mental health consumers presenting to ED frequently have physical health comorbidities, which need to be considered when weighing risks and benefits of interventions such as physical restraint and sedation.

Given the prevalence of presentations of this nature, nurses need to have the knowledge and skills necessary to care for people who exhibit suicidal behaviours in a safe and therapeutic manner, which minimises the potential for further harm, both physical and psychological.

Reflection

1. Consider what knowledge, skills and attitudes you have learned, which you may be able to apply to your care of people who do not obviously exhibit problems with their mental or emotional health.
2. What policy and legal requirements exist in your workplace which may need to be considered and adhered to when considering the need for physical or chemical restraint in the ED?

Useful websites

Australian Institute of Health and Welfare (AIWH). Suicide and self-harm monitoring: www.aihw.gov.au/suicide-self-harm-monitoring

Australian Broadcast Corporation (ABC). You Can't Ask That, Series 2. 'Suicide Attempt Survivors': iview.abc.net.au/video/LE1617H003S00-First-hand accounts from consumers with a lived experience of suicide attempt

References

Alarcon Manchego P, Knott J, Graudins A et al 2015. Management of mental health patients in Victorian emergency departments: A 10-year follow-up study. Emergency Medicine Australasia 27:529–36.

Australian Bureau of Statistics (ABS) 2020. Causes of death, Australia, 2019. Cat. no. 3303.0. ABS, Canberra. Online. Available: www.abs.gov.au/statistics/health/causes-death/causes-death-australia/2019#media-releases.

Australian Bureau of Statistics (ABS) 2019. Causes of death, Australia, 2018. Cat. no. 3303.0. ABS, Canberra.

Australian Institute of Health and Welfare (AIHW) 2021. Suicide and self-harm reporting, data. Deaths by suicide over time. Online. Available: www.aihw.gov.au/suicide-self-harm-monitoring/data/deaths-by-suicide-in-australia/suicide-deaths-over-time.

Australian Institute of Health and Welfare (AIHW) 2019. Australian burden of disease study: Impact and causes of illness and death in Australia 2015. AIHW, Canberra.

Australian Institute of Health and Welfare (AIHW), Pointer SC 2019. Trends in hospitalised injury, Australia, 2007–08 to 2016–17. AIHW, Canberra.

Borges G, Bagge CL, Cherpitel CJ et al 2017. A meta-analysis of acute use of alcohol and the risk of suicide attempt. Psychological Medicine 47(5):949–57.

Carroll R, Metcalfe C, Gunnell, D 2014. Hospital presenting self-harm and risk of fatal and non-fatal repetition: Systematic review and meta-analysis. PloS one 9(2):e89944.

Carter G, Spittal MJ 2018. Suicide risk assessment: Risk stratification is not accurate enough to be clinically useful and alternative approaches are needed. Crisis: The Journal of Crisis Intervention and Suicide Prevention 39(4):229–34.

Chesney E, Goodwin GM, Fazel S 2014. Risks of all-cause and suicide mortality in mental disorders: A meta-review. World Psychiatry 13(2):153–60.

Dickson JM, Cruise K, McCall CA et al 2019. A systematic review of the antecedents and prevalence of suicide, self-harm and suicide ideation in Australian Aboriginal and Torres Strait Islander youth. International Journal of Environmental Research And Public Health 16(17):3154.

Franklin C 2015. An update on strengths-based, solution-focused brief therapy. Health and Social Work 40(2):73–6.

Franklin C, Zhang A, Froerer A et al 2016. Solution-focused brief therapy: A systematic review and meta-summary of process research. Journal of Marital and Family Therapy 43(1):16–30.

Gibson M, Stuart J, Leske S et al 2021. Suicide rates for young Aboriginal and Torres Strait Islander people: The influence of community level cultural connectedness. Medical Journal of Australia 214(11):514–18.

Hill NTM, Witt K, Rajaram G et al 2021. Suicide by young Australians, 2006–2015: A cross-sectional analysis of national coronial data. Medical Journal of Australia 214(3):133–9.

Jorm AF 2020. Lack of impact of past efforts to prevent suicide in Australia: A proposed explanation. Australian and New Zealand Journal of Psychiatry 54(6):566–7.

Kennedy A, Adams J, Dwyer J et al 2020. Suicide in rural Australia: Are farming-related suicides different? International Journal of Environmental Research and Public Health 17(6):2010.

NSW Ministry of Health 2015. Management of patients with acute severe behavioural disturbance in emergency departments. North Sydney. Online. Available: www1.health.nsw.gov.au/pds/ActivePDSDocuments/GL2015_007.pdf.

Parnas S, Isobel S 2017. Navigating the social synapse: the neurobiology of bedside manner. Australasian Psychiatry 26(1):70–2.

Perera J, Wand T, Bein KJ et al 2018. Presentations to NSW emergency departments with self-harm, suicidal ideation, or intentional poisoning, 2010–2014. Medical Journal of Australia 208(8):348–53.

Rayner G, Blackburn J, Edward K-l et al 2019. Emergency department nurse's attitudes towards patients who self-harm: A meta-analysis. International Journal of Mental Health Nursing 28(1):40–53.

Reeves E 2015. A synthesis of the literature on trauma-informed care. Issues in Mental Health Nursing 36(9):698–709.

Ryan CJ, Large M, Gribble R et al 2015. Assessing and managing suicidal patients in the emergency department. Australasian Psychiatry 23(5):513–16.

Santangelo P, Procter N, Fassett D 2018. Mental health nursing: Daring to be different, special and leading recovery-focused care? International Journal of Mental Health Nursing 27(1):258–66.

Shea SC 2017. Psychiatric interviewing: The art of understanding, 3rd edn. Elsevier.

Slade T, Johnston A, Teesson M et al 2009. The mental health of Australians 2: Report on the 2007 national survey of mental health and wellbeing. Department of Health and Ageing, Canberra.

Soole R, Kõlves K, De Leo D. Suicides in Aboriginal and Torres Strait Islander children: analysis of Queensland Suicide Register. Australia and New Zealand Journal of Public Health 2014; 38:574–8.

Too LS, Spittal MJ, Bugeja L et al 2019. The association between mental disorders and suicide: A systematic review and meta-analysis of record linkage studies. Journal of Affective Disorders 259:302–13.

Tran QN, Lambeth LG, Sanderson K et al 2020. Trend of emergency department presentations with a mental health diagnosis in Australia by diagnostic group, 2004–05 to 2016–17. Emergency Medicine Australasia(32):190–201.

Wand T 2015. Recovery is about a focus on resilience and wellness, not a fixation with risk and illness. Australian and New Zealand Journal of Psychiatry 49(12):1083–4.

Wand T, D'Abrew N, Acret L et al 2016. Evaluating a new model of nurse-led emergency department mental health care in Australia: Perspectives of key informants. International Emergency Nursing 24:16–21.

CHAPTER 3.8

Assessing and responding to someone presenting with panic

Justin Chia and Timothy Wand

KEY POINTS

- Anxiety and panic symptoms are a common reason for people to present to the Emergency Department (ED)
- Most often these symptoms are driven by psychological processes, but can also be due to substances or an underlying physical health condition
- Ruling out an underlying physical cause is important and can reassure the person
- Non-pharmacological approaches to managing anxiety and panic are preferred
- Information provided to people with anxiety and panic on self-care and self-management strategies can assist greatly and normalise their experience.

LEARNING OUTCOMES

This chapter will assist you to:

- identify the cardinal symptoms of anxiety and panic
- understand the pathophysiology associated with anxiety and panic
- have knowledge of screening questions, investigations and physical health conditions to consider
- have ideas on strategies and suggestions to provide individuals with anxiety and panic on self-care and self-management.

Lived experience comment
by Helena Roennfeldt

TAKEN SERIOUSLY

For people in mental distress, being listened to, given time and taken seriously are associated with more positive experiences. This is evident by nurses advocating on our behalf, providing reassurance and offering follow-up. It can be imperative for people who have presented repeatedly to the ED to be taken seriously and treated with kindness. Nurses who remember our name and story are appreciated, rather than continually needing to repeat these details. Relational and human aspects of care can, in part, override the negative effects of the cold, physical environment in ED. Significantly, kindness and someone who will listen may reduce the need for coercive or unnecessary pharmacological treatment.

INTRODUCTION

Anxiety is normal and can be good for us; for example, improving our performance and keeping us alert. However, pronounced anxiety against a backdrop of constant fear and worry can be debilitating (Andrews et al 2018). Anxiety and panic symptoms are widespread in the general population. Data from the Australian Institute of Health and Welfare (AIHW) reports that 14.4% of the population have an anxiety-related condition (AIHW 2018). Moreover, it is identified that 35–50% of adults will experience a panic attack at some point in their lives. In 2016–17 'neurotic, stress-related, and somatoform disorders' accounted for 26.7% (73 837) of mental health-related presentations to Australian emergency departments (EDs) (AIHW 2018). Mental health-related presentations accounted for 3.6% of all ED presentations; however, this is most likely an underestimation due to difficulty in coding these presentations (AIHW 2018).

'Panic disorder' is one of the less common anxiety-related conditions; however, it often presents with high levels of severity. It has high comorbidity with other mental health conditions such as depression (Andrews et al 2018; Baldwin et al 2014) and is strongly correlated with suicidal ideation, planning and dying by suicide. 'Panic disorder' is linked to higher rates of help-seeking due to both the accompanied fear of medical illness-linked attacks causing high rates of presentation to medical services during and after attacks (Elders 2020, p. 165).

STRESS, FEAR AND ANXIETY

'Stress, fear and anxiety are normal internal experiences that occur in response to a stressor' (Elders 2020, p. 157). The term 'stressor' describes either an internal or external stimulus that promotes the stress response. From an evolutionary perspective, stress, fear and anxiety make sense – they are part of an inbuilt mechanism which enables us to recognise danger early and primes us physiologically and behaviourally for a self-preservation response. Human brains have the capacity to learn and store the information that's required to ensure a timely response to threats or danger. Our stress response system shapes human behaviour and is implicated in the development of anxiety disorders and many other mental health conditions (Elders 2020).

The acute symptoms of anxiety and panic are manifestations of the fight-or-flight response. These symptoms are the result of both an increase in release of catecholamines and a consequence of hyperventilation, which have overlapping symptom profiles. During the fight-or-flight response, catecholamines are released from the adrenal medulla and the sympathetic nerve terminals, which precipitates behavioural and physiological changes that prepare the body to overcome a stressor.

The catecholamines adrenaline (epinephrine) and noradrenaline (norepinephrine) play a vital role in the fight-or-flight response, acting as both neurotransmitters and hormones, producing cardiovascular, respiratory and metabolic effects. They increase two- to tenfold during times of stress and act as powerful cardiac stimulants, raising the heart rate and increasing the force of myocardial contraction and coronary blood flow.

Another manifestation of the fight-or-flight response is increased respiration, which occurs via connections between the limbic system and hypothalamus to the brainstem respiratory centre. Hyperventilation is one of the physiological responses most frequently seen in panic attacks.

During hyperventilation, individuals exhale excessive carbon dioxide, precipitating an acute respiratory alkalosis with a drop in arterial partial pressure of carbon dioxide ($PaCO_2$) and an elevation in pH. Patients who chronically overbreathe may develop a compensated respiratory alkalosis with near normal pH and a decrease in bicarbonate (HCO_3^-).

Alkalosis increases calcium binding to albumin and a decreased ionised calcium, as well as shifting potassium into cells, leading to serum hypokalaemia. This hypocapnia-induced respiratory alkalosis produces a variety of symptoms. Increased neuro-excitability as a result of hypocalcaemia causes paraesthesia (tingling in lips and extremities) and carpopedal spasm.

Tachycardia can result from the physiological changes that occur in respiratory alkalosis including hypokalaemia and increased sympathetic activity. Chest pain may be caused by coronary vasospasm or decreased myocardial oxygen delivery and may also be the result of overuse of chest wall muscles in overbreathing, rather than using the diaphragm, as in normal breathing. Feeling hot, flushed and sweaty is attributed to hyperventilation, leading to increased work in breathing. Gastrointestinal symptoms occur in acute respiratory alkalosis, including nausea, vomiting and increased gastrointestinal motility. Peripheral and central nervous system symptoms include dizziness, vertigo, anxiety, forgetfulness and clumsiness.

The physical manifestations of anxiety and panic commonly account for people presenting to EDs. It is therefore important for ED clinicians to be informed of the numerous causes of anxiety and panic and equipped to respond effectively.

'PANIC DISORDER'

'Panic disorder' is characterised by unpredictable experiences of intense, episodic surges of anxiety that occur in the form of panic attacks. The person experiences the intense physiological anxiety symptoms described above (tachycardia, sweating, shaking, dyspnoea, chest pain, dizziness, nausea, tingling), along with a sense of depersonalisation (feeling detached from oneself). Panic attacks can occur outside of 'panic disorder' in relation to other presentations of anxiety; however, higher frequency, non-selective triggering environments and anticipatory anxiety helps differentiate 'panic disorder' from other types of anxiety disorder (Elders 2020).

Panic attacks reach a peak of severity within approximately 10 minutes and can last up to 45 minutes (Baldwin et al 2014). It is common to experience catastrophic cognitions during panic attacks due to the surge of physiological symptoms. These can include a sense of imminent death ('I'm going to have a heart attack and die'), mental health deterioration ('I'm going to lose my mind'), or a negative outcome regarding fear of losing consciousness ('I'll pass out and something will happen to me when I'm unconscious'). As a result, people engage in rapid safety behaviours during panic attacks in order to seek help (e.g. phoning emergency services), escape the attack (e.g. sit down) and further monitor symptoms (e.g. body scanning, taking one's pulse) (Elders 2020).

As the panic attack begins to abate, the person obtains a false impression that: a) they were on the brink of a catastrophic event; and b) their safety behaviours prevented the imminent catastrophe that was occurring during the attack. This signals a major misinterpretation of anxiety symptoms (e.g. 'I could have a panic attack and die'), leading to scanning for a further attack and greater anticipatory anxiety. A number of preventive safety behaviours develop to avoid future attacks and reduce perceived risk should one occur, for example, becoming dependent on others to go out, body hypervigilance (body scanning for symptoms) and avoiding potential triggering/high-risk situations. These safety behaviours can lead to agoraphobia in approximately two-thirds of cases (Baldwin et al 2014; Royal Australian and New Zealand College of Psychiatrists 2003) and vicious cycles of panic attacks, anxiety and ever-increasing safety behaviours. See Fig. 3.8.1, which illustrates Clark's cognitive model of 'panic disorder' (Elders 2020).

With reference to a common scenario, this chapter describes the underlying pathophysiology of the physical symptoms of anxiety and panic and differential diagnoses to consider. Organic conditions that are associated with symptoms of anxiety and panic are highlighted. Brief interventions are provided for ED clinicians to use when explaining symptoms, and to promote individual self-care and self-management.

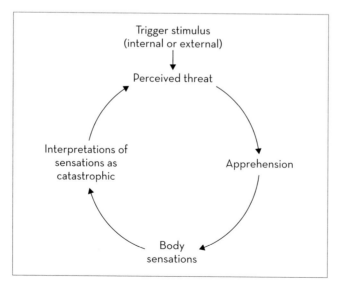

Fig. 3.8.1 Clark's cognitive model of 'panic disorder'

SCENARIO 3.8.1

Yasmina

Yasmina is a 40-year-old woman of Turkish background. She has presented to the ED several times over a two-week period reporting dizziness, palpitations, shortness of breath, dry mouth, tingling in the fingers and gastrointestinal discomfort. She has undergone numerous investigations during her ED visits including vital signs, ECGs, a chest x-ray, full blood count and thyroid function. Yasmina has also been referred to the neurology outpatient 'dizzy clinic'.

Yasmina is a non-smoker and does not consume alcohol or any illicit substances, such as cannabis or amphetamines. She drinks minimal coffee and tea and does not consume 'energy drinks', which also have a high caffeine content. Yasmina is referred to the mental health nurse in the ED for a review.

With little prompting, Yasmina recognises that stress has played a role in her symptoms. She has a supportive husband, two small children and works full-time as a community pharmacist. Yasmina acknowledges that she tends to worry, especially about her children. She often fears that something bad, such as an illness or accident, will happen to them. Yasmina explains that her mother died from cancer when she was 10 and that her father died from a heart attack when she was 16. Yasmina was essentially raised by her grandmother, whom she describes as highly anxious and 'overprotective'. Recently, Yasmina's grandmother was admitted to intensive care in a hospital in Turkey and was not expected to survive. Yasmina flew to Turkey to see her grandmother; however, she had panic symptoms during the flight over. She had never experienced any difficulty flying in the past. The hospital where she visited her grandmother was the same hospital in which her mother was treated and died. Returning to that hospital and seeing her grandmother in the ICU caused great distress for Yasmina. She also missed her husband and children and decided to fly home only two days after arriving in Turkey.

RED FLAGS

- Panic symptoms can mimic many medical conditions, including cardiovascular and respiratory conditions, hyperthyroidism and others.
- Comorbid cardiac and respiratory conditions also increase with panic.
- Many of the symptoms associated with coronary artery disease are common with panic.
- Even if a history of anxiety is known, clinicians should not discount the potential for comorbid coronary disease.
- For people presenting with chest pain, a focused history, physical examination, ECG and judicious use of diagnostic tests should occur to rule out acute life-threatening conditions.

PROTECTIVE FACTORS

- Yasmina has a supportive husband and family.
- She is educated, has full-time employment, stable housing and no financial stress.
- Her diet and lifestyle do not predispose her to any serious physical conditions.
- Yasmina is seeking help and recognises that stress plays a role in her symptoms.

KNOWLEDGE

- On presentation, the majority of individuals experiencing panic symptoms will identify with current life stressors associated with the onset of their panic state. This may be a single significant event, or it may be due to numerous cumulative life stressors.
- A history of childhood adversity and instability and numerous forms of psychological trauma are all strongly associated with mental health challenges such as anxiety and panic. This may be particularly the case for people from refugee backgrounds, where trauma experiences are common.
- Anxiety and panic symptoms may also be associated with physical conditions, such as acute or chronic pain.
- Numerous substances, both licit and illicit, are also linked with anxiety and panic symptoms, including caffeine, alcohol, nicotine, amphetamine, cocaine and cannabis.
- It should also be noted that symptoms and expressions of anxiety and panic can be variable and are also influenced by cultural factors. In some cultures, symptoms might present more somatically than in others, e.g. physical symptoms such as pain experienced throughout the body.

ATTITUDES

- It is important that symptoms are not dismissed, even if due to psychological stress.
- The person should be reassured that they are deserving of care.

MENTAL HEALTH SKILLS

- General screening questions can support consumers to disclose anxiety that is becoming problematic. Questions should be simple, time-specific and identify the experience of heightened anxiety and behavioural responses (like avoidance). For example, questions such as 'Over the past few weeks, how much have you been bothered by feeling nervous, worried, frightened, anxious or on edge? Feeling panicked or frightened? Avoiding situations where you feel anxious? (Elders 2020)
- Physical symptoms experienced should be validated in an empathetic, reassuring manner, while emphasising the relationship between mental and physical health.
- Hearing of common fears associated with anxiety and panic can provide reassurance and normalise the person's experience. For example, people who experience panic attacks often report that they are 'going mad', or 'losing control'. Reassurance that this is a fear held by many people who experience panic attacks can be immensely therapeutic.

NURSING ACTIONS AND INTERVENTIONS

- General supportive nursing actions and interventions are required and will help alleviate anxiety. Introducing yourself, presenting a calm demeanour, providing reassurance and explaining all procedures, being sure that the person understands.
- Performing tests such as an ECG have a dual benefit. They rule out serious underlying physical health causes for the symptoms and also act as reassurance for the person. However, these tests should not be undertaken repeatedly unless indicated.
- Anxiety may be present with substance intoxication or withdrawal. It is important to screen for substances associated with anxiety and panic, such as cocaine, methamphetamine and cannabis, or non-illicit substances such as caffeine, nicotine and alcohol.
- Symptoms may also result from prescribed medications, including herbal medicines (e.g. St John's Wort, ginseng, guarana), salbutamol, steroids, ADHD drugs, phenytoin, thyroxine, Parkinson's disease medications, and recent commencement of antidepressants.

- Brief interventions consisting of a simple explanation of symptoms and suggestions for self-management should be encouraged in the emergency care setting, as this also has great potential for circumventing repeated presentations. For example, demonstrating, then talking the person through a simple breathing technique can help the person understand that they have some agency in addressing their symptoms.

RELEVANT TREATMENT MODALITIES AND CONSIDERATIONS

- The recommended approaches for resolving anxiety and panic symptoms are non-pharmacological.
- Providing health information (verbal and printed) can be a powerful therapeutic tool in helping people alleviate the distress associated with anxiety disorders and helps improve engagement, treatment outcomes and a person's psychosocial functioning.
- People should be encouraged to engage in activities and interests that they find relaxing and shift attention from their physical and cognitive symptoms; for example, yoga, meditation or gardening.
- Metabolism-altering exercise (e.g. brisk walking, running, swimming or cycling) has proven effective for discharging the nervous energy associated with anxiety and panic, thereby reducing symptoms.
- There is mounting evidence that walking in nature, or simply exposure to natural settings, has a positive impact on mental and emotional wellbeing (Frumkin et al 2017; James et al 2015; Keniger et al 2013; Tucker et al 2015). Nature is even being 'prescribed' by doctors in the United States and the United Kingdom.
- Referral to a mental health professional such as a psychologist can be helpful for ongoing support and skill development. Therapies such as cognitive behaviour therapy (CBT), acceptance and commitment therapy (ACT) and solution-focused therapy (SFT) can be helpful.

SUMMARY

The physical and psychological symptoms of anxiety and panic are real, uncomfortable and distressing, often leading to an emergency presentation. Therefore, it is important that symptoms are taken seriously and that an adequate history and physical exam are undertaken to rule out medical causes. Once a diagnosis of anxiety or panic is made, suitable interventions or referrals should be instigated. Brief interventions such as information on lifestyle factors, slow breathing exercises, relaxation techniques, and promoting activities, interests and exercise are well suited to the ED context. There is a good prognosis for those individuals who are willing to experiment with a range of non-pharmacological approaches to improve self-management.

Reflection

1. How might cultural factors play a role in the manifestation of anxiety and panic symptoms with Yasmina?
2. In Yasmina's situation, what suggestions and strategies would you recommend that she consider trying to better manage her symptoms?

Useful websites

Beyond Blue: www.beyondblue.org.au/the-facts/anxiety/types-of-anxiety/panic-disorder

Stop, Breathe and Think App by Reach Out – free app for iOS that provides coaching for deep-breathing exercises: au.reachout.com/tools-and-apps

Black Dog Institute: www.blackdoginstitute.org.au/resources-support/anxiety/help-support/
Head to Health: www.headtohealth.gov.au
Health Direct: www.healthdirect.gov.au/anxiety
Mind Spot Clinic: mindspot.org.au

References

Andrews G, Bell C, Boyce P et al 2018. Royal Australian and New Zealand College of Psychiatrists clinical practice guidelines for the treatment of panic disorder, social anxiety disorder and generalized anxiety disorder. Australian and New Zealand Journal of Psychiatry 52(12): 1109–72.

Australian Institute of Health and Welfare (AIHW) 2018. Mental health services in Australia. Online. Available: www.aihw.gov.au/reports/mental-health-services/mental-health-services-in-australia/report-contents/hospital-emergency-services.

Baldwin DS, Anderson IM, Nutt DJ et al 2014. Evidence-based pharmacological treatment of anxiety disorders, post-traumatic stress disorder and obsessive-compulsive disorder: A revision of the 2005 guidelines from the British Association for Psychopharmacology. Journal of Psychopharmacology 28(5):403–39.

Elders A 2020. Anxiety. In: Foster K, Marks P, O'Brien J et al Mental health in nursing: Theory and practice for clinical settings, 5th edn. Elsevier Australia, Sydney.

Frumkin H, Bratman GN, Breslow SJ et al 2017. Nature contact and human health: A research agenda. Environmental Health Perspectives 125(7):075001.

James P, Banay R, Hart J et al 2015. A review of the health benefits of greenness. Current Epidemiology Reports 2(2):131–42.

Keniger LE, Gaston KJ, Irvine KN et al 2013. What are the benefits of interacting with nature? International Journal of Environmental Research and Public Health 10 (3):913–35.

Tucker A, Norton CL, DeMille SM et al 2015. The impact of wilderness therapy: Utilizing an integrated care approach. Journal of Experimental Education 39(1):15–30.

Assessing and responding to someone presenting with an eating disorder

Rea Nolan and Tegan Louttit

KEY POINTS

- Eating disorders are potentially lethal illnesses – anorexia nervosa has the highest rate of mortality of any psychiatric illness due to its physiological and psychological effects.
- Eating disorders are generally characterised by disordered eating and overvaluation of body weight, size and shape.
- Eating disorders can occur in anyone regardless of their BMI, age or gender.

LEARNING OUTCOMES

This chapter will assist you to:
- identify the signs and symptoms of an eating disorder
- develop an understanding of the risk factors and complications associated with malnutrition and eating disorders
- explore the nursing interventions involved in assessing and treating people with eating disorders
- understand the requirement for both medical and mental health intervention
- value the role of the family/carers/ support persons in mental health care.

Lived experience comment
by Helena Roennfeldt
HOLISTIC CARE

Accessing emergency care for an eating disorder can be challenging and further compounded by experiences of self-harm and feelings of suicide. Having an eating disorder also sits in a liminal space where we need medical and mental health support, and sometimes it feels like we don't fit into either the mental health or medical boxes. Holistic and person-centred care is crucial to ensure that neither medical nor mental health needs are overlooked. Often, people with eating disorders feel misunderstood and judged. If we have presented frequently to the ED, it can feel like staff stop listening and instead refer to our history. Not feeling believed can compound feelings of humiliation and reduce our having personal agency. Similarly, long wait times and not being provided with information can send a message about our value. Conversely, the relational and human aspects of care can spark hope and contribute to future recovery.

INTRODUCTION

Eating disorders are potentially life-threatening illnesses and can impact on every organ and system in the body (National Eating Disorders Association 2021). Anorexia nervosa has the highest mortality rate of all the psychiatric illnesses (Watson et al 2019) and people with anorexia nervosa, bulimia nervosa and binge eating disorder all have heightened suicide risk in comparison to the general population (Smith et al 2018). Eating disorders can have profound acute and long-term consequences for the individual and place significant stress on their loved ones and support systems. Early identification and intervention can be critical to recovery.

EPIDEMIOLOGY

There is no single known cause of eating disorders; their development is multifactorial and influenced by sociocultural, biological, psychological and genetic factors (Mayhew et al 2018). Deloitte Access Economics (2015) estimate that approximately 1 million Australians (around 4%) have an eating disorder. While the most well-known eating disorders are anorexia nervosa (AN) and bulimia nervosa (BN), these occur in less than 1% of the total population. In contrast, the most prevalent eating disorders are binge eating disorder (BED) and other specified feeding and eating disorders (OSFED), which affect 6% and 5% of the total Australian population respectively. See Box 3.9.1, which outlines the common eating disorders.

People of all genders, nationalities, ethnicities and cultural backgrounds are affected by eating disorders (Butterfly Foundation 2020). Common risk factors include genetic predisposition, trans or female gender, trauma, age (adolescence, menopause), gastrointestinal problems, diabetes/withholding insulin and weight concerns. Perhaps the most significant risk factor for developing an eating disorder is disordered eating and weight suppression (Gorrell et al 2019; Stice et al 2020). The majority of people with an eating disorder (excluding those with AN) have normal to higher BMI (Dooley-Hash et al 2019). Therefore, screening for weight concerns and disordered eating should occur in the emergency department (ED), particularly for high-risk groups (e.g. teenagers and women) and those presenting with symptoms of malnutrition or mental health concerns.

EATING DISORDER PRESENTATIONS TO EMERGENCY DEPARTMENTS

A 2019 US study found that, irrespective of the reason for presentation, nearly 16% of adults aged 21–65 presenting to EDs who were screened using the SCOFF questionnaire (Luck et al 2002; see Box 3.9.2) identified as positive for a potential eating disorder

Box 3.9.1 The different types of eating disorders

- Anorexia nervosa (AN): oral restriction, weight loss and low body weight resulting from concern about body weight of shape, fear of fat and intense fear of weight gain, and persistent behaviour that interferes with weight gain. Two types – restricting type (oral restriction, fasting and or exercise) and binge/purge type (intermittent bingeing and or purging).
- Bulimia nervosa (BN): Episodes of binge eating followed by shame and compensatory behaviours (vomiting, laxatives, overexercise and/or oral restriction).
- Binge eating disorder (BED): Ingesting large amounts of food in a short period of time with a sense of lacking control, often not in response to hunger cues. The individual may also experience self-disgust and shame in association with the behaviour.
- Other specified feeding or eating disorders (OSFED) includes: Atypical anorexia; missing only a single key criterion for diagnosis of AN (such as underweight), but with the presence of weight loss and behaviour interfering with weight gain. Atypical bulimia nervosa; missing a single key criterion for diagnosis of BN, such as the presence of weight change or body image concerns.
- Avoidant restrictive food intake disorder (ARFID): Significant restriction of nutritional range (20 or less foods) due to poor appetite, sensory characteristics of foods and fear of choking, vomiting or other negative reactions with associated weight loss, reliance on supplements for nutritional needs or impacting on social functioning.
- Rumination disorder: regurgitation and re-chewing or spitting out previously ingested food, in isolation of any other eating disorder.
- Pica: repeated oral ingestion of items with no nutritional value (most commonly occurs in childhood).

American Psychiatric Association 2013; World Health Organization 2020.

Box 3.9.2 SCOFF Questionnaire – Assessment Tool

THE SCOFF QUESTIONS*

S Do you make yourself **S**ick because you feel uncomfortably full?
C Do you worry you have lost **C**ontrol over how much you eat?
O Have you recently lost more than **O**ne stone in a 3-month period?
F Do you believe yourself to be **F**at when others say you are too thin?
F Would you say that **F**ood dominates your life?

*One point for every 'yes'; a score of ≥2 indicates possible anorexia nervosa or bulimia nervosa

A further two questions have been shown to indicate a high sensitivity and specificity for bulimia nervosa. These questions indicate a need for further questioning and discussion.

1. Are you satisfied with your eating patterns?
2. Do you ever eat in secret?

Luck et al 2002; Adapted from https://insideoutinstitute.org.au/assets/scoff-questionnaire.pdf

(Dooley-Hash et al 2019). Given that up to nearly 80% of people with an eating disorder may be undiagnosed and untreated (Hart et al 2011), this finding highlights the importance of identifying and responding to the illness in the ED. In particular, children and young people become medically unstable more quickly than adults, so thorough physiological screening and early intervention is required.

The SCOFF is a simple and effective screening tool, that is particularly relevant for the screening of AN and BN in young women (Kutz et al 2020). Other commonly utilised screening tools include the Eating Disorder Examination (objective semi-structured interview) or the Eating Disorder Examination Questionnaire (subjective self-report), which can be used to assess four key areas, including dietary restraint, eating, shape and weight concerns (CREDO n.d.).

People with eating disorders most commonly present to the ED with pathophysiological complications. As eating disorders can affect all physiological systems; the physical symptoms they may present with are varied. Common complaints on presentation include chest pain, abdominal pain, palpitations and syncope (Ismail & Nunez 2020). The most serious complications of eating disorders are cardiac arrest and suicide. Half of all deaths in patients with AN are thought to be of medical origin (Gibson et al 2019). Cardiac dysrhythmias and chest pain are often related to diminished cardiac muscle mass and electrolyte imbalances (Gibson et al 2019), and may be an indicator for sudden cardiac death risk. Low blood pressure and bradycardia are common and often due to an increase in vagal tone (Gibson et al 2019).

People with type 1 and type 2 diabetes are at an increased risk of a comorbid eating disorder and endocrinological dysregulation (Winston 2020). Those with type 1 diabetes may be up to twice as likely to develop an eating disorder (Goebel-Fabbri et al 2019). Warning signs for comorbid eating disorder with diabetes may include recurrent hypoglycaemia or ketoacidosis, poor glycaemic control or medication non-concordance (Goebel-Fabbri et al 2019). Hypoglycaemia may also be observed in individuals without diabetes and may cause sudden death. The frequency of hypogylcaemic episodes increases as malnutrition worsens (Gibson et al 2019). Due to the depletion of glycogen stores (which self-regulate insulin and blood sugar balances), patients with grossly inadequate oral intake may be at risk of refeeding syndrome when nutrition is re-commenced. If not monitored for and managed appropriately, this condition can also be lethal (Bioletto et al 2021).

Many compensatory behaviours of eating disorders, such as vomiting, the use of laxative and/or diuretics and excessive or compulsive exercise, have irreversible, life-changing and potentially fatal consequences, including but not limited to: dental damage, mallory weis tears, loss of normal gut function, bowel obstruction, kidney failure, osteoporosis, impaired fertility, growth and immunological compromise (Gibson et al 2019). In addition to the physiological complications, many features of eating disorders impact negatively on a person's quality of life and psychosocial functioning (van Hoeken & Hoek 2020).

PSYCHOLOGICAL IMPACTS

Eating disorder behaviours can begin as a way to achieve feelings of self-control and to manage negative or overwhelming emotions (Golan & Mozeikov 2021). Alternatively, a sequela of biological symptoms can develop following a period of malnutrition (this may be relating to dieting, illness or food scarcity), which perpetuate disordered eating behaviours and cognitions. Regardless of the origin of the malnutrition, findings from the Minnesota Starvation Study of 1950 (Keys et al), demonstrate that the symptoms and features of starvation are consistent and can cause (among others) social isolation and withdrawal, emotional dysregulation and cognitive rigidity, which can perpetuate the disease duration (Agüera & Jiménez-Murcia 2020).

Understanding and empathy towards people with eating disorders is commonly poor, with reactions that may vary between trivialised or normalised responses (i.e. 'Congratulations on your weight loss! You must tell me your diet tips') to critical or stigmatised responses (i.e. 'It's a choice, they did this to themselves'). People with eating disorders are often reluctant to present to a healthcare setting, including the ED, or disclose their illness behaviour to anyone. This can be due to previous negative experiences, discrimination, stigma, or fear of having their physical and mental health concerns invalidated or misunderstood (Williams et al 2018).

Motivation to change or recover is often a challenging issue for this patient group due to the cognitive impacts and perceived function of the eating disorder and is the core feature of ambivalence. However, evidence indicates that even brief interventions assist patients to move towards a readiness for change and engagement in ongoing treatment (Denison-Day et al 2018). Pugh (2020) discusses how eating disorder voices can become integrally enmeshed with an individual's identity to the point where the person may even grieve the separation from their eating disorder during recovery stages.

The approach, sensitivity and empathy displayed by ED staff can vastly improve (or worsen) the experience of the person with an eating disorder presenting to services and influence their likelihood of being open to and receiving effective treatment.

EVIDENCE-BASED TREATMENT

Intervention in the ED is just one step in the course of treatment for eating disorders. Ideally, medical and nutritional resuscitation and stabilisation occur in the hospital setting, while the psychological treatment occurs in the community (Hay et al 2014).

The use of evidence-based treatment (EBT) is essential to reduce the morbidity and mortality of the illness and improve patient outcomes (Brockmeyer et al 2018). In outpatient or community settings, the evidence base for adolescent treatments differs somewhat to that for adults, and the evidence for different treatments depend on the type of eating disorder the person is experiencing (Hay 2020):

- Family-based therapy (FBT) is most suited to young people (children, adolescents and young adults living at home) with AN or BN – delivered up to 40 sessions.
- Adolescent-focused therapy for eating disorders is an alternative to FBT used for young people with AN who cannot engage in FBT (i.e. living independently or with limited supports), and when FBT has been ineffective or following FBT completion.
- Cognitive behavioural therapy for eating disorders (CBT-E) is indicated for young people with a diagnosis of BN or BED, and adults with AN, BN, BED, OSFED or Atypical AN – 20–40 sessions depending on the diagnosis and severity of illness.
- Specialist supportive clinical management (SSCM) is indicated for any adult with an eating disorder diagnosis.
- Maudsley model of anorexia treatment in adults (MANTRA) is indicated for adults with AN.

- Other elements to ongoing treatment include promoting support and education for the person's family/support persons and ongoing supportive meal therapy (SMT) access (Treasure et al 2020).
- Social connectedness and access to the recovery stories of others or lived experience peer support can also be beneficial.

Medicare has extended the mental health care plan to include an eating disorders treatment and management plan, which provides up to 40 psychological and 20 dietetic sessions per financial year for people with some eating disorders (Australian Government 2019).

In Australia, there are several national and statewide guidelines and frameworks (Hay et al 2014; NSW Ministry of Health 2021; Queensland Health 2020), created to support the delivery of evidence-based treatment for people with eating disorders. These pathways and guidelines support clinicians to identify and respond to the physical and psychological complications of eating disorders in hospital and community settings. The efficacy of guidelines to improve patient care and outcomes relies on their successful implementation and application into clinical practice (Burgers et al 2020). It is therefore important that all nurses are aware of their local emergency management guidelines and how, when and why to implement these.

SCENARIO 3.9.1

Sarah

Sarah is a 23-year-old female brought in by her mother to the emergency department, following a syncopal episode with chest pain at the gym this morning. Sarah has a history of anxiety (for which she sees a psychologist) and was previously treated for bulimia nervosa at 15 years old. Sarah denies any vomiting and reports that her GP has advised she is 'not skinny enough' to have an eating disorder relapse. Her mother and psychologist have expressed increasing concern about her deteriorating mental state and weight loss. Her current weight is 62 kg (BMI 24.5) and she reports 6 kg weight loss in 6 weeks. Sarah started a new 2 hour per day gym routine to lose weight for an upcoming wedding; her goal weight is 45 kg (BMI 17.8). She last had her period 3 months ago. Sarah denies any recent stressors and attends full-time university studies and part-time work in retail.

On triage, Sarah's BGL is 3.2 mmol and she has reluctantly accepted a sweet biscuit to correct this. Her postural physical observations show postural hypotension of 25 mmHg and postural tachycardia of 36 bpm. Her mother reports Sarah 'barely eats anything' and has been more irritable and argumentative than usual. Sarah has just been advised that she requires admission under a medical team for further assessment and treatment. Sarah tells you she didn't want to attend the ED and is voicing frustration and reluctance about needing to stay.

RED FLAGS

- Chest pain and syncope.
- Postural hypotension and postural tachycardia.
- Amenorrhea.
- Hypoglycaemia.
- Rapid weight loss of 6 kg in 6 weeks.

Box 3.9.3 Other complications of disordered eating

- Cardiac complications: e.g. cardiomyopathy, heart valve injury, cardiac arrhythmias
- Gastrointestinal problems: e.g. Mallory Weiss tear, gastro-oesophageal reflux disease (GORD), constipation, malabsorption, diminished motility, superior mesenteric artery (SMA) syndrome
- Endocrine complications: Amenorrhoea or irregular menses in women, and decreased libido in men, hypoglycaemia
- Skin conditions: Dry skin, hair loss, lanugo, acrocyanosis
- Metabolic disorders: e.g. osteoporosis, reduced fertility, euthyroid sick syndrome, diabetes, dyslipidaemia
- Hepatologic/immunologic: Anaemia, neutropenia, leukopenia, thrombocytopenia
- B_{12} or folate deficiency, other vitamin deficiencies
- Electrolytes and renal problems: Hypophosphatemia, renal insufficiency, nephrolithiasis, hypokalemic nephropathy, Pseudo-Bartter syndrome
- Dental: Swelling around the cheeks or jaw, calluses on knuckles, dental decay, bad breath
- Neuromusculoskeletal: Cognitive decline, grey and white matter atrophy, peripheral neuropathy, altered consciousness, muscular weakness, lethargy
- Physical symptoms: Dizziness, syncope, shortness of breath or chest pain, cold sensitivity or intolerance, pallor

Note: List is not exhaustive

Gibson, et al 2019.

- Excessive exercise.
- History of anxiety and eating disorder.
- Concerned mother and psychologist.
- Poor understanding of medical risk.
- Reluctance to accept treatment and minimising of current symptoms.
- GP's reported statement about weight and BMI.
  (see Box 3.9.3 for additional potential complications)

PROTECTIVE FACTORS

- Supportive mother.
- Engaged with a psychologist.
- Attending a GP.
- Previous recovery from an eating disorder.
- Engaged in work and study, and is future focused.
- Attended ED, despite reluctance to do so.
- Accepted physical intervention for BGL management (sweet biscuit).

KNOWLEDGE

- People with eating disorders have a heightened risk of death from cardiac complications associated with eating/starving behaviours. Chest pain, syncope and postural changes are indictors of cardiac stress. It is important to check postural physical observations – postural HR and BP – lying and standing completed 2 minutes apart – ECG and other cardiac monitoring may be required.

- Refeeding syndrome is a rare but potentially fatal metabolic/clinical complication of starvation that can occur within the first few weeks of commencing refeeding. Clinical signs include confusion (an early sign), chest pain, sensory disturbances, glucose disturbance, neuromuscular weakness, arrhythmias, fluid retention and oedema. Those at risk include people who are malnourished, who have lost weight rapidly, who purge and/or who have concurrent medical condition.
- BMI is not an independent indicator of risk – people within the healthy weight range can experience the serious physical complications described above.
- Local and national guidelines relating to treatment pathways for malnutrition, hypoglycaemia, rehydration, thiamine deficiency, electrolyte imbalance and/or eating disorders exist and should be used.
- Patient rights and responsibilities, capacity assessment and associated legislation. If Sarah wishes to leave hospital prior to completed assessment or treatment, local escalation pathways should be used.

ATTITUDES

- Clinician's own beliefs and biases about body image, weight and shape, as well as perceptions and stereotypes around eating disorders, may impact delivery of supportive and non-judgemental care.
- Each individual has their own beliefs, attitudes and cultural influences on ideal body weight and shape.
- Eating disorders can occur in anyone regardless of their BMI, age, cultural background, socioeconomic status or gender.
- Eating disorders are a mental and medical illness, not a personal choice.
- Treatment for eating disorders is more complex than to 'just eat'.
- Consider the value in obtaining collateral from family and community supports and significance of their concerns.
- Ambivalence, shame and secrecy are features of eating disorders and patients may fear judgement from others which may impact disclosure, as well thoughts of being 'not sick enough', 'not thin enough', 'not deserving enough' of treatment.

MENTAL HEALTH SKILLS

- Building rapport with the person requires the use of active listening skills and a supportive approach. Remember that feelings of guilt, shame, fear or disgust around eating behaviours are common, so a supportive and non-judgemental approach when screening and assessing the person is essential to ensure the person feels comfortable to disclose openly.
- Supporting the person using de-escalation techniques and anxiety management-focused strategies can help. Ambivalence about treatment or the concept of recovery is part of the illness and should be expected. Using a motivational approach can enhance engagement and help to increase adherence to treatment recommendations.
- Assessment of mental state and assessment of risk (medical compromise, cardiac risk, risk of disengagement with services) is essential. This includes capacity assessment and knowledge of associated legislation as required.
- Engaging the family. Family and loved ones often feel anxious, guilty, judged and blamed; it is important to engage with and support family members who have a key role to play in the person's recovery.
- Psychoeducation and de-stigmatisation of mental health issues with other staff members are important roles for all health professionals.

NURSING ACTIONS AND INTERVENTIONS

In the first instance
- Remain calm and empathetic (role-modelling desired behaviour).
- Acknowledge Sarah and her mother's fears and frustrations.
- Provide psychoeducation to Sarah and her mother around the symptoms and risks of malnutrition and identify that the treatment is the same regardless of origin.
- Provide psychoeducation around the warning signs, risks and importance of addressing hypoglycaemia (cardiac arrest, decreased level of consciousness), postural hypotension (dizziness, weakness, fainting), postural tachycardia (falls, fainting).
- Minimise mobilisation to reduce energy expenditure, fall and cardiac risks.
- Consider increased supervision or 1:1 nursing if required.
- Follow fast-acting carbohydrate with long-acting carbohydrate, repeat BGLs as per clinical pathways.

When attending to cares
- Attend to postural physical observations and BGLS as clinically indicated.
- Attend and record patient's height and weight (as self-reports may be inaccurate).
- Supervise and record all food and fluid intake (as self-reports may be inaccurate).
- Observe and enquire about physical symptoms (e.g. dizziness, fainting, shortness of breath, chest pain) and safety (e.g. thoughts of self harm or suicide).
- Screen intensity, frequency and duration of physical activity and other compensatory behaviours (i.e. vomiting, laxative/ diuretic use, oral restriction).
- Collect a thorough history as appropriate (including substance use, medical history, mental health and trauma history), consider offering assessments with mother and Sarah separately.
- Explore recent medication history (including supplements, laxatives, oral contraceptive pills and over-the-counter medications).
- Screen for nutritional intake leading up to admission, to assist in assessing refeeding syndrome risk.
- Administer medications as prescribed and also consider the need for multivitamin, thiamine and electrolyte supplementation as required.
- Monitor for distress, as these discussions may be confronting. Consider ways to redirect Sarah from distress (i.e. during mealtimes/enteral feeding) or engaging in unhelpful or harmful behaviours (i.e. exercise, vomiting).
- Negotiation or changes to prescribed nutrition/enteral feeding are not to occur. (Patients may state they will eat if you give them food, but their physiologically compromised state indicates their inability to adequately nourish themselves for an extended period and they now require carefully prescribed nutrition to reduce risk of refeeding syndrome).

Documentation
- Document food and fluid intake, BGL, bowel chart and medications.
- Document clinical findings, interventions taken and outcomes of these.
- Document observed compensatory behaviours and interventions for these.
- Collateral from family and community supports.
- Document supportive behaviours or activities that Sarah finds helpful.

RELEVANT TREATMENT MODALITIES AND CONSIDERATIONS

In hospital
- Screening and early identification improves recovery rates.
- Diagnostic clarification to inform treatment plan.
- Dietetic assessment and refeeding pathway.
- Psychiatric assessment.

- Support services and ongoing education for mother and patient (as this illness affects the whole family).
- Consideration of mental health admission following medical stabilisation (to support re-introduction of adequate and regular oral intake).
- Monitoring for and treatments to reduce risk of refeeding syndrome.

In the community
- Evidence suggests recovery is most likely with the combination of GP medical monitoring, psychological and dietetic interventions.
- Evidence-based interventions/treatments may include: supportive meal therapy, counselling/psychology, cognitive behaviour therapy enhanced (CBTe) or specialist supportive clinical management (SSCM).
- Local mental health legislation and the importance of involving substitute decision-makers if the patient is deemed to not have capacity due to illness.
- Stage of change impacts the indicated treatment.
- Consider collateral from GP, who will continue and coordinate community care.

SUMMARY

In this chapter we explored the physical complications related to eating disorders and demonstrated how to recognise this illness in an emergency setting. We identified the red flags and risk factors associated with malnutrition and discussed the nursing responses required. The value of comprehensive assessment and collateral were noted, while reflecting on the attitudes and biases associated with eating disorders is essential. The evidence-based treatment interventions were discussed and applied to the clinical scenario with consideration of individual protective factors and supports.

Nurses have an important role in the identification, monitoring, support and provision of treatment to patients with eating disorders. The value of their investment in identifying, understanding and treating this illness can contribute to significantly improved patient outcomes.

Reflection

1. BMI is not individually indicative of cardiac health or of an eating disorder diagnosis. What are your predisposed ideas of what a person with an eating disorder looks like?
2. What is an 'appropriate' response from a concerned family member? What would your reaction be if you were worried a loved one was dying or not being taken seriously in an emergency situation and what would make you feel better?
3. Are eating disorders a mental illness or a medical issue? Whose responsibility is it to manage the risks and complications of an eating disorder in a hospital setting?

Useful websites

Australia and New Zealand Academy of Eating Disorders: www.anzaed.org.au/
Butterfly Foundation: butterfly.org.au/
Centre for Clinical Interventions: www.cci.health.wa.gov.au/
Centre of Excellence in Eating Disorders: https://ceed.org.au/
InsideOut Institute (formerly Centre for Eating and Eating Disorders): https://insideoutinstitute.org.au/treatment-services
National Eating Disorders Collaboration: https://nedc.com.au/

References

Agüera Z, Jiménez-Murcia S 2020. Advances in eating disorders. Journal of Clinical Medicine 9(12):4047.

American Psychiatric Association (APA) 2013. Diagnostic and statistical manual of mental disorders (DSM-5), 5th edn. APA, Arlington VA.

Australian Government 2019. Upcoming changes to MBS items – eating disorders. Online. Available: www.mbsonline.gov.au/internet/mbsonline/publishing.nsf/Content/Factsheet-EatingDisorders.

Bioletto F, Pellegrini M, Ponzo V et al 2021. Impact of refeeding syndrome on short-and medium-term all-cause mortality: A systematic review and meta-analysis. The American Journal of Medicine 134(8):10009–18.

Brockmeyer T, Friederich HC, Schmidt U 2018. Advances in the treatment of anorexia nervosa: A review of established and emerging interventions. Psychological Medicine 48(8):1228–56.

Burgers J, van der Weijden T, Grol R 2020. Clinical practice guidelines as a tool for improving patient care. In: Wensing M, Grol R, Grimsaw J (eds) Improving patient care: The implementation of change in health care. Wiley, Oxford.

Butterfly Foundation 2020. The reality of eating disorders in Australia. Butterfly Foundation, Sydney. Online. Available: butterfly.org.au/wp-content/uploads/2020/12/The-reality-of-eating-disorders-in-Australia-2020.pdf.

Centre for Research on Eating Disorders at Oxford (CREDO) n.d. The eating disorder examination (EDE). Online. Available: www.credo-oxford.com/1.1.html.

Deloitte Access Economics 2015. Investing in need: Cost-effective interventions for eating disorders. Report commissioned for Butterfly Foundation. Butterfly Foundation, Sydney. Online. Available: butterfly.org.au/wp-content/uploads/2020/06/FULL-REPORT-Butterfly-Foundation-Investing-in-Need-cost-effective-interventions-for-eating-disorders-report.pdf.

Denison-Day J, Appleton KM, Newell C et al 2018. Improving motivation to change amongst individuals with eating disorders: A systematic review. International Journal of Eating Disorders 51(9):1033–50.

Dooley-Hash S, Adams M, Walton MA et al 2019. The prevalence and correlates of eating disorders in adult emergency department patients. International Journal of Eating Disorders 52(11):1281–90.

Gibson D, Workman C & Mehler PS 2019. Medical complications of anorexia nervosa and bulimia nervosa. The Psychiatric Clinics of North America 42(2):263–74.

Goebel-Fabbri A, Copeland P, Touyz S et al 2019. Eating disorders in diabetes: Discussion on issues relevant to type 1 diabetes and an overview of the Journal's special issue. Journal of Eating Disorders 7(1):1–3.

Golan M, Mozeikov M 2021. Eating disorders, emotion regulation, and mentalization: addressing the gap between theory and practice. Journal of Psychology and Neuroscience. Online. Available: unisciencepub.com/articles/eating-disorders-emotion-regulation-and-mentalization-addressing-the-gap-between-theory-and-practice/.

Gorrell S, Reilly EE, Schaumberg K et al 2019. Weight suppression and its relation to eating disorder and weight outcomes: A narrative review. Eating Disorders 27(1):52–81.

Hart LM et al 2011. Unmet need for treatment in the eating disorders: A systematic review of eating disorder specific treatment seeking among community cases. Clinical Psychology Review 31(5):727–35.

Hay P 2020. Current approach to eating disorders: A clinical update. Internal Medicine Journal 50:24–9.

Hay P, Chinn D, Forbes D et al 2014. Royal Australian and New Zealand College of Psychiatrists clinical practice guidelines for the treatment of eating disorders. Australian and New Zealand Journal of Psychiatry 48(11):977–1008.

Ismail A, Nunez J 2020. Points and Pearls: Emergency department management of eating disorder complications in pediatric patients. Pediatric Emergency Medicine Practice 17(2):e1–2.

Keys A, Brožk J, Henschel A et al 1950. The biology of human starvation. University of Minnesota Press, Minneapolis.

Kutz A, Marsh A, Gunderson CG et al 2020. Eating disorder screening: A systematic review and meta-analysis of diagnostic test characteritics of the SCOFF 35(3):885–93.

Luck AJ, Morgan JF, Reid F et al 2002. The SCOFF questionnaire and clinical interview for eating disorders in general practice: comparative study. British Medical Journal 325(7367): 755–6.

Mayhew AJ, Pigeyre M, Couturier J et al 2018. An evolutionary genetic perspective of eating disorders. Neuroendocrinology 106(3):292–306.

National Eating Disorders Association 2021. Common health consequences of eating disorders. Online. Available: www.nationaleatingdisorders.org/health-consequences.

NSW Ministry of Health 2021. NSW Service plan for people with eating disorders 2021–2025. Online. Available: www.health.nsw.gov.au/mentalhealth/resources/Publications/service-plan-eating-disorders.pdf.

Pugh M 2020. Understanding 'ED': A theoretical and empirical review of the internal eating disorder 'voice'. Psychotherapy Section Review 65 Winter. Online. Available: www.researchgate.net/publication/346448575_Understanding_%27ED%27_A_theoretical_and_empirical_review_of_the_internal_eating_disorder_%27voice%27.

Queensland Health 2020. Assessment and treatment of children and adolescents with eating disorders in Queensland. Online. Available: www.health.qld.gov.au/__data/assets/pdf_file/0040/956569/qh-gdl-961.pdf.

Smith A, Ortiz S, Forrest L et al 2018. Which comes first? An examination of associations and shared risk factors for eating disorders and suicidality. Current Psychiatry Reports 9;20(9):77.

Stice E, Rohde P, Shaw H et al 2020. Weight suppression increases odds for future onset of anorexia nervosa, bulimia nervosa, and purging disorder, but not binge eating disorder. The American Journal of Clinical Nutrition 112(4):941–7.

Treasure J, Parker S, Oyeleye O et al 2020. The value of including families in the treatment of anorexia nervosa. European Eating Disorders Review 29(3):393–401.

van Hoeken D, Hoek HW 2020. Review of the burden of eating disorders: mortality, disability, costs, quality of life, and family burden. Current Opinion in Psychiatry 33(6):521.

Watson HJ, Yilmaz Z, Thornton LM et al 2019. Genome-wide association study identifies eight risk loci and implicates metabo-psychiatric origins for anorexia nervosa. Nature Genetics 51(8): 1207–14.

Williams EP, Russell-Mayhew S, Ireland A 2018. Disclosing an eating disorder: A situational analysis of online accounts. The Qualitative Report 23(4):914–31.

Winston AP 2020. Eating disorders and diabetes. Current Diabetes Reports 20(8):32.

World Health Organization (WHO) 2020. International classification of diseases and health related problems (11th rev.). Online. Available: icd.who.int/browse11/l-m/en.

CHAPTER 3.10
Assessment and management considerations working with women experiencing a mental health perinatal emergency in remote Australia

Fergus Gardiner, Breeanna Spring and Mathew Coleman

KEY POINTS

- Rural and remote Australia have high chronic disease prevalence coupled with lower provision of healthcare per population as compared to major city areas.
- Due to limited local birthing options, many rural and remote women are advised by their rural general practitioner to relocate to an inner-regional or major city area with a large birthing unit prior to their expected due date. Medical emergencies, such as threatened pre-term labour are managed by aeromedical or road ambulance transfer.
- In addition to having low maternity, obstetrics and gynaecology, these areas also have limited mental healthcare provision. As such, a remote clinician must be comfortable in the initial management of a complex patient presentation (often as the only clinician).

LEARNING OUTCOMES

This chapter will assist you to:
- understand the complexities faced by remote clinicians and promote ongoing education in the management of perinatal mental health presentations in remote Australia
- recognise risk factors for postnatal depression, including history of psychiatric illness, family history of affective and anxiety disorders, isolation or low level of supports for the mother and partner
- recognise symptoms of postnatal depression and when a presentation is a psychiatric emergency requiring transfer, such as suicidal thoughts and/ or attempts
- understand the management principles of trauma-informed care in the postpartum period
- recognise when safe transportation is required to a specialist mother and baby unit for definitive care.

KEY POINTS—cont'd

- Perinatal mental health presentations can be psychiatric emergencies. Clinicians must be prepared to respond to acute deteriorations in mental states,

KEY POINTS—cont'd

and be able to work within multi-disciplinary teams, with remote specialist clinicians and aeromedical services.

Lived experience comment
by Helena Roennfeldt

PEER SUPPORT

How can you be prepared for the shock of the life change that comes with becoming a mother? Being away from your usual support system, not having a family to rely on, social isolation and mental distress make this experience even more challenging. Shame is one of the most pervasive challenges associated with having disturbing thoughts, not feeling like you are coping and experiencing feelings of suicide. Shame causes us to keep our thoughts and emotions hidden behind closed doors. However, much of our healing comes from learning from others who have also experienced these challenges. Linking mothers and fathers to peer support groups, including warmlines and online groups, can help people to feel less lonely. Peer support is essential in giving hope by providing ongoing support and encouragement that is uniquely informed by lived experience.

INTRODUCTION

The Royal Flying Doctors Service (RFDS) is the largest aeromedical service in the world, providing primary evacuation and intra-hospital transfer by road and air throughout Australia's 7.69 million square kilometres. Most of the Australian population ($n = 24\,992\,860$) in 2018 lived in major cities ($n = 18\,003\,544$; 72.0%), or inner-regional areas ($n = 4\,445\,356$; 17.8%), with the remainder in outer-regional ($n = 2\,052\,366$; 8.2%), remote ($n = 291\,213$; 1.2%), and very remote areas ($n = 200\,381$; 0.1%) (ABS 2018). The majority of rural and remote Australia have low population concentrations distributed over vast distances, which is often termed the 'tyranny of distance' (Brown et al 1999) when it comes to service provision.

Service provision in rural and remote Australia is significantly lower per 1000 population compared to major city areas (Gardiner et al 2018). As such, many rural and remote patients are often required to travel to access healthcare, or forgo treatment until a visiting service comes to their geographical area (Gardiner et al 2021).

PERINATAL MENTAL HEALTH

Perinatal mental health can include any of the mental health disorders. Symptoms can predate conception, commence or continue during, or develop after pregnancy and delivery, and can have a major impact on maternal and fetal/infant mental and physical morbidity and mortality. More formally, the perinatal period is considered from the time of conception to one year postpartum (RANZCOG 2015). Previous approaches to perinatal mental health predominantly focused on the postpartum period, in particular postnatal depression. However, more recent studies have identified that antenatal depressive symptoms are as common; depression often commences in the antenatal period, and anxiety disorders are as common as depression perinatally (Austin 2004; Austin & Priest 2005).

In Australia, mental health disorders are a leading cause of indirect mortality, particularly for women who experience severe postpartum disorders, including depression, psychosis, and mania. In the longer term, mental illness can also have a longer lasting negative impact on a woman's occupational and social functioning (Austin et al 2013). Mental disorders and symptoms can have a significant impact on all aspects of a woman's life, and consequently on infants, other family members and significant others. In addition to the significant changes that occur for a woman during her pregnancy, delivery and then caring for a newborn child, social networks can be disrupted and increased isolation and stress can result. Risk factors for difficulties during the perinatal period can include a history of mental health problems, lack of support, previous trauma, including physical, emotional or sexual abuse, isolation (physical, mental, cultural), stressful life events, and a history of drug or alcohol abuse (RANZCOG 2015). For women living in regional, rural or remote communities, the need to give birth away from their communities, can lead to extra financial costs, lack of practical and emotional support, isolation, lack of integrated care between systems, inappropriate or culturally unsafe health care, and temporary separation from older children (Austin et al 2013).

BABY BLUES

Up to four in five mothers experience the 'baby blues' 3–5 days after giving birth, which is usually transient and self-limiting, remitting within 10 days. However, in Australia up to 16% of women (and 10% of fathers) can experience more significant symptoms indicative of a depression (RANZCOG 2015).

POSTPARTUM DEPRESSION

Postpartum depression is the most common disorder observed in the postpartum period. It is characterised by pervasive depressed mood, disturbances of sleep and appetite, low energy, anxiety and suicidal ideation. Additionally, feelings of guilt or inadequacy about the new mother's ability to care for the infant, and a preoccupation with the infant's wellbeing or safety severe enough to be considered obsessional. Anxiety symptoms can co-occur with depressed mood, but the overriding presentation is one of hopelessness, guilt and low mood. Onset can range from days after delivery through to many months after, usually within 6 months (Henshaw et al 2003).

More serious forms of depression, including puerperal psychosis (or postpartum depression with psychotic features) occurs in around 1 in 1000 woman, and should be considered a psychiatric emergency. Other forms of postpartum depression may be associated with bipolar affective disorder or other mental health disorders, such as post-traumatic stress disorder.

Detecting symptoms in the postpartum period improves outcomes for women. A number of tools have been evaluated for effectiveness in identifying depression in the perinatal period: the Edinburgh Postnatal Depression Scale (EPDS); Postnatal Depression Screening

Scale (PDSS); and the Kimberley Mums Mood Scale (Marley et al 2017). The most commonly used scale, the EPDS, suggests a score of ≥ 12 or ≥ 13 for detecting possible major depression, or at least a red flag requiring closer follow-up. Australian clinical practice guidelines suggest all women should complete the EPDS at least once, preferably twice, in both the antenatal period and the postnatal period (ideally 6–12 weeks after the birth). Administration of the EPDS can be readily integrated with existing routine antenatal and postnatal care (Austin et al 2013).

The development of suicidal ideation, and, less often, infanticidal ideation, must be considered standard in women who experience depressed mood or anxiety in the pastpartum period. They should be asked about their suicidal thinking, planning and self-harm behaviour and any past suicide attempt. Enquiring into suicidal thinking does not induce thoughts of suicide (Hall 2002). Rather, it provides an opportunity to ensure the safety of the woman and her baby and arrange appropriate follow-up care.

PUERPERAL PSYCHOSIS

Puerperal psychosis is an important, but rare, presentation that must be considered in any woman with disordered mental state in the postpartum period. Risk is elevated in women who have had a past experience of postpartum psychosis or bipolar disorder. Onset is unexpected and rapid, usually occurring within 48 hours to 2 weeks after giving birth, but may occur up to 12 weeks after birth (Austin et al 2013). Mood swings, confusion, strange beliefs, disrupted sleep, hallucinations and a dramatic change in previous functioning are key signs and symptoms of this psychiatric emergency.

The management of postpartum mental health emergencies requires the full assessment of the mother, the safety of her circumstances and the availability of expert assistance and input. Care pathways need to be adapted to individual circumstances and local resources, and informed by clinical judgement. Management must be considered in the context of being culturally safe for the diverse communities and populations throughout Australia; they must incorporate and understand the individual woman's context, take a family-centred approach and be trauma-informed. The optimal care is provided with a multidisciplinary approach that focuses on maternal and infant safety, culturally, socially, medically and psychiatrically.

When emergency postnatal mental health events arise, containment and referral to specialist mental health mother and baby unit may be required. Safely managing, transporting and caring for both mother and infant may be required for women in a rural and remote location. Assessing and managing an agitated patient in a remote location with limited specialist healthcare provision or resources can be extremely difficult. Many remote or very remote locations do not have healthcare provision (Gardiner, Bishop et al 2021); however, those that do are generally staffed by remote area nurses with telehealth support and visiting medical services, such as the RFDS (Gardiner, Richardson et al 2021). As such, a single psychiatric emergency presenting to a remote clinic or regional emergency department (ED) places considerable strain on available resources and capacities, especially if the patient requires supervision and/or containment after hours. In these situations, aeromedical retrieval is often required. To ensure patient and staff safety an adequate preflight assessment is required (Le Cong et al 2015).

SCENARIO 3.10.1

Jane

Jane is a 27-year-old woman living on a broad acre farm 90 km from a small rural community. She recently returned home, having given birth to her first child at a major Australian city hospital. She attended the emergency department (ED) of her local hospital by herself because she had been excessively tearful, wasn't eating and had stated she 'didn't want to go on'.

Jane had a relatively uncomplicated, planned vaginal delivery in the state capital city, approximately 650 km away 3 weeks prior. Her local town hospital had limited maternity services and she was anxious throughout the antenatal period, and had decided to have her first child in a private facility in the city. Her husband Rob, who worked on the family farm, was supportive and present for the delivery.

Jane had limited local social supports. She met Rob 4 years ago and moved interstate to live with him on his family's farm. She joined a local hockey team and made several friendships. She described bouts of depression and anxiety during late adolescent years, but had never sought help or treatment. She complained of feeling anxious throughout the pregnancy, particularly during the first trimester, which was complicated by morning sickness, and in the third trimester as delivery drew nearer.

Jane was physically fit, a non-smoker/no illicit substances, who drank alcohol on weekends, occasionally to excess before becoming pregnant, when she ceased drinking alcohol altogether. Although the pregnancy was unplanned, it was very much welcomed by her and Rob. Jane had a termination of pregnancy in her early 20s as she was single, had only just left home and had just started a career in local council administration.

After a 3-day confinement period following delivery of her child, a boy named Jack, Jane returned home to the farm. She had noted a deterioration in her mood, particularly in the last 48 hours. No longer anxious, she described feeling overwhelmed with a sense of worthlessness and guilt that she would never be a good mum to Jack. She had difficulty with breastfeeding, found Jack's attachment to the nipple painful, but was committed to continue. Jack was taking up to 2 hours to feed, resulting in Jane feeling exhausted and 'barely able to think straight'.

Rob returned to work harvesting, and Jane felt very lonely. She didn't tell him she was attending the ED. She reported having thoughts about ending her life over the preceding week, including thoughts of drinking one of the pesticides on the farm that had a warning label indicating it was dangerous and fatal if consumed. She had never previously harmed herself, but admitted to having fleeting thoughts that perhaps Jack would be better off dead too; however, she became instantly distressed with feelings of guilt and worthlessness when this occurred. 'How could I think such a thing . . . I must be the most horrible mother ever!'

Jane denied experiencing hallucinations, but admitted she thought Rob may be watching her closely because she 'just couldn't be trusted to do the right thing for Jack' – but she wasn't sure if this was true. She burst into tears when questioned further. Jane sat slumped in a chair throughout the ED interview, which was conducted by the local remote area nurse. She didn't make eye contact and held Jack in her arms without looking at him. However, she would not let anyone take him from her for weighing or examination. By the time the local on-call GP arrived, she refused to talk at all, partly because she was inconsolable, but also because she kept repeating: 'I must be the worst! I just have to leave. I don't deserve to be here anymore'.

Continued

A call to Rob revealed he had been very concerned about Jane over the last 48 hours. He knew she had been 'a bit depressed', but had become argumentative, irritable and erratic in what she said and did. 'I can't get anywhere near her or Jack … It's been really worrying me, but I've been so busy on the farm. I was thinking about driving her back to the city to see her obstetrician, but she refused and accused me of trying to harm her.'

Jane had to be prevented from leaving the local ED in a distressed, inconsolable and non-communicative state. Simple assertive redirection to her bed in the ED was effective. The GP consulted with the capital city women's hospital, where it was agreed that Jane should be transported by air to the mother and baby unit (MBU). Jane refused to be driven by Rob, intimating that she would jump out of the car if made to go and refused to be separated from Jack. Jane was ambivalent regarding accepting help and initially declined transfer to the MBU for ongoing care and management of her depressed mood. In consultation with the on-call psychiatrist at the MBU, and after discussing the situation with Rob, it was decided to transfer Jane under the Mental Health Act as she was unwell, had declined less restrictive treatment and there were significant risks to herself and her baby. Jane was assessed as lacking capacity to believe and weigh up information. After informing Jane of the need for transfer to the MBU, she agreed to transfer as long as she could travel with her baby. Rob arrived soon after and was supportive of the decision and requirement for definitive treatment at the MBU.

RED FLAGS

- Safety: Undertaking a risk assessment and safety plan in these situations requires a comprehensive approach, taking into consideration static risk factors (e.g. past history of mental illness, substance use, suicidal behaviour, medical conditions, social circumstances) and dynamic risk factors (current medical and perinatal circumstances, mental state, suicidal ideation, social supports). The risk assessment and safety plan must extend to the infant (current health status, maternal infanticide ideation, neglect, etc).
- Jane's suicidal ideation is consistent with her depressed mood; however, her erratic behaviour, withdrawal and paranoid thinking may escalate the chances of her impulsively or erratically harming herself and her baby.
- Could this be an emerging puerperal psychosis or postnatal mania?
- Capacity to contain and manage any risks/safety in the local environment.
- Are there any medical issues that may be contributing to the presentation?
- What is the best (safest) mode of transport to the mother and baby unit?

PROTECTIVE FACTORS

- A possible mental health history; however, no evidence of previous psychosis, puerperal psychosis or bipolar affective disorder.
- No past history of deliberate self-harm or suicidal behaviour.
- No current substance use.
- A supportive partner.

KNOWLEDGE

- When assessing perinatal mental health in rural and remote areas, particularly emergency presentations, staff may not have the appropriate knowledge, skills or confidence to undertake comprehensive mental health assessments and knowledge of how to manage a woman's care. In these instances, a GP (preferably the woman's GP) should be included.

- Jane presents with antenatal risk factors for developing postnatal depression. Her circumstances of difficulty feeding, poor sleep and exhaustion, combined with a past history of a termination of pregnancy, social isolation with tenuous social supports, all point to a formulation that provides explanations for her presentation.
- Her deterioration in the last 48 hours may herald the onset of a more significant and serious mental illness, but may also be a culmination of poor sleep and exhaustion in someone already depressed. Her location and care environment must be included in safety planning.
- Women may decline specialist referral for a plethora of reasons, including, although not limited to, a background of trauma, fear of authorities, lack of money, and lack of trust or knowledge (Austin et al 2013).
- When a woman's needs are urgent, particularly when presenting with severe symptoms or suicidal ideation, the use of general or preferably perinatal mental health emergency pathways should be followed.

ATTITUDES

- Perinatal mental health is a major contributor to mother morbidity and mortality in Australia.
- Postnatal mental health conditions can be a psychiatric emergency.
- Risk assessments need to be comprehensive and take into consideration static and dynamic risk factors for mothers and babies.
- Trauma-informed care principles help to improve outcomes for women.

MENTAL HEALTH SKILLS

- Establish a rapport with the patient, explain the process of the transfer, what will occur and timeframes.
- Facilitate open communication and address any fears or concerns the person may have; imparting that the medical team is advocating for her and supporting her needs will help keep the patient calm and comfortable in-flight.
- A trauma-informed approach to care is essential. This includes developing trust and transparency; collaboration and mutuality; fostering empowerment, choice and control; ensuring safety; and working in partnership (Austin et al 2013). Recognising Jane's past experiences of a termination of pregnancy, social isolation, expectations of breastfeeding etc, can help to improve the therapeutic relationship, engage her in assessment, planning and further management, and will improve outcomes.
- In cases where a referral is declined by the woman, close attention to maintaining a good therapeutic relationship is particularly important. Actively talking about the advantages of an assessment and the aspects of referral and follow-up are key.
- Reassurance and emotional support could include cognitive–therapeutic interventions, as well as empathy and strategies for coping with stress (Boscarino et al 2010).

NURSING ACTIONS AND INTERVENTIONS

- Prior to departure, an RFDS medical officer should conduct a comprehensive history and patient assessment with the senior referring staff member, ether via telehealth or telephone.
- The flight nurse combines a number of roles, including mental health nurse and midwifery skills, starting with checking the medical assessment and familiarising yourself with all elements. An assessment on the tarmac before departure includes a baseline postpartum check (fundus, vaginal loss, breasts) and full vital sign observations, including a Richmond Agitation Sedation Scale (RASS) and temperature.

- Provide medical crew with key information:
  - person's background, medical history, potential risks which may need to be mitigated in-flight
  - a full list of sedation provided prior to transfer and identification of how effective these have been in keeping the patient safe and comfortable, mitigating any distress or self-harm. (This helps the medical team to anticipate care required in-flight; and prepare sedation if needed for severe distress. Anxiety or psychotic thoughts are typically exacerbated when transferring a patient requiring monitoring and containment in a small aircraft.)
- For perinatal transfers, ensuring the baby is safe and well, with the in-flight care being on the onus of the caretaker (preferably a next of kin or relative), adds complexity.
- If the mother is breastfeeding, this needs to be considered – for example, facilitating a feed prior to transfer. Maintaining normality and a sense of self and safety for the patient during the transfer is essential.
- If the patient is to be transferred under the Mental Health Act, all paperwork must be checked to ensure validity and remain with the patient at all times, along with the police officer escort if required.
- Ensure the patient has had normal meals prior to transfer; if not, take a blood glucose level. If indicated, provide the patient with oral or intravenous glucose. If a long transfer is anticipated, prepare meals for transit.
- If a long flight is anticipated, an indwelling catheter is desirable due to the requirement for physical containment for inflight care and safety.
- Patient is to be positioned comfortably on a stretcher with four secure restraints, which remain in place for the flight duration, ensuring the patient is physically stable.
- Preparations made for the flight are for the worst-case scenario, to ensure optimal patient and staff safety during transit. Patient access inflight is difficult, so intravenous sedation access must be prepared and readily available. A long line with sedation prepared should be attached to the patient prior to transfer for use if required. Two peripheral intravenous cannulas are essential.
- If the patient has a support person, the treating team secures the passenger within their seat and conducts a pre-flight safety briefing.

Inflight
- Maintain patient dignity and comfort.
- An aeromedical retrieval can cause secondary trauma, so it is important to reassure and support the patient emotionally.
- The patient would typically be located on the front stretcher, with the medical officer at the head of the bed near the airway equipment, in anticipation of deterioration requiring any airway support or adjuncts.
- In transit, full monitoring should be readily available and applied with any sedation, including electrocardiogram monitoring, oxygen saturations, RASS scores and end tidal carbon monoxide monitoring ($ETCO^2$) via combination nasal prongs and $ETCO^2$ (RFDSW 2018).
- Treating team conduct neurovascular observations during flight.
- If any sedation is required, calculate and document clearly for accepting team.

RELEVANT TREATMENT MODALITIES AND CONSIDERATIONS

If a patient requires aeromedical retrieval from a remote area for ongoing care in a metropolitan centre, patient and staff safety are the primary concerns. During retrieval, especially in the case of a mother and her baby, the least restrictive means of restraint, and care aimed at enabling optimum patient safety, are used.

In the management of acute agitation, the following minimum criteria should be adopted to avoid/minimise the risk of an in-flight emergency:

- *Management of acute agitation:* As a first line measure, treat and exclude reversible cause of agitation, such as (although not limited to) pain, emotional distress, and sustained sleep deprivation (Puryear 2018). Acute arousal can be treated with pharmacological sedation, aimed at reducing patient and staff in-flight risk.
- *Medical monitoring:* Sedation may be required; however, acute sedation carries many risks. As such, continuous electrocardiographic monitoring and pulse oximetry should be undertaken prior, and during transportation, along with blood pressure recordings. A non-invasive capnography should be used, with oxygen supply, and a suction device and basic airway equipment available during the flight.
- *Aeromedical retrieval to a higher level of care:* Pharmacological sedation and mechanical restraints may be required in the event of unpredictable agitation in such a high-risk environment. This could include ketamine sedation as a second-line drug when emergency sedation is required, and oral and parenteral first-line agents have not achieved reduce arousal. When given as a sedative infusion, it allows for safe transport and handover to psychiatric care.

SUMMARY

Perinatal mental health presentations can be challenging and complex. Postnatal depression is the most common perinatal mental health condition, with up to 16% of Australian women experiencing this disorder. Notable risk factors exist for women, including a history of psychiatric illness, a family history of affective and anxiety disorders, isolation or low level of supports for the mother and partner (including intimate partner violence, psychosocial stresses, a past history of childhood abuse and low education/low socioeconomic status). Symptoms usually develop within the first few months after delivery, and can also be experienced by fathers. More severe forms of postnatal depression can be associated with the risk of suicide, and rarely infanticide. Screening plays an important role in identifying women presenting with postnatal depression, and measures that are culturally appropriate are available and continue to be developed in Australia. The management measures usually include GPs to exclude organic causes, and involve multidisciplinary professionals, including psychologists, social workers, child development nurses and psychiatrists. When indicated, referral to specialist inpatient mother and baby units can be required. The safe transportation of rural and remotely located women and their infants can be undertaken, safely and in a trauma-informed manner.

Reflection

1. In what ways can perinatal mental health conditions be a psychiatric emergency?
2. What are the principles to ensure trauma-informed care for women who present to emergency settings with perinatal mental health problems requiring transfer to mother and baby units?

Useful websites

Beyond Blue: Understanding perinatal depression and anxiety: www.beyondblue.org.au/docs/default-source/resources/bl0940-understanding-perinatal-depression-and-anxiety-brochure_acc.pdf?sfvrsn=631946eb_2

Centre of Perinatal Excellence: www.cope.org.au/

PANDA: www.panda.org.au/

SANE Australia. Perinatal mental health issues: www.sane.org/information-stories/facts-and-guides/perinatal-mental-illness

References

Austin M-P 2004. Antenatal screening and early intervention for 'perinatal' distress, depression and anxiety: Where to from here? Archives of Women's Mental Health 7(1):1–6.

Austin M-PV, Middleton P, Reilly NM et al 2013. Detection and management of mood disorders in the maternity setting: The Australian Clinical Practice Guidelines. Women and Birth 26(1):2–9.

Austin MP, Priest S 2005. Clinical issues in perinatal mental health: New developments in the detection and treatment of perinatal mood and anxiety disorders. Acta Psychiatrica Scandinavica 112(2):97–104.

Australian Bureau of Statistics (ABS) 2018. Population estimates by age and sex, regions of Australia. Australian Bureau of Statistics, Canberra. Online. Available: www.abs.gov.au/AUSSTATS/abs@.nsf/DetailsPage/3235.02018?OpenDocument.

Boscarino JA, Adams RE, Figley CR 2010. Secondary trauma issues for psychiatrists. Psychiatric Times 27(11):24–6.

Brown WJ, Young AF, Byles JE. Tyranny of distance? 1999. The health of mid-age women living in five geographical areas of Australia. Australian Journal of Rural Health 7(3):148–54.

Gardiner F, Bishop L, Graaf Bd et al 2020. Equitable patient access to primary healthcare in Australia. The Royal Flying Doctor Service of Australia, Canberra.

Gardiner F, Gale L, Ransom A, Laverty M 2018. Looking ahead: Responding to the health needs of country Australians in 2028 – the centenary year of the RFDS. The Royal Flying Doctor Service, Canberra.

Gardiner F, Richardson A, Roxburgh C et al 2021. Characteristics and in-hospital outcomes of patients requiring aeromedical retrieval for pregnancy, compared to non-retrieved metropolitan cohorts. The Australian and New Zealand Journal of Obstetrics and Gynaecology 61(4):519–27.

Gardiner FW, Rallah-Baker K, Santos AD et al 2021. Indigenous Australians have a greater prevalence of heart, stroke, and vascular disease, are younger at death, with higher hospitalisation and more aeromedical retrievals from remote regions. EClinical Medicine 42:101181.

Hall K 2002. Suicide prevention topic 7: Does asking about suicidal ideation increase the likelihood of suicide attempts? NZHTA Report. Online. Available: nzhta.chmeds.ac.nz/publications/topic7.pdf

Henshaw C 2003. Mood disturbance in the early puerperium: A review. Archives of Women's Mental Health 6(2):s33–42.

Le Cong M, Finn E, Parsch CS 2015. Management of the acutely agitated patient in a remote location. Medical Journal of Australia 202(4):182–3.

Marley JV, Kotz J, Engelke C et al 2017. Validity and acceptability of Kimberley mum's mood scale to screen for perinatal anxiety and depression in remote aboriginal health care settings. PLOS ONE 12(1):e0168969.

Puryear LJ 2019. Acute psychiatric conditions in pregnancy. Critical care obstetrics, 6th edn. Wiley, Hoboken NJ.

Royal Flying Doctors Service (RFDS) 2018. Western Operations. Part 1 Clinical guidelines. Online. Available: www.flyingdoctor.org.au/assets/magazine/file/Part_1_-_Clinical_Manual_-_January_2018_-_Version_8.0_-_FINAL.pdf.

The Royal Australian and New Zealand College of Obstetricians and Gynaecologists (RANZCOG) 2021. Best practice statement: Mental health care in the perinatal period. RANZCOG, Melbourne. Online. Available: https://ranzcog.edu.au/RANZCOG_SITE/media/RANZCOG-MEDIA/Women%27s%20Health/Statement%20and%20guidelines/Clinical-Obstetrics/Mental-Health-Care-in-the-Perinatal-Period-(C-Obs-48).pdf?ext=.pdf.

CHAPTER 3.11

Assessment and management considerations working with someone experiencing psychosis in a PACER team community setting

Fiona l'Anson and Catherine Daniel

KEY POINTS

- Most people diagnosed with psychotic disorders can experience recovery if they are supported in ways they identify as most valuable to themselves (Raeburn & Ball 2020).
- It is important to avoid the risk of diagnostic overshadowing and/or allowing personal attitudes or stigma associated with the person or their presentation to influence the approach to clinical assessment and risk management.
- Collateral information from family members/carers/others is essential to completing a more holistic clinical assessment, which enables more robust and effective risk assessment, management and care planning.
- It is important to use effective inter-personal strategies, communication and verbal de-escalation skills to assist with managing a person's distress and reduce the use of restrictive clinical practice.

LEARNING OUTCOMES

This chapter will assist you to:

- identify the skills and knowledge required to conduct a psychiatric mental state examination and clinical risk assessment
- discuss potential contributing factors to a person's deterioration in mental state
- understand the challenges associated with conducting comprehensive mental state and clinical risk assessments and effective care planning in complex and evolving situations and environments
- describe the importance of effective communication, inter-agency collaboration and interpersonal strategies in effective care of a person experiencing an acute psychiatric crisis
- discuss the concepts of person-centred, trauma-informed and recovery focused care.

Lived experience comment
by Helena Roennfeldt

IMPACT OF CRISIS RESPONSES

The chapter highlights the prevalence of negative perceptions of people with mental illness by underscoring stereotypes of dangerousness and the lack of evidence to support this belief. The experience of psychosis and receiving mental health crisis care can be complicated by police involvement, increasing public stigma and criminalisation of mental illness. Police involvement can further exacerbate distress and cause fear and humiliation. Feeling like we are being punished can be compounded by restrictive practices such as physical and mechanical restraint and forced medication. Being listened to, shown genuine care and being involved in decision-making reduce negative impacts and increase the likelihood of future help-seeking.

INTRODUCTION

The term 'psychosis' is used to describe phenomena in which people experience a move away from regular perception into an inner world in which patterns of thinking, feeling and behaving have become distorted. These experiences commonly occur early in a person's adult life and can affect perception, behaviour, mood, thinking ability and social and occupational functioning. Many people experience psychosis as confusing, bizarre and frightening. For others, however, psychosis can actually be more bearable than their 'real world' (Raeburn & Ball 2020).

Psychosis and schizophrenia-related phenomena affect around 1% of the population. Aetiology is probably due to a melange of causes, including social, environmental, psychological and biological factors: all are current foci of research and theory development. People in lower socio-economic groups (Burns et al 2014), those who are homeless (Ayano et al 2019) and people in prison are more likely to be experiencing psychosis than someone in the general community (Korobanova et al 2021). Many people fear that experiencing a psychotic episode means they will inevitably be burdened with a lifetime diagnosis of schizophrenia, but this is not correct. Long-term studies have shown that more than 70% of people with a diagnosis of schizophrenia experience recovery (Raeburn & Ball 2020; Vita & Barlati 2018; Zipursky & Agid 2015).

Despite their prevalence and impact, psychosis and schizophrenia-related phenomena have yet to be fully understood. They continue to be erroneously associated with 'split personality' or 'multiple personality', and people who are diagnosed with schizophrenia or psychotic disorders are often mistrusted, feared and discriminated against. Often, psychosis is not only strange for the person who experiences it, but also becomes confusing for people around them. Unfortunately, fear created by the confusion then leads people who receive diagnoses to be treated in discriminatory ways. People who have experienced psychosis feel the effects of stigma – which can be as bad or worse than the effects of psychosis itself. People diagnosed with conditions such as schizophrenia are often considered unpredictable and dangerous. In fact, the reverse is true: people who experience psychosis have far higher chance of being victims of crime and violence (Khalifeh et al 2015; Raeburn & Ball 2020).

Psychotic disorders such as schizophrenia are currently understood as being characterised by one or more of the following five types of symptoms:

- **Delusions:** fixed beliefs that are not amenable to change in light of conflicting evidence. Content may include a variety of themes (e.g. persecutory, referential, somatic, religious, grandiose). For example:
    - paranoid delusions, such as the belief the person is being followed or monitored e.g. 'My neighbour is plotting to kill me'
    - grandiose delusion, where a person may believe they have special abilities or 'powers', e.g. 'I have the ability to fly' or 'I'm on a mission from God'
    - thought broadcasting, which is the belief that the person's thoughts are being broadcast to or heard by others
    - thought withdrawal, which is the belief that thoughts are being placed in the person's mind against their will (Raeburn & Ball 2020).
- **Hallucinations** refer to distortions in perception. People with psychosis may experience hallucinations in any of the five senses: hearing, seeing, feeling, smelling or tasting sensations that do not appear to be real. Common hallucinations include:
    - auditory hallucinations commonly include but are not limited to hearing voices (talking to or about the person), hearing music and other noises when there is no sound (e.g. hearing someone call their name when home alone)
    - visual hallucinations include seeing things that are not there, or seeing things in a strange way (e.g. seeing unusual shapes, colours or lights, or seeing an image of a person)
    - somatic hallucinations involving feeling something touch or happen in your body when there is nothing there (e.g. feeling as though ants are crawling on your skin)
    - olfactory hallucinations, which involve smelling things when there are no smells around (e.g. smelling rotting fish in the house, even though there are no fish there)
    - gustatory hallucinations, which refer to tasting things in a strange way (e.g. tasting metal in the mouth) (Raeburn & Ball 2020).
- **Disorganised thinking** is inferred from a person's speech. It is commonly characterised as including speech that switches rapidly from one topic to another; this may be described as ' derailment' or 'loose associations'. A person may reply to questions with answers that are tangential, which means they are oblique or unrelated. Sometimes speech may be incomprehensible, and it may be described as incoherent or 'word salad'. Mildly disorganised speech can impact effective communication and make conversation difficult to follow. This may be further complicated if there is cultural and linguistic diversity. Speech may include:
    - 'neologisms' use of words that don't exist
    - 'echolalia' – repeating words/phrases used by other people in conversation
    - 'perseveration' the person uses excessive continuation/repetition of single response or idea (Raeburn & Ball 2020).
- **Disorganised behaviour** may be exhibited in a variety of ways, including chaotic or erratic behaviour and agitation. This may impact goal-orientated daily activities. Catatonic behaviour is a significant decrease in response or reaction to the environment. This can include:

- ○ resistance to instructions or requests (negativism)
- ○ maintaining a rigid, inappropriate or bizarre posture
- ○ absence of any verbal and/or motor response to stimuli (e.g. mutism)
- ○ extreme restlessness and excessive motor activity without obvious cause or purpose (catatonic excitement).

Other examples are repeated movements, including staring or grimacing. Catatonia is traditionally associated with schizophrenia; however, people may experience catatonic symptoms with other mental disorders or medical conditions (Raeburn & Ball 2020).

- **Negative symptoms** are absences or reductions of thought processes, emotions and behaviours that were present prior to the onset of the illness, but have since diminished or are absent following the onset of the illness. Common examples include reductions in the expression of emotions in the face, eye contact, intonation of speech, and movements of the hand, head, and face that normally give an emotional emphasis to speech. These symptoms are substantial in schizophrenia, but less common in other psychotic disorders (Raeburn & Ball 2020).

Symptoms of psychosis often contribute to deterioration in interpersonal relationships. Heightened levels of anxiety are experienced as the person identifies a perceived conflict between what is and what should be. Anger may occur when others appear to disregard what the person acknowledges as their reality and attempts are made to refocus and address reorientation. The person may feel their need for safety and security is threatened by their attempt to cope with an 'alien world'.

It is important to remember that the signs and symptoms described above are the opinion and view of the American Association of Psychiatrists, who constructed the *Diagnostic and Statistical Manual of Mental Disorder* (DSM-5). Such descriptions are therefore layered with cultural understandings from a US/Western point of view and lack objective scientific evidence. There are no laboratory tests or other diagnostic procedures that can confirm or refute a diagnosis of a 'psychotic' type disorder. Making psychiatric diagnoses therefore relies heavily on detailed history-taking, behavioural observation and opinion (Raeburn & Ball 2020).

Common diagnostic terms currently used to describe psychotic disorders in modern healthcare include:

- substance-induced psychotic disorder
- brief intermittent psychosis
- delusional disorder
- schizophreniform disorder
- schizophrenia
- schizoaffective disorder (Raeburn & Ball 2020).

The above introduction to psychosis has been adapted from existing text by Raeburn and Ball 2020.

ABOUT PACER*

The Police, Ambulance and Clinical Early Response (PACER) service provides a dedicated joint police and mental health response activated by police and targeted to times of greatest demand. It provides on-scene comprehensive mental health triage and assessment, crisis intervention, care planning and telephone assistance in the community. The service aims to provide appropriate and seamless trauma-informed care, reducing the need for transport to emergency departments (EDs) and increasing out-of-hospital referral capabilities, while streamlining the transport, mental health triage/assessment, handover and admission process for those requiring hospital treatment.

PACER differs from traditional emergency mental health care pathways, given that the mobile emergency mental health response acts as a secondary police response, informed by current police and mental health background information, and facilitating the opportunity to assess the person close to the time of crisis.

PACER assistance can be requested for:

- onsite clinical assessment of a person's mental health status
- onsite or telephone advice on mental health referral options
- advice on appropriate transport options
- advice on de-escalation strategies and options
- design of intervention strategies for frequent users of emergency services.

Note: The implementation, scope of practice and the use of the Mental Health Act within the PACER initiative may differ between states and territories. The description above and subsequent sections denoted with an asterisk (*) are based on the service model initially developed and implemented in November 2018 at the PACER pilot site in South Eastern Sydney Local Health District at St George Hospital and Community Mental Health Services, Kogarah. This model has since been adopted in multiple locations in the state of New South Wales.

Why was PACER established?

PACER has been established in some parts of Australia, including New South Wales, Victoria, Queensland, Western Australia and Northern Territory, in direct response to the increasing number of mental health presentations to EDs under the Mental Health Act brought in by police and ambulance. Different states and territories have adapted the model to meet their local service requirements.

The PACER service has been well received by consumers, carers and police and ambulance services, with some of the benefits outlined below (Henry & Rajakaruna 2018; McKenna et al 2015).

Benefits of PACER for consumers and carers*

PACER provides consumers, their carers, relatives and friends with more immediate clinical intervention for their mental health crisis, using a least restrictive community-based approach, therefore increasing the likelihood of better outcomes (Evangelista et al 2016). PACER also assists in the streamlining of the transport, mental health triage/assessment, handover and admission process for those requiring hospital treatment.

Benefits of PACER for police*

- Improved collaboration and inter-agency work between police, ambulance and health services.
- Improved knowledge and understanding of mental health diagnoses and management, and associated reduction in stigma.
- Reduced time on-scene for mental health events – average of 45 minutes (as of June 2020).

- Reduced demand on NSW police to transport involuntary mental health consumers.
- Increased capacity to provide mental health assessments for people in custody.

Benefits of PACER for ambulance*

- Eliminates the need for ambulance attendance for persons where ED is not required.
- Reduced demand on ambulance service for transport of mental health consumers.
- Improved information-sharing with ambulance, police and health service for better use of agency time and resources.

What skills and experience are needed?

PACER clinicians are experienced mental health nurses/clinicians with specialist postgraduate qualifications in mental health and extensive experience working in the field of mental health nursing in various acute settings, including in EDs and in the community. PACER clinicians have the skills and training required to detain a person under the Mental Health Act.

What are the challenges of working as a PACER clinician with police in the community?

The challenges of the PACER clinician role differ from those in other emergency settings, e.g. the ED.

- Working alongside police (primarily) and ambulance services. Challenges include:
  o different organisational cultures
  o differing perspectives on risk and risk management (i.e. in mental health the use of least restrictive care is an underlying tenet versus police need to comply with different protocols and procedures to ensure safety)
  o increased emphasis on communication, collaboration and inter-agency relationships; these are critical for effective service provision.
- Providing crisis clinical intervention in varied community-based settings (e.g. homes, schools, public places, such as parks, train stations) rather than the contained clinical environment of a hospital setting.
- Operating as a lone-working clinician, making time-critical clinical judgements close to the time of crisis, in constantly evolving situations (i.e. while PACER clinicians do have access to a consultant psychiatrist on call, immediate risk assessment and clinical decision-making is highly autonomous).
- Though not directly applicable to this scenario, a frequent call type made to 000 is in response to concerns for the welfare of a person experiencing an emotional crisis, having voiced suicidal ideation. Using traditional care pathways, pre-PACER implementation, such a person would immediately be transported to the ED by police for mental health assessment and would often be discharged a few hours later. With PACER, time spent conducting the assessment and subsequently coordinating care plans and follow-up, provides the context for the therapeutic intervention required to avoid mental health admission. This is the advantage of the PACER initiative, to avoid transport to the ED for those that do not require psychiatric admission. However, the challenge of the PACER role is to coordinate care plans and follow-up in a community setting while ensuring a safe and timely conclusion to the event.

SCENARIO 3.11.1

John

John is a 38-year-old man with an established diagnosis of schizophrenia, polysubstance use and a history of non-adherence with prescribed medication. John's mental state has been stable for 3 years. He lives at home with his mother Mary, who is his primary carer, and he receives a disability pension. John has had a part-time job delivering newspapers twice a week for the last 3 years. He is currently under the care of the local community mental health team, who have recently discussed a change to his treatment plan with him. John has agreed to transition from daily oral antipsychotic medication to a monthly depot injection, as he agrees this will help him with medication adherence. He is required to continue with oral medication while the therapeutic dose of the depot is established.

Current situation
Mary called 000 to request police assistance at the home address due to concern about a sudden deterioration in John's mental state. The police radio broadcast historical risk alerts from past interactions for the attention of police due to respond to the event, including John's history of aggression towards police; his previous attempts to grab police guns; his numerous previous drug-related offences; and that he was previously scheduled under the Mental Health Act by police.

Police attend John's home and conduct an initial assessment of the situation. Mary reports that John arrived home late last night, appearing agitated and preoccupied, and has not slept since then. She became increasingly concerned when she discovered John had punched a hole in the wall, causing an injury to his hand. John appears suspicious of police and says he won't speak with them, but is willing to speak with a mental health clinician. The police contact the PACER clinician to attend the scene.

The PACER clinician Kate conducts a mental health assessment and assists police with identifying a safe and appropriate management plan. Kate advises police that John appears to be acutely psychotic and is expressing paranoid ideas. He will probably require transport to hospital – a request is made for ambulance assistance made (to reduce possible delays).

Collateral from Mary (John's mother, on scene prior to speaking with John)
Mary says that John has been taking his oral medication as prescribed by the community mental health consultant psychiatrist (in a reducing regimen). However, she found an empty packet of illicit drugs in John's room, which hadn't been there previously. She would like to support John at home as she has done in the past, but she is currently concerned that he is acutely unwell. She is also fearful for her own safety, given John's expressed belief that she is conspiring with police and that she has installed cameras in the house to enable police surveillance. Mary is concerned, given John's past behaviour when unwell that his physical aggression may escalate from damaging property (i.e. punching the wall) to harming her.

On interview and assessment of John
Kate observes that John appears to be distracted by auditory and/or visual hallucinations and can be observed to be responding to unseen stimuli.

Kate approaches John to introduce herself, showing her hospital ID and explaining her role. When asked what led up to his mother calling 000, John reports that he punched the wall because 'there was a camera in there and she (pointing to his mother) is helping the police monitor me. They're just waiting to arrest me!' John continues to verbalise paranoid ideas

Continued

and persecutory delusions regarding his mother, and becomes increasingly distressed and agitated when talking about the police. He expresses fear that police will arrest him or take him to hospital; he has previous negative experiences of both. John denies having used any illicit substances recently and reports that he is still taking his oral medication as directed. During the discussion, John continues to respond to unseen stimuli and became unable to provide further answers to questions posed during the assessment, therefore, the interview is terminated.

Risk assessment conducted to explore the need for use of the Mental Health Act, risks to others, himself and further deterioration

Decision-making

Kate explains to John that it seems likely the reduction in his medication has resulted in an increase in psychotic symptoms. Kate advises John that everyone is concerned about his current mental state and that it is currently not safe to continue with community treatment at this time. John is advised that he needs to go to hospital, for both his mental health and to have his injured hand assessed and treated. John refuses to accept this explanation and declines to go to hospital. Following her assessment, Kate deems that John does not have the capacity to make a decision about his current care and at that point, she determines that John will need to be treated under the Mental Health Act. The outcome is discussed with police on scene.

Potential escalation point

The ambulance arrives and Kate leaves John to provide a clinical handover outside, including discussing John's need for medication and the possibility of physical restraint if he becomes physically aggressive. A joint clinical discussion between Kate, the ambulance crew and police identify an appropriate strategy to ensure a safe and effective outcome. The police stay with John and he becomes increasingly agitated; however, when Kate re-enters the room he appears to calm slightly. Kate uses verbal de-escalation techniques with some success. While John still does not agree that he needs to go to hospital, he is agreeable to taking some oral sedative medication to help ease his distress, and physical restraint is not required. After a short period, John's level of distress and agitation has reduced and he responds to verbal encouragement. He is able to move himself onto the ambulance stretcher for transport to the ED (appropriate to medical needs, given sedation administered).

RED FLAGS

- Level of agitation/aggression – safety and appropriateness of intervention in community.
- Possible illicit substance use – considerations:
  - Level of intoxication.
  - Associated and/or other physical health concerns – consider/assess the need to prioritise medical treatment dependent on acuity.
  - Capacity for mental health assessment dependent on level and type of intoxication
  - And/or escalation of risk of harm associated with substance use.
- Level of insight/capacity around current mental state and willingness to engage.
- Paranoid ideas about police – possibility that police presence may escalate level of agitation.
- Possible risk of harm to mother given John's belief she is conspiring with police.
- Pain related to hand injury.

PROTECTIVE FACTORS

- Active support network, e.g. mother, community mental health team:
  - Current engagement with community mental health team.
  - Stable accommodation with his mother who is also engaged in his care.
  - Has maintained regular employment for 3 years.
- Level of insight/capacity and willingness to engage (if these are present).
- John usually engages with nurses when they take time to explain the role and show their ID (i.e. differentiating health role from police), despite expressing some paranoid ideas about others around him.

KNOWLEDGE

- It is important to remember that a mental health assessment should never be a mental illness assessment. Assessment can be helpful or unhelpful. It is a process, not a single event – and it can be considered as an intervention in itself (Raeburn & Ball 2020).
- A psychiatric mental state examination (MSE) is a standard component of a comprehensive mental health/psychiatric assessment. It is used in conjunction with other types of information to identify likely disorders or conditions that a person may be experiencing. It also allows the health professional to monitor a person's progress and response to treatment over time.
- Consider that key aspects of assessing 'insight' and 'judgement' of a person can delegitimise their experience. Instead, assessment should focus on principles of mutual learning and sharing the experience of being human (Raeburn & Ball 2020).
- A comprehensive psychiatric risk assessment should include historical, current and longitudinal risk of harm (see below for more information).
- Knowledge around issues of capacity and consent are essential in an acute/emergency setting to inform decision-making and need for restrictive interventions and the Mental Health Act.
- Collateral information from others is important to verify or contradict the information provided by the person.
- When it is unclear what the cause of an acute deterioration in mental state is, it is important to consider all the possible options:
  - The use of illicit substances can impact on a person's mental health presentation, e.g. levels of agitation/increased psychotic symptoms.
  - Physical health conditions, such as intoxication, delirium, acquired brain injury, that may be presenting as or exacerbating psychiatric symptoms.
  - Potential interactions with medication.
- It is appropriate to prioritise immediate medical treatment over mental health in some instances. Examples for consideration include the person's level of substance intoxication, their level of sedation and the existence of any physical injury.
- Pharmacological treatment, impact of cross-titration, side effects and adverse reactions which may affect a person's medication adherence or decision to switch medications.
- Consideration of the impact of stigma and the influence of knowing historical risk alerts from past interactions on the management of the current scenario.

ATTITUDES

- It is important to remain open-minded and non-judgemental when caring for people with a mental illness to avoid bias when considering assessment outcome.
- Perceptions regarding people with a mental illness always perpetrating violence need to be challenged. In reality, people with a mental illness are more likely to be the victims rather than perpetrators of violence due to increased vulnerability (Callaghan & Grundy 2018).

- An individual nurse's previous acquaintance with the individual can provide a sense of familiarity for the person and reduce the need to repeat questions and build on existing rapport previously established.
- A nurse's prior experience of managing similar events may reduce tolerance and accumulate stress and burnout.
- Police attitudes towards people with mental illness – consideration of their personal prior experience of dealing with the individual, similar events and possible job-related trauma from adverse outcomes on other occasions. This may lead attending police to have a more risk-averse approach to managing the current situation.

MENTAL HEALTH SKILLS

- Establishing trust and rapport to build an effective therapeutic relationship, i.e. active listening, non-verbal and verbal communications in a respectful and kind manner.
- Effective communication with John and his mother, i.e. provide privacy, explain the assessment process and patient journey.
- Effective communication and inter-agency collaboration (i.e. police/ambulance/ED) and collaborative care planning.
- Verbal de-escalation techniques, i.e. remain calm, listen and allow time and space to focus on the person's needs, so they feel validated; ensure personal space is maintained and body language is non-threatening.
- Timely risk assessment and management – to decrease distress to John and his mother, maintain the safety of everyone on scene and ensure prompt access to appropriate care and treatment.
- Decision-making regarding the use of the Mental Health Act and appropriate form of transport, considering the local memorandum of understanding between police, ambulance and health services.
- Providing trauma-informed care with an awareness of past trauma, interactions with police and emergency services and previous experiences with use of restrictive care to achieve a positive outcome for John.
- Ability to work flexibly in changing environments and conditions and respond appropriately.

Nursing actions and interventions

- Liaise with police prior to arrival on scene – appropriate information sharing regarding known history/diagnosis/risks and current presentation.
- Plan approach, e.g. consider that hospital transport may be a likely outcome – request ambulance attendance to reduce delays.
- Police must first establish safety of the scene before PACER clinician can commence intervention.
- Introductions made – PACER role explained and consent received (Note: dependent on insight/capacity and acuity of risks, risk management overrides need for consent). Refer to the Useful websites section for further information, noting that guidance between states and territories may differ. Clinicians must familiarise themselves with the local policy.
- Conduct comprehensive mental health assessment/triage.
- Consider required treatment/management in a timely manner.
- Provide immediate carer support to John's mother and advice regarding sources of ongoing assistance.
- Handover to the ED:
  - Liaison with consultant psychiatrist, registrar, clinical nurse consultant (mental health), bed manager/after hours nurse manager, ED doctor.

- o   Handover to ED triage nurse, treating ED team (nurse/doctor).
- o   Considerations for ED (access to food, notifying next-of-kin (if indicated), check/search belongings).
- o   Timely documentation of PACER clinician assessment to expedite John's journey through the ED.
- Post-event debrief with police – provide psychoeducation regarding assessment, process and outcome.

RELEVANT TREATMENT MODALITIES AND CONSIDERATIONS

Consider the available options for care and treatment, utilising the least restrictive appropriate option available.

- Frustration with diagnostic systems such as the DSM-5, has led people working within allied health professions and people with lived experience of mental illness to develop a range of emerging, alternative approaches to understanding experiences currently labelled as psychosis and schizophrenia. For example, Open Dialogue Therapy (ODT) is a therapeutic technique developed in Scandinavia for treatment of psychosis. The primary goal of ODT is the increased engagement of a person's social network/family in therapy, with a view to creating a more open dialogue about experiences related to psychosis in the home environment (Raeburn & Ball 2020).
- Ongoing treatment in the community:
  - o   Does John currently have the insight into his current mental state and capacity to agree to engage in community treatment?
  - o   Is it currently safe for John to remain in the community?
- Transfer and admission to hospital on a voluntary basis:
  - o   Does John have the capacity to agree to a voluntary hospital presentation? Review resources listed in the Useful websites section.
  - o   Transfer and admission to hospital under the Mental Health Act.
- Risk assessment and considerations:
  - o   Historical risk – informing current risk assessment, safety planning and risk management strategies.
  - o   Current risk – suicidal ideation, plan or intent, risk of self-harm, misadventure, risk of harm to others, risk of harm from others. Chronic risk vs acute risk.
  - o   Longitudinal risk – risk of harm to reputation, risk of further deterioration in mental state without assertive assessment and treatment.
- Use of sedation – to be considered, dependent on level of distress, aggression or risk of harm to others if verbal de-escalation proves insufficient.

SUMMARY

This chapter demonstrates the role of mental health nurses (PACER clinicians), working with police, to manage a mental health crisis, where someone is experiencing an acute psychotic episode and paranoid ideation in the community. It has identified the skills and knowledge required to conduct a mental state examination and clinical risk assessment, exploring contributing factors to a person's deterioration in mental state. Conducting a comprehensive mental health assessment and clinical risk assessment can be complex and challenging – particularly in evolving situations. Therefore, gaining collateral information from family members, carers or others involved in the person's care is essential for effective risk assessment, management and care planning. It is important to avoid the risk of diagnostic overshadowing and/or allowing personal attitudes or stigma associated with the person or their presentation to influence the approach to clinical assessment and risk management.

The **PACER** clinician role is a senior nursing position which focuses on providing mental health assessments at the point of crisis and exploring alternative pathways to the emergency department and increasing referral options in the community. Informal education is a significant part of the role and supports emergency services staff, who are the first point of contact in a crisis situation, to provide more effective intervention and understand the importance of person-centred, trauma-informed and recovery-focused care. Effective care of a person experiencing an acute psychiatric crisis is underpinned by the use of effective communication, inter-agency collaboration and interpersonal strategies. Collaboration and communications with the person, including verbal de-escalation skills can assist with managing a person's distress and reduce the use of restrictive clinical practice.

Reflection

1. Reflect on the scenario and the description of the role of the PACER clinician.
   a. What elements of the scenario caused you to reflect on your own practice in the emergency setting?
   b. What mental health nursing skills do you need to develop?
   c. What knowledge do you need to help you provide more holistic care to all clients who present for emergency care, assessment and treatment?
2. What is the impact of stigma on the person's behaviour and treatment during a crisis/emergency situation?
3. Arriving at the ED with police can be a distressing time for the person.
   a. What engagement strategies have you seen your colleagues use?
   b. Which were effective?
   c. What is your approach to establishing rapport?

Useful websites

Informed Consent. State Government of Victoria 2017–2020: www2.health.vic.gov.au/mental-health/practice-and-service-quality/mental-health-act-2014-handbook/recovery-and-supported-decision-making/informed-consent,

Presumption of Capacity. State Government of Victoria 2017–2020: www2.health.vic.gov.au/mental-health/practice-and-service-quality/mental-health-act-2014-handbook/recovery-and-supported-decision-making/presumption-of-capacity.

References

Parts of this chapter (denoted with *) have been compiled from information developed internally by Angela Karooz (General Manager, Mental Health Services in South Eastern Sydney Local Health District) in collaboration with the PACER Team, led by the author of this chapter, Fiona I'Anson at St George Hospital, Community Mental Health Services, in conjunction with St George Police Area Command, Kogarah, Sydney. Material utilised has not been formally published.

Ayano G, Tesfaw G, Shumet S 2019. The prevalence of schizophrenia and other psychotic disorders among homeless people: A systematic review and meta-analysis. BMC Psychiatry 19:370.

Burns JK, Tomita A, Kapadia AS 2014. Income inequality and schizophrenia: Increased schizophrenia incidence in countries with high levels of income inequality. International Journal of Social Psychiatry 60(2):185–96.

Callaghan P, Grundy A 2018. Violence risk assessment and management in mental health: A conceptual, empirical and practice critique. The Journal of Mental Health Training, Education, and Practice 13(1):3–13.

Evangelista E, Lee S, Gallagher A et al 2016. Crisis averted: How consumers experienced a police and clinical early response (PACER) unit responding to a mental health crisis. International Journal of Mental Health Nursing 25(4):367.

Henry P, Rajakaruna N 2018. WA Police Force mental health co-response evaluation report. The Sellenger Centre for Research in Law, Justice and Social Change.

Khalifeh H, Johnson S, Howard L et al 2015. Violent and non-violent crime against adults with severe mental illness. The British Journal of Psychiatry 206(4):275–82.

Korobanova D, Spencer S-J, Dean K 2021. Prevalence of mental health problems in men and women in an Australian Prison sample: comparing psychiatric history taking and symptom screening approaches. International Journal of Forensic Mental Health 21(1):89–105.

McKenna B, Furness T, Brown S et al 2015. Police and clinician diversion of people in mental health crisis from the Emergency Department: A trend analysis and cross comparison study. BMC Emergency Medicine15:14.

Raeburn T, Ball M 2020. Chapter 12: Psychosis and schizophrenia. In: Foster K, Marks P, O'Brien A et al (eds) Mental health in nursing: Theory and practice for clinical settings, 5th edn. Elsevier Australia, Sydney.

Vita A, Barlati S 2018. Recovery from schizophrenia. Current Opinion in Psychiatry 31(3):246–55.

Zipursky RB, Agid O 2015. Recovery, not progressive deterioration, should be the expectation in schizophrenia. World Psychiatry 14(1):94.

CHAPTER 3.12

Assessment and management considerations working with people presenting with mood disorder in the pre-hospital (paramedic) practice setting

Louise Roberts

KEY POINTS

- A range of challenges can be associated with the pre-hospital presentation of people experiencing mental health concerns due to the acute nature of the presenting complaint, the unpredictable physical environment of the home and public spaces, the presence of family members or bystanders, the confined nature of the ambulance and the time required to access and obtain further support, if required, and the limited alternative pathways for care and referral.
- The workload for those working in the emergency medical provision of mental health care in the pre-hospital setting can range from 20% to 30%.
- Providing mental health care in the pre-hospital setting entails comprehensive basic assessment skills,

LEARNING OUTCOMES

This chapter will assist you to:

- critically discuss the factors that are relevant to mental health assessment and apply these to the pre-hospital environment
- discuss and reflect on the characteristics of bipolar disorder and how a person experiencing bipolar disorder may present in the pre-hospital setting
- discuss the relevance of ambulance workloads in the care of those experiencing mental health concerns
- discuss the role and priorities of paramedics in delivering acute and primary mental health care in the pre-hospital setting.

KEY POINTS—cont'd

communication skills and empathy as a corner stone to practice and the ability to combine mental health care and physical care in time-limited circumstances.

- As a clinician, providing mental health care in the pre-hospital setting can be positive and satisfying – you enable access to further care, provide a unique assessment (first on scene, observe the person in their home environment and in the acute stages of the condition) and can be the first health professional that the person connects with
- Developing rapport and ensuring a safe therapeutic environment are essential parts of the approach in the pre-hospital setting.

Lived experience comment
by Helena Roennfeldt

RESPONSES TO A CRISIS CAN IMPACT FUTURE HELP-SEEKING

When experiencing mental health crises, what we value most is emotional support and human connection. Relational skills are critical in providing support in ways that validate our distress and maximise our autonomy and choice. A holistic approach to mental health crisis care is needed right from the beginning. This includes first responders acknowledging contextual factors and asking about circumstances and trauma that may have contributed to our experience, such as homelessness, poverty, relationship breakdown, job loss, substance use, parenting, family violence, childhood abuse – a whole range of potential issues that are much, much more than just a clinical response. All mental health treatment, including responding to mental health crises, aims to support personal recovery and quality of life, including ways to help people make sense of their experiences, make decisions and control their treatment. It is crucial to reduce any adverse impact of treatment (particularly coercive treatment) and be mindful of the laws that protect our rights if we are being involuntarily treated for mental illness, including rights to privacy and other human rights. Significantly, responses to a crisis can impact future help-seeking and how we engage in future treatment.

INTRODUCTION

Paramedics are frontline service providers for both emergency and non-emergency presentations of people experiencing mental health and/or alcohol and other drug (AOD) issues. They provide immediate treatment, initial assessment and transport or referral for those in need (McCann et al 2018).

As public health needs and demands change, and prevalence of chronic medical conditions including mental health concerns and illness increase in the community, paramedic practice in Australia, New Zealand and internationally has slowly moved towards models of primary and community care, at the same time maintaining traditional emergency service provision (Eaton et al 2019; Evashkevich & Fitzgerald, 2014; Elliott & Brown 2013) and crossing boundaries between emergency medical care, primary and tertiary care. As one of only a few professions that attend individuals in their home and in the community, paramedics are in a privileged position to advocate for and assist those experiencing mental health concerns (Roggenkamp et al 2018). From this unique position, during a crisis paramedics offer immediate support and gather essential information that no one else may have witnessed or be present for.

Paramedics work collaboratively across multidisciplinary health provisions, can advocate for the individual to access further care and be integral in the development of alternative care pathways for those who need mental health support. The advent of online support and information (e.g. Beyond Blue, HeadSpace, Black Dog Institute, Sane) increases the expectation and need for paramedics to engage in psychoeducation, be aware of clinical standards of care for those with mental health needs and professional requirements to collaborate with mental health services to help the person engage (or re-engage) with treatment and support.

REGISTRATION AND STANDARDS OF CARE

As registered professionals, paramedics are required to demonstrate competency in assessment and clinical care, including mental health care. This includes:

a. assessing the patient or client, taking into account their history, views and an appropriate physical examination where relevant; the history includes relevant psychological, social and cultural aspects.

b. formulating and implementing a suitable management plan (including providing treatment and advice and, where relevant, arranging investigations and liaising with other treating practitioners).

c. facilitating coordination and continuity of care (Paramedicine Board of Australia 2018).

To provide competent care in the pre-hospital setting for those with mental ill-health, paramedics need to be able to approach the person with empathy, compassion and employ keen observational skills. They need to conduct and document a relevant and comprehensive mental state examination (MSE), including objective observation of the person's appearance, behaviour, conversation and speech, thought flow and content, the person's perception, affect and mood, and cognition. The resulting clinical decisions on the person's insight and capacity, and their judgement, have significant implications for patient outcomes and care provision. Table 3.12.1 outlines the key features of assessment for paramedics.

TABLE 3.12.1 Key features of assessment for pre-hospital presentations where mental health concerns are identified

Approach	
Danger/scene evaluation and awareness	• Observations of physical hazards and potential risks • Exits and egress • Who else is around? • Watch and observe how the person is interacting with their environment and with others if they are on scene • What are they doing and saying? • How are they reacting to your presence?
Response	• Observe the person's body language and tone, volume, pace and pitch of their voice • What is the context of the distress and what history can you obtain? • Is substance use involved or any other medical conditions that might be relevant to the change in behaviour?
Communication/ empathy	• Actively listen • Be genuine and present when interacting with the person • Watch and communicate through your own words, body language and voice
Mental State Examination	
Appearance and behaviour	• Self-care and hygiene, posture, clothing, physical features, any tattoos or piercings or other distinguishing features, build, movement (psychomotor activity), mannerisms, gait
Speech and conversation	• What is the person saying and how are they saying it? • Rate, volume, flow, pitch and frequency (cadence) e.g. pressured, loud or soft, disjointed or mumbled
Thought form and content	• Presence of disorganised thoughts, continuity of ideas, disturbance of language or meaning • Presence of delusions, suicidal thoughts, obsessions or phobias
Perception	• How does the person see themselves and what is their view of the world? • Note any changes in sensory perception, e.g. hallucinations, dissociation, derealisation or depersonalisation
Cognition	• Orientation, memory, concentration and abstract thinking
Clinical decision-making insight, capacity and judgement	• Based on the mental state examination. • Consider the person's understanding of their own situation, current behaviour, emotions and feelings • Is the person able to take in information, process that information and make decisions regarding their own health care based on information provided and discussed?

Modified from Roberts 2021, p. 906.

MENTAL HEALTH WORKLOAD IN THE PRE-HOSPITAL SETTING

Paramedics and ambulance services provide acute crisis care for those with mental health conditions, but also serve as the link between those with primary mental health care needs and community services. Increasingly, paramedics are required to assess and make clinical

Box 3.12.1 National Ambulance Surveillance System (NASS)

Currently it is difficult to get comprehensive data on non-fatal suicidal and self-harming behaviours in the community because hospitalisation data and clinical data from emergency departments only tend to report on those presenting with serious physical and mental health issues who are admitted for further treatment. In addition, classification of mental health and self-harm is not currently well defined in the International Classification of Disease, which leaves a gap in knowledge. To fill this knowledge gap, the National Ambulance Surveillance System (NASS) was established. NASS is a public initiative by the Commonwealth Government, Turning Point Drug and Alcohol Centre, Monash University and jurisdictional ambulance services across Australia to monitor self-harm behaviours across participating states and territories. The project is a world-first public health system to monitor and capture data about mental health and self-harm behaviours. The data from NASS is used to identify trends, determine community need and to support planning for resource and service provision.

decisions around the need for hospital and intensive mental health care, or to evaluate the appropriateness of alternative referral to community mental health services. In addition, ambulance services provide key data, enabling a more complete picture on community mental health needs, non-suicidal self-harm and suicidal behaviours in the Australian community to be established (e.g. see Box 3.12.1).

For data collection purposes, mental health and self-harm related ambulance attendances are defined as those where the person presents with mental health symptoms, or where self-harm occurred during the preceding 24 hours or during paramedic attendance. These presentations do not denote a diagnosis, but a diagnosis may be evident in the history gained from the person or significant others. In research by Lubman and colleagues (2020), mental health symptoms were identified from ambulance data under the following broad categories:

* anxiety: 'overwhelming and intrusive worry, and/or panic attack symptom profile'
* depression: 'symptom profile consistent with depression, such as low mood, feelings of hopelessness, despair, worthlessness, anhedonia, change in sleep and/or appetite'
* psychosis: 'presence of hallucinations or delusions'
* other mental health symptoms: 'mental health symptoms not otherwise unspecified' (Lubman et al 2020).

    Self-harm-related ambulance attendances were defined and coded as:
* self-injury (non-fatal intentional injury without suicidal intent) (Klonsky et al 2016)
* suicidal ideation (thinking about killing oneself without acting on the thoughts)
* suicide attempt (non-fatal intentional injury with suicidal intent, regardless of likelihood of lethality)
* suicide (fatal intentional injury with suicidal intent).

    Suicide, suicide attempt and suicidal ideation are considered mutually exclusive; however, self-injury could be simultaneously coded with any other self-harm case category.

In 2020 ambulances attended 33 000 incidents involving suicidal behaviours (suicidal ideation, suicide attempt, death by suicide) in new South Wales, Victoria, Queensland,

Tasmania and the ACT (AIHW 2021). In line with population distribution, over one-third (36%) of attendances occurred in NSW (AIHW 2021). The rate of ambulance attendances for suicidal ideation ranged from about 280 attendances (52.0 per 100 000 population) in Tasmania to over 8400 attendances (103.3 per 100 000 population) in NSW (AIHW 2021). Attendance rates to suicide attempts in comparison to suicide ideation were lower across all jurisdictions and ranged from about 250 attendances (46.1 per 100 000 population) in Tasmania to around 3700 attendances (72.4 per 100 000 population) in Queensland (AIHW 2021).

CHANGES IN MOOD: CARING IN THE COMMUNITY

Approximately one in 40 adults in Australia experience bipolar disorder each year (Malhi et al 2020). Bipolar disorder is a recurrent illness commonly characterised by episodes of depression and hypomania/mania (elevated mood and increased psychomotor movement). These mood-related episodes have a significant effect on the person's ability to function and socially engage. Family members and significant others will often be the first to notice and become concerned about the person's mood changes. Multiple studies suggest that the mean age of onset for bipolar appears to be in the late teens and early 20s, although findings vary between 20 and 30 years (Rowland & Marwaha 2018; Malhi et al 2021). People with bipolar disorder are 30 to 60 times more likely than the general population to die by suicide (Malhi et al 2021).

There have been studies exploring the relationship between sociodemographic factors, such as economic status, employment type, relationship status and creativity, with the development of bipolar disorder. Results are mixed, with some studies suggesting that there is some evidence of higher rates in low income, unemployed and unmarried groups, but others finding that higher socioeconomic status and higher occupational level, as well as creativity, have been associated with higher prevalence of bipolar disorder (Rowland & Marwaha 2018). Other key factors implicated in the development of bipolar disorder are genetic factors, which involve multiple genes, their interaction with the environment and psychological stress or significant life events (e.g. childhood trauma, neglect and abuse, infection).

The following scenario is used to demonstrate the knowledge, attitudes and mental health skills required in the pre-hospital setting when working with someone who is experiencing disturbance in mood.

SCENARIO 3.12.1

Samuel

An ambulance is dispatched at 20.00 hours to a residential address for a 36-year-old male (Samuel). Sam has accidently broken a beer bottle and has cut his right hand during an evening family gathering. The family is concerned for Sam, who doesn't seem to realise what has happened.

On arrival: The house is clean, well maintained with clear entry and egress. Sam's family seems to be supportive. Paramedics are met by Sam's sibling (Jess) and Sam's oldest child (Jonas, 14 years old) and directed to the backyard (outdoor area) where Sam is moving around the backyard, talking in a stream of sentences as though trying to get a point across (pressured speech). Sam has a kitchen tea towel wrapped around his hand to manage the bleeding. (The shattered bottle has been cleaned up. On quick inspection, the wound does not appear to be large or deep and the bleeding has been brought under control.) Sam seems to be alternating between an irritated and astonished response to the fuss that is being made of a 'small cut and an accident' to laughing, wanting to just get back to the gathering, continue drinking and to finish off the evening. Sam is currently employed, but has told his sister Jess that it is 'full on' and stressful, and he is thinking about looking for a new job.

Jonas tells you that his dad has not slept for the past week and he has heard him wandering around their house at all hours of the night. He knows his dad has had periods of low mood (depression) previously, but things seem to have been worse since their mum left around 7 months ago. He has only seen his dad this 'hyper' (hyperactive, moving around, speaking rapidly) once before when he was around 11 years old. Jonas is currently being cared for by his father, who has custody.

Sam is very reluctant to speak with you; he has begun drinking another beer while you have been assessing the scene and trying to engage with him. He does not want you to touch him or to take any vital sign observations. You observe his distress increasing, and he is becoming louder in his tone of voice, stating he 'just wants to leave'.

RED FLAGS

- Safety of the clinicians, the patient and others.
- The open backyard and home environment are a potential risk.
- The increased psychomotor movement, lability of Sam's mood and his decreasing engagement with his family and clinicians when they try to assist or intervene.
- The physical injury and potential for infection, need for further review and treatment.
- The previous history of low mood (depression), and recent changes in sleeping patterns, periods of increasing irritability and recent personal relationship breakdown.
- Potential effects on behaviour from the consumption of alcohol.
- Consider potential interactions between mental health medications such as mood stabilisers, antidepressants and alcohol and other substances that Sam may have consumed.
- Consider Sam's son Jonas and his safety at home, his role as potentially being a young carer and how this may have impacted his life (e.g. how have things been at home, how does he feel about his own safety, what supports does he have, does he have a relationship with his mother etc?). Depending on the circumstances, Child Protection Services or other support services may need to be considered (HeadSpace, BeyondBlue, COPMI (Children of Parents with Mental Illness), community mental health services).

PROTECTIVE FACTORS

- The scene has been made safe by the family and they appear to be a positive support network.
- Jonas, the son, appears to be particularly concerned and supportive of his father and able to corroborate information.
- Although increasingly agitated, Sam is still engaging and responsive to your questions.
- Sam appears to be currently oriented to time, place and person; he recalls why you have been called and can articulate what happened.
- Currently employed and caring for his son.

KNOWLEDGE

- Scene awareness, assessment and mitigation of scene dangers are the first consideration and are essential to the safety of paramedics and others at the scene. This may be particularly relevant at parties or gatherings where people may be intoxicated, or in situations where the environment itself is unsafe.
- A broad understanding of risk and risk assessment is required, e.g. physical risk, social networks, changes in participation in activities, isolation and withdrawal, help-seeking, what personal and external resources the person has access to, presence of suicidal ideation, behaviours or intent, recent significant life events. Consider if there is a potential for deterioration in the person's behaviour and wellbeing (e.g. if they are intoxicated, or the person has other comorbidities that might put them at further risk of deterioration).
- There are a range of features that can indicate mania, e.g. inflated self-esteem or grandiosity, a decreased need for sleep (e.g. feels rested after only 3 hours of sleep). The person may be more talkative than usual and their speech may demonstrate that they are experiencing a flight of ideas, or they might state the subjective experience that their thoughts are racing. When people are manic they are often highly distractible, i.e. their attention is easily drawn to unimportant or irrelevant external stimuli, and there may be a marked increase in goal-directed activity (either socially, at work or school, or sexually) or psychomotor agitation (i.e. purposeless non-goal-directed activity). Some people also demonstrate excessive involvement in activities that have a high potential for painful consequences which may constitute 'harm to self' legally (e.g. engaging in unrestrained buying sprees, sexual indiscretions or foolish business investments).
- Depression is more than just feeling sad or flat; when someone is experiencing depression, they can feel worthless, struggle to think or concentrate or make decisions, and experience depressed mood or irritability most of the time. Depression can also have physical impacts, such as appetite and weight changes, insomnia or hypersomnia, and fatigue or low energy. The person will probably experience marked disinterest in things that they usually enjoy and some people experience thoughts of death, suicidal ideation, a suicide plan or attempt.
- It is important to consider the needs of the person's family, and in particular, the children of people who are experiencing a change in their mental health and who may need their own support, especially if they are a primary carer.
- It is always important to consider other potential causes for the labile mood, e.g. substance use, electrolyte changes, hypoxia.

ATTITUDES

- Paramedics often work with people experiencing crisis situations, where rapid development of a therapeutic relationship between clinician and patient is required in order to be able to provide care. Studies have suggested that the development of a strong and genuine therapeutic interaction, even if only over a short period of time, has a significant effect on a person's willingness to engage with care, follow up with further mental health care, and on recovery and patient outcome (Kondrat & Teater 2012).
- While paramedics have been found to have lower empathy scores towards people experiencing substance use and mental health emergencies (Kus et al 2019), empathy is essential to paramedic practice.
- Paramedics work with people from varied socioeconomic circumstances, cultural and family backgrounds, health status and living environments. They also provide care to groups and individuals who are vulnerable, are often subject to stigma and discrimination, and are often directly impacted by healthcare decisions that result in poor patient outcomes (Lindgren et al 2018). There is a potential to judge and make assumptions regarding the person based on what is seen and heard as paramedics arrive on scene, as

such, paramedics have a responsibility to ensure a non-judgemental, non-discriminatory approach. An open mind and awareness of one's own biases and understandings are essential to remaining professional when attending any patient, but especially when developing a therapeutic rapport.

MENTAL HEALTH SKILLS

- Mental state and related risk assessment are essential parts of paramedic practice and relevant to all health professionals working in emergency settings, including the pre-hospital environment. To do this well, communication skills are required – it's not just about the *what,* it's about the *how*. Talking and developing a therapeutic rapport is key – in these instances communication is both a treatment and an intervention.
- Concepts of listening, empathy, and 'understanding the subjective experience' of the person are seen as important interpersonal skills in acute psychiatric healthcare settings and arguably are also highly relevant for healthcare professionals working in the pre-hospital setting (Schmidt et al 2020). Being genuine and present in the moment are essential to establishing meaningful and caring interactions with patients. Active listening means encouraging the person to speak and attending to what they say. It includes paraphrasing and summarising what they have said to allow for clarification and expansion on their lived experience and indicates you have listened and gathered meaning from what they have said.
- There are many risk assessment tools that feature in the emergency setting. One example is the START risk assessment tool, which assesses seven dynamic risks (violence to others, suicide, self-harm, being victimised, substance abuse, self-neglect, unauthorised absences (alternatively, help-seeking behaviour)) and treatability, and can be used as a guide to determine a level of engagement and risk when attending those with mental health concerns.
- Several emergency departments use specific risk assessment tools which have been validated, such as: STAMP (Staring and eye contact, Tone and volume of voice, Anxiety, Mumbling and Pacing) (Chapman et al 2009; Luck 2007), and well recognised tools such as the Brøset Violence Checklist (BVC), all of which describe behaviours and factors to alert staff to potential violence, such as confusion, irritability, boisterousness, physical and verbal threats and attacking objects (Lorettu et al 2020).
- De-escalation techniques include the use of verbal statements, tone and body language to acknowledge the person, being non-confrontational and non-judgmental in tone, rate and rhythm of speech, and the use of open body language that is non-threatening. Be conscious of personal space and aware of verbal (tone of voice, rate and rhythm, pitch and frequency) and non-verbal communication (non-verbal – facial expressions, body position and posture and movements) – yours and theirs. According to Bowers (2014), the key features of de-escalation involve controlling your own responses and behaviours, working with empathy and respect, delimiting the situation by making it safe for you and the person, clarifying the problem with the person and then trying to take steps to address or resolve the situation.
- Engage with the person's family/friend/primary carer, who will have a unique insight into their loved one's experience and who needs information, support and to be involved in decision-making and care planning.

PARAMEDIC ACTIONS AND INTERVENTIONS

- Scene evaluation and risk mitigation. Make the space safe for you, others and the person.
- Watch and listen. Before attempting to establish a therapeutic rapport with the person, assess and gather information from the environment, the person's interactions with others, and how they move and interact with their environment. (This reflects how are

they seeing themselves, others and the space they are in.) Are they frightened? Are they angry? etc.

- Modify your approach. Consider the personal space required for someone who is displaying increased arousal and emotions (e.g. pacing, pressured speech, flight of ideas and the potential for changes in perception and reality testing (hallucinations and or delusions).
- Ensure you observe for and manage any injuries and assess for alternative causes for change in behaviour, e.g. substance use, hypoglycaemia, dehydration (especially in older adults).
- Act to ensure that the person feels safe and heard – use open and closed questions, active listening, de-escalation strategies and calm/open body language to gain rapport.
- Consider early activation of support and use mental health services/connections to assist in care provision, e.g. mental health triage, mental health community teams, operation (ambulance services) clinical liaisons and support.
- Obtain vital sign observations as appropriate and assess/manage any injuries. It might not be possible to obtain any vital signs (heart and breathing rate, blood pressure, electrocardiograph, blood sugar level) depending on the level of arousal and agitation the person is experiencing; establishing a strong rapport with the person will help increase the possibility that this will occur.
- Gather and take note of the history obtained (previous episodes, recent and past help-seeking, medications, social and personal supports, changes in behaviour and social interaction and how that has impacted functioning for the person and significant others in their life).

RELEVANT TREATMENT MODALITIES AND CONSIDERATIONS

- People experiencing bipolar disorder are generally managed using a combination of pharmacological management, psychotherapies (e.g. cognitive behavioural therapy, motivational interviewing, psychoeducation, family-focused therapy, mindfulness-based interventions) and peer support (Malhi 2021).
- The management of depressive symptoms tends to focus on the restoration of regular and restorative sleep patterns, healthy diet and regular exercise patterns, as well as psychotherapies and antidepressants.
- Paramedics should have a baseline understanding of SSRIs, SNRIs and TCAs to be able to ask about potential side effects and potential overdose. Common antidepressants seen by paramedics in the community include selective serotonin reuptake inhibitors (SSRIs) (escitalopram, citalopram, fluoxetine, fluvoxamine, paroxetine, sertraline), serotonin-norepinephrine reuptake inhibitors (SNRIs) (venlafaxine, duloxetine, desvenlafaxine, levomilnacipran, milnacipran), and, although not as common, tricyclic antidepressants (TCAs) (amitriptyline, clomipramine, dosulepin, doxepin, imipramine, nortriptyline) (Malhi 2021).
- A major consideration in the community setting is serotonin syndrome, which results from increases in serotonin at the $5HT_{2A}$ receptors in the central nervous system and is a potential complication associated with all drugs having a serotonergic effect. This can occur with high doses of single agents or when combinations of serotonergic agents are used, or when changing from one antidepressant to another without an appropriate washout period, potential drug interactions or drug overdose. What to look for and if present indicates a need for early/urgent transport:
  - Neuromuscular movement disorders: hyperreflexia, tremors, twitching loss of muscle coordination with hypertonia and clonus (involuntary rhythmic contractions) being symmetrical and often appearing more significant in lower limbs.
  - Autonomic: hyperthermia, fever, shivering, sweating, tachycardia, hypertension, flushing, dilated pupils, diarrhoea.
  - Cognitive effects: confusion, agitation, restlessness, hypomania, hyperactivity.
- Mania is generally managed with the use of mood stabilisers (lithium and valproate), which can be used on their own or in combination with second generation antipsychotics.

- A key consideration when attending someone who is on lithium is the potential for lithium toxicity as it has a small therapeutic range (Tobita et al 2021). Signs and symptoms to be aware of are:
  - feeling weak, having a worsening tremor, feeling unbalanced or uncoordinated (ataxia), poor concentration, diarrhoea, headache (Tobita et al 2021).
- As part of the initial assessment and care, paramedics can potentially offer sedation to manage agitation (e.g. benzodiazepines or antipsychotics – depending on clinical level, scope of practice, other drug interactions and level of agitation)
- When the person is presenting in the acute phases of mania and/or depression and presents with an increased risk to self, others, and the history-taking and assessment suggest decreased social engagement, decrease in help-seeking, lack of personal and external resources and the potential for deterioration, then transport for further assessment should be considered.
- As a last resort, if de-escalation has not been effective and the person is at risk of harm, consideration may be given to the use of paramedic powers under the relevant Mental Health Act.
- If mechanical or chemical restraint is implemented then appropriate care needs to be taken to protect the person's dignity, airway, breathing and circulation with adequate attention taken to monitoring and assess the person's level of sedation if chemical restraint is used (Cole et al 2018; Nambiar et al 2020).

SUMMARY

This chapter outlines the importance and value of understanding paramedic workload in the area of mental health care. The chapter explores key aspects of the mental state assessment and examination, communication and approach to a person who has increased psychomotor movement, agitation, pressured (rapid) speech and changes in behaviour. The changes in behaviour in the scenario have been noticed and deemed concerning enough for family members to call for paramedic care. Often the role of the family is key to gathering relevant history and background to assist in gaining rapport and gaining 'common' ground to build the caring relationship.

Reflection

1. What de-escalation strategies would you use with Samuel? Consider how you would use your body language, voice and recognition of emotions and context to gain a therapeutic rapport.
2. Would you consider offering oral or other (depending on scope of clinical practice) medication to manage Samuel's increased labile mood and agitation? Would you consider using your powers under the Mental Health Act? What factors would be relevant?

Useful websites

Bipolar description/resources: www.blackdoginstitute.org.au/resources-support/bipolar-disorder/
Brøset Violence checklist: www.frenzs.org/bvc-broset-violence-checklist/?gclid5EAIaIQobChMI7o K1q-rm8wIVw5JmAh3ZiwArEAAYASAAEgIbgfD_BwE
Children of Parent with Mental Illness: www.copmi.net.au/
Health Direct: www.healthdirect.gov.au/bipolar-disorder
National Alliance on Mental Illness (NAMI): www.nami.org/About-Mental-Illness/Mental-Health-Conditions/Bipolar-Disorder

References

Australian Institute of Health and Welfare (AIHW) 2021. Suicide and self-harm monitoring: Ambulance attendances. Online. Available: www.aihw.gov.au/suicide-self-harm-monitoring/data/ambulance-attendances.

Bowers, L 2014. A model of de-escalation. Mental Health Practice 17(9):36–7.

Chapman R, Perry L, Styles I et al 2009. Predicting patient aggression against nurses in all hospital areas. British Journal of Nursing 18:476–83.

Cole JB, Klein LR, Nystrom PC et al 2018. A prospective study of ketamine as primary therapy for prehospital profound agitation. The American Journal of Emergency Medicine 36(5): 789–96.

Eaton G, Wong G, Tierney S. et al 2021. Understanding the role of the paramedic in primary care: A realist review. BMC Medicine 19:145.

Elliott R, Brown, P 2013. Exploring the developmental need for a paramedic pathway to mental health. Journal of Paramedic Practice 5(5):264–70.

Evashkevich M, Fitzgerald M 2014. A framework for implementing community paramedic programs in British Columbia. Ambulance Paramedics of British Columbia. ResearchGate DOI: 10.13140/RG.2.1.1611.5445.

Klonsky ED, May AM, Saffer BY 2016. Suicide, suicide attempts, and suicidal ideation. Annual Review of Clinical Psychology 12:307–30.

Kondrat DC, Teater B 2012. Solution-focused therapy in an emergency room setting: Increasing hope in persons presenting with suicidal ideation. Journal of Social Work 12(1):3–15.

Kus L, Henderson L, Batt AM 2019. Empathy in paramedic practice: an overview. Journal of Paramedic Practice 11(4):1–5.

Lindgren BM, Svedin CG, Werkö S 2018. A systematic literature review of experiences of professional care and support among people who self-harm. Archives of Suicide Research 22(2):173–92.

Lorettu L, Nivoli AM, Milia P et al 2020. Violence risk assessment in mental health. In: Carpiniello B, Vita A, Menacci C (eds) Violence and mental disorders. Springer Nature, Switzerland.

Lubman DI, Heilbronn C, Ogeil RP et al 2020. National Ambulance Surveillance System: A novel method using coded Australian ambulance clinical records to monitor self-harm and mental health-related morbidity. PLoS ONE 15(7):e0236344.

Luck L, Jackson D, Usher K 2007. STAMP: Components of observable behaviour that indicate potential for patient violence in emergency departments. Journal of Clinical Nursing 59:11–9.

Malhi G, Bell E, Bassett D et al 2021. The 2020 Royal Australian and New Zealand College of Psychiatrists clinical practice guidelines for mood disorders. Australian & New Zealand Journal of Psychiatry 55(1):7–117.

McCann TV, Savic M, Ferguson N et al 2018. Paramedics' perceptions of their scope of practice in caring for patients with non-medical emergency-related mental health and/or alcohol and other drug problems: A qualitative study. PLoS ONE 13(12):e0208391.

Nambiar D, Pearce JW, Bray J et al 2020. Variations in the care of agitated patients in Australia and New Zealand ambulance services. Emergency Medicine Australasia 32(3):438–45.

Paramedicine Board of Australia 2018. Code of conduct for registered health practitioners (interim) June 2018. Online. Available: www.paramedicineboard.gov.au/Professional-standards/Codes-guidelines-and-policies.aspx.

Roberts L 2021. Mental health conditions. In: Williams B, Ross L (eds) Paramedic principles and practice: A clinical reasoning approach, 2nd edn. Elsevier Australia, Sydney.

Roggenkamp R, Andrew E, Nehme Z et al 2018. Descriptive analysis of mental health-related presentations to emergency medical services. Prehospital Emergency Care 22(4): 399–405.

Rowland TA, Marwaha S 2018. Epidemiology and risk factors for bipolar disorder. Therapeutic Advances in Psychopharmacology 8(9):251–69.

Schmidt M, Stjernswärd S, Garmy P et al 2020. Encounters with persons who frequently use psychiatric emergency services: Healthcare professionals' views. International Journal of Environmental Research and Public Health 17(3):1012.

Tobita S, Sogawa R, Murakawa T et al 2021. The importance of monitoring renal function and concomitant medication to avoid toxicity in patients taking lithium. International Clinical Psychopharmacology 36(1):34–7.

CHAPTER 3.13

Assessment and management considerations for supporting asylum seekers and refugees

Monica McEvoy

KEY POINTS

- People with refugee/asylum seeker experience are likely to have experienced multiple traumatic events prior to and during their attempts to seek asylum in Australia, and this results in increased risk factors for deteriorating mental health.
- The psychological impact of trauma during immigration detention may result in pervasive refusal syndrome, with profound and long-term effects on the mental health of young people held in these circumstances.
- Prolonged uncertainty of insecure visa status directly results in high levels of hopelessness and fear, with a subsequent increase in deliberate self-harm and suicidal ideation and behaviour.
- Nurses and other health professionals working in emergency care settings play an important role in assessing the mental state of asylum seekers and

LEARNING OUTCOMES

This chapter will assist you to:

- understand the psychological impacts of immigration detention on the mental health of children and young people, including pervasive refusal syndrome (PRS) and post-traumatic stress disorder (PTSD)
- identify the role of nurses in assessing deteriorating mental health with specific reference to the complexities experienced by people who are asylum seekers
- describe how to work with an interpreter in assessing mental health.
- describe the interpersonal strategies that will assist a young asylum seeker to manage emotional distress and suicidal behaviour
- describe a trauma-informed response to this escalation in psychological distress.

KEY POINTS—cont'd

people with refugee backgrounds who present experiencing suicidal ideation, and in ensuring that the safety planning process occurs in a safe and supportive environment.

Lived experience comment
by Helena Roennfeldt

WHAT HAPPENED TO YOU?

The question 'What happened to you?' rather than 'What is wrong with you?' is powerful because it allows for context and reduces the risk of individualising problems arising as a consequence of experiences and exposure to trauma. Trauma events themselves are harrowing, but how trauma is responded to also significantly shapes our trauma experience, e.g. silencing, disbelief, minimising and isolation afterwards can be just as traumatic – maybe even more – than the events. Healing from trauma is often ongoing, messy, and requires physical and emotional safety. Notably, trauma affects us all differently. There are often understandable reasons for behaviour such as self-injury if someone takes the time to listen, and nothing replaces a trusting relationship to enable disclosure and to begin the journey of healing from trauma.

INTRODUCTION

As of mid-2021, the United Nations Refugee Agency (UNHCR) estimates there are more than 84 million people forcibly displaced globally: 48 million internally displaced by war and persecution, 26.6 million refugees, 4.4 million asylum seekers and 4.3 million stateless people world wide (UNHCR 2022). Sixty-eight per cent of all refugees originate from Syria, Venezuela, Afghanistan, South Sudan and Myanmar. However, given 6.7 million refugees have fled Ukraine since 24 February 2022 (as at 27 May 2022) in response to the Russian invasion and 5.7 million Afghans have fled Afghanistan since the Taliban took control in 2021 (Operational Data Portal 2022), it is likely that these statistics will significantly shift and increase in coming months and years. Conversely, there was a 54% decrease in the number of permanent resettlement places globally in 2017 compared to 2016 (UNHCR 2019), reflecting the move from the provision of permanent settlement of refugees to a policy of temporary protection in a number of countries, including Australia.

Over the past 75 years, Australia has provided humanitarian refugee resettlement to some 900 000 people. As at 31 August 2021, there were 38 513 people seeking asylum here, including 31 122 people known in public policy as the 'legacy caseload', which includes those who arrived by boat on or after 13 August 2012, those who arrived prior to that date but hadn't had their claims processed by that date, as well as babies born in Australia to people in the legacy caseload. There are 1380 people still subject to harsh offshore processing policies, and 19 000 people are subject to either a temporary protection visa (TPV), which allows them to live in the community for 3 years, or a Safe Haven Enterprise Visa (SHEV), which offers 5 years temporary protection and requires people to spend some of this time in regional Australia. In addition, there are just over 1220 asylum seekers living with transitional visas, of whom 276 are children (Refugee Council of Australia 2021a). This allows them to live in the community with the expectation that they will transit back to their country of origin, or to another country to seek asylum, within 6 months.

With the change of government in Australia in May 2022, it is likely there will be some reforms to refugee policy and practice – including the abolition of temporary protection visas to enable refugees to settle permanently in Australia, progressive expansion of the Refugee and Humanitarian Program to 27 000 places per year, and community sponsorship program for 5000 people. In addition, the previous government's commitments to offer 16 500 additional places to Afghanis seeking asylum and enabling 3 years of humanitarian protection to Ukrainians displaced by the Russian invasion, will be honoured. However, the offshore processing policy is set to continue (Refugee Council of Australia 2022).

People with refugee and asylum seeker backgrounds may present to emergency settings for physical or mental health treatment. When undertaking a health and/or mental health assessment, understanding the complexities associated with the refugee/asylum seeker experience is crucial. The multifaceted interaction of past and ongoing traumas, uncertainty relating to visa status, cultural understandings and expressions of distress, and the impacts of displacement on identity development, represent multiple risk factors for this vulnerable population. The individual's personal, cultural, political and social worlds need to be considered for a useful, accurate and relevant assessment. It is also important to understand the restrictions of the visas people have been granted (and/or were living under for some time) and the impact of their legal status on the health, mental health and wellbeing.

IMMIGRATION DETENTION AND CAUSAL LINKS TO MENTAL HEALTH

The literature consistently reports negative impacts of immigration detention on the mental health of asylum seekers (von Werthern et al. 2018). The most common disorders reported include high levels of anxiety, depression and post-traumatic stress disorder (PTSD), and poor quality of life. Pervasive refusal syndrome (PRS) has been identified as a serious risk for children living in immigration detention, and the experience of living with unending uncertainty has been closely linked with a sense of lethal hopelessness, leading to high levels of suicidal thoughts (Procter et al 2018; von Werthern et al 2018). Exposure to trauma experienced in the person's country of origin is associated with higher levels of these disorders in the context of immigration detention (Kaplan 2020). While the detention of children is not common, until 2018 Australia had a policy of offshore immigration processing of all asylum seekers, including children (see below). This practice has been found to have profound and long-term effects on the mental health of asylum seekers in general, and children in particular (von Werthern et al 2018). For younger children, the effects include developmental regression and dysregulated behaviour, while older children have been found to experience symptoms of PTSD, anxiety and depression (von Werthern 2018). The detention environment may leave parents struggling with their own mental health concerns and undermine their capacity to provide the support necessary for their child's healthy development (von Werthern 2018).

TRAUMA

Trauma is common, resulting from experiencing an event, or series of events, that are physically and psychologically harmful or life-threatening, and which can have lasting adverse effects on the person's wellbeing (Kaplan 2020). A trauma response can occur after experience of abuse, neglect, violence, persecution, war, disaster, loss or other psychologically damaging events. The majority of asylum seekers will have experienced many forms of trauma in their search for safety, and the offshore immigration detention practices implemented by the Australian Government between 2013 and 2022 have proved to be traumatising and re-traumatising for both children and adults (von Werthern et al 2018).

Trauma-informed practice involves recognising the widespread impact of trauma in the general population and the high likelihood that asylum seekers and refugees entering emergency care settings will have experienced one or more traumas. It requires recognition that the symptoms of trauma are adaptations to traumatic events, confidence in responding to the person experiencing the symptoms, and the active resistance of practices or approaches that may be re-traumatising or which expose the person to ongoing trauma (Isobel et al 2021).

POST-TRAUMATIC STRESS DISORDER

Studies indicate that a significant proportion of refugee young people experience post-traumatic stress disorder (PTSD) (Reavell & Fazil 2017). PTSD can be a consequence of experiencing a traumatic event, and symptoms include hyperarousal, flashbacks and re-experiencing traumatic events, and behaviours resulting in the avoidance of triggers. Experiences of violence during the flight from the country of origin and in refugee camps have been found to be stressors for refugee children, and there is a relationship between the number of stressors and the severity of PTSD symptoms (Reavell & Fazil 2017). Experiences of trauma and violence have also been linked with the diagnosis of pervasive refusal syndrome, as experienced by young asylum seekers in immigration detention settings (Newman et al 2020). There are a number of co-morbidities that occur alongside complex reactions to trauma such as PTSD; these include depression, anxiety and dissociative disorders (Kaplan 2020).

THE IMPACT OF UNCERTAINTY

In 2012, Australia's policy of offshore processing for all asylum seekers who arrived by boat, whereby they would never be resettled in Australia, even if recognised as refugees, resulted in 122 children being detained in Nauru for up to 5 years (Refugee Council of Australia 2021b). In 2018 there was a strong push from the community to transfer all asylum seeker children to Australia. These young people and their families were placed in community detention before being given what was then known as a Final Departure Bridging Visa E (Subclass 051), which entitled them to lawfully stay in Australia for 6 months while making arrangements to leave Australia (Department of Immigration and Border Protection 2017).

Although the Labor government elected in May 2022 has committed to abolish TPVs, during the years that the previous Coalition government was in power, people subject to a TPV or SHEV (described above) were able to apply for another temporary visa, but not a permanent visa. This meant that with protracted processing of visa applications, people could be living on temporary visas for many years (e.g. 8+ years), and as a result, experience significant mental distress and deterioration due to living with such uncertainty (Procter 2018). While policies may soon change, people subjected to years of continued uncertainty will continue to experience the impacts of these policies on their mental health, on their confidence and their ability to engage with life and the community, as well as on cognitive functioning, such as concentration and memory. In addition, complexities around visa status and work entitlements have meant that many people in the community are not eligible to work and are therefore reliant on charities for food and shelter. Living with uncertainty is a 'trauma-related stressor' and has been shown to significantly impact working memory capacity in refugee adolescents (Mirabolfathi et al 2020). The uncertainty of insecure visa status has also been strongly linked with suicidality and serious mental deterioration among people seeking asylum in Australia (Nickerson et al 2019).

LETHAL HOPELESSNESS

The term *lethal hopelessness* has been used to describe the asylum seeker experience of living with unending uncertainty (Procter et al 2018). Having to reiterate their traumatic experiences in successive interviews can also trigger trauma symptoms and increases the risk of suicidal thinking and deliberate self-harm (Procter et al 2018). The social withdrawal associated with lethal hopelessness can lead to relationships within the family becoming fractured and people having less opportunity to express their inner distress. Where an asylum seeker presents with thoughts of suicide, it is important for all health professionals, in their interactions with the person and their family, to bear witness to the distress and sense of injustice they are experiencing with solicitude and understanding (Procter et al 2018).

Safety planning with refugees and asylum seekers experiencing suicidal thoughts and deliberate self-harm needs to be:
- inclusive of cultural understandings of mental health and suicidality
- include the important people in the person's life – those who help to relieve or ameliorate their distress, and
- focus on the activities that provide some relief from the distress.

The aim of safety planning is for the person to reconnect to moments of hopefulness in their life and to highlight ways of being that promote this, as opposed to those that embed the fixed idea that death is the only solution.

PERVASIVE REFUSAL SYNDROME

Pervasive refusal syndrome, sometimes termed traumatic withdrawal syndrome, is a rare, potentially life-threatening psychiatric condition in which a young person, generally between the ages of 7 and 15 years, pervasively refuses to eat, drink, walk, talk or care for themselves over a period of several months to the point where hospitalisation is required. The diagnostic criteria also include the active and angry refusal of help and rejection of encouragement, as well as social withdrawal and school refusal (Ngo & Hodes 2020).

PRS has been more recently described as presenting in asylum-seeking children with high levels of trauma experienced in their home country, on the journey to the host country, and in immigration detention (Ngo & Hodes 2020). The experience of multiple rejections of asylum applications and living with the persistent threat of deportation has the effect of re-traumatising the child, resulting in significant mental health consequences.

For children who lived in immigration detention in Nauru, this involved not only the loss of liberty but constant experiences of bullying and harassment from locals, and exposure to violence from fellow detainees. For many asylum seekers, such experiences are reminiscent of what they experienced in their country of origin, where their human rights were denied or abused. Depression and PTSD, which are common among asylum-seeker young people, are seen as potential differential diagnoses for PRS (von Werthern 2018).

There is no known evidence-based treatment for PRS. However, inpatient care is usually required with a multidisciplinary team approach involving re-feeding and activity-based interventions, and for some young people, long-term psychological treatment (Nunn et al 2014). There is a limited role for medication, and family involvement can relieve anxiety.

In 2018 at least 30 young asylum seekers living in detention in Nauru were diagnosed with symptoms of PRS, and transferred to Australia or the United States for treatment (Ngo & Hodes 2020). When assessed in Australia, 15 of these young people were found to have PRS (Newman et al 2020). While these young people and their families were happy to be in Australia, after discharge from hospital they remained in community detention until late 2020, with limitations on their movement and no work rights or welfare payments for their parents. The prolonged uncertainty has resulted in an inevitable deterioration in their mental health (Procter et al 2018). Their recent release into the community highlights a need for all health practitioners, and particularly those working in emergency settings, to become more aware of PRS and other issues that impact on people with traumatic personal asylum-seeking histories.

The scenario below demonstrates some of the issues for consideration that nurses and other health professionals in emergency care settings need to be cognisant of when working with people who are refugees or asylum seekers.

SCENARIO 3.13.1

Nathisan

Nathisan is 16-year-old young Tamil man who came to Australia by boat with his parents seeking asylum in 2013 (when he was 8 years old) and who subsequently spent 5 years in immigration detention on Nauru. Nathisan has been brought to the paediatric emergency department of a major metropolitan children's teaching hospital by ambulance, accompanied by a school counsellor, after telling the counsellor he was going to jump in front of a train and disclosing deliberate self-harm.

While on Nauru, Nathisan witnessed the self-immolation of another asylum seeker, made two serious suicide attempts and was diagnosed with pervasive refusal syndrome prior to being transferred with his family to Australia for treatment in 2018. In August 2020, the family were placed on a final departure Bridging Visa E (BVE), which enables temporary residence in the Australian community while arrangements are made to leave Australia. Under this visa, there is no entitlement to government welfare, accommodation or income support, which in Nathisan's situation, means the family have had to rely on charities for food and rent. The visa is due to expire in 2 weeks and the family has been told that they are expected to return to their country of origin.

Nathisan has been well engaged at school, enjoying learning and spending time with his peers playing cricket and soccer. He has been seeking support from the school counsellor when he finds it difficult to concentrate in class and complete assignments. His help-seeking has increased over the last month.

Nathisan is withdrawn and lying in bed with a sheet covering him. His parents have arrived, and his distressed father is demanding loudly with limited English that his son be seen immediately by a doctor, while his mother is sitting in a chair near Nathisan weeping quietly. His father says that Nathisan's moods have been swinging at home, and he has been expressing a lot of anger towards his parents, blaming them for the family's current situation. His father has been trying to get work, but has been unsuccessful.

Nathisan's cuts to his left forearm have been assessed and cleaned and no further medical intervention is required. You approach Nathisan and introduce yourself as the nurse allocated to him, but he turns away. You request consent to undertake basic observations such as pulse and blood pressure and he nods his agreement.

RED FLAGS

- Prior suicide attempts increase the risk of future attempts.
- Living with the uncertainty of insecure visa status has been causally linked with poor mental health outcomes.
- Trauma exposure prior to leaving Sri Lanka, during the journey to Australia, and in immigration detention for 5 years in Nauru.
- Previous diagnosis of pervasive refusal syndrome.
- The imminent expiry of their current Bridging Visa E and uncertainty over their future will result in severe anxiety for all family members. This, combined with the above red flags, significantly increases the risk of a serious deterioration in mental health, including suicidality.

PROTECTIVE FACTORS

- Nathisan has a supportive family.
- Nathisan's school is also supportive, and he is enjoying learning and spending time with friends.
- Nathisan enjoys playing sport with his friends.
- He has developed a supportive relationship with the school counsellor.

KNOWLEDGE

- It is important to understand the impacts of trauma and immigration detention on young people. The underlying question in a trauma informed response moves from 'What is wrong with you?' to 'What has happened to you?'. It provides space for the person to describe the issues they are experiencing in their own words, embracing alternative idioms of distress. It looks to develop a deeper understanding of the problem, to redefine it in another way, providing ways to move forward that include connection to others and purposeful activity.
- The impact of living with indefinite uncertainty challenges family relationships, particularly for families who have experienced multiple traumas. This can lead to feelings of disconnection and isolation, and result in an increased risk of drug and alcohol misuse, interpersonal violence and self-harm.
- The biological markers of trauma are those that sit within the body. The physical signs of trauma can include pain, headaches, sleep disturbance, abdominal discomfort and

appetite changes. During your assessment, ask about the presence and frequency of nightmares, flashbacks and anxiety.

- Safety planning for asylum seekers presenting with suicidal thoughts and self-harm should include identifying feelings of safety within the emergency care setting itself. People who have been held in immigration detention may experience high levels of anxiety and mistrust in unfamiliar environments, so providing information about (and encouraging them to ask about) procedures and processes that are occurring can provide some relief, as can asking directly if the person is feeling safe, and if not, whether there is anything you can do to support increased feelings of safety. Providing an explanation for any noise that is occurring in the environment is also important, as this may be frightening and decrease the person's sense of safety.

- Bearing witness to the distress of others in circumstances when there is no certainty is difficult. Research reveals that Australian immigration policies impact on clinician wellbeing more than exposure to traumatic narratives (Posselt et al 2019).

ATTITUDES

- All health professionals need to reflect on their own attitudes towards refugees and asylum seekers, people from different cultural backgrounds and people presenting with suicidal ideation and/or self-harm. Our attitudes impact on our practice and our ability to help.

- There are many myths surrounding refugees and asylum seekers; for example, relating to people's motivations for leaving their country of origin and the nature of national and international processes surrounding seeking asylum. Organisations such as the Refugee Council of Australia and the Asylum Seeker Resource Centre provide information that help to increase understanding of the issues and reflect the complexities associated with the asylum seeker/refugee experience of seeking safety.

- Engagement will be enhanced by ensuring that all actions demonstrate understanding of the person's experience, e.g. carefully introducing yourself, paying attention to the nature of the environment in which the assessment is taking place, considering previous experiences the person may have had with previous service providers while in detention, and acknowledging aspects of the environment that may be triggering for the young person and their family.

- Validating the experience of the young person and their family demonstrates an attitude of acceptance and a non-judgemental approach.

- Respectful curiosity relating to cultural understandings and idioms of distress.

MENTAL HEALTH SKILLS

- Empathic interpersonal engagement skills (engage with both Nathisan and his parents) using a trauma-informed approach are required. For example, asking, 'Can you tell me what has been happening for you?' provides an opportunity for Nathisan to speak about the issues that are relevant to him and in language that makes sense to him. It is important to use the words he uses to describe what is happening for him in any further questions. A trauma-informed approach provides an opportunity for Nathisan to speak about the story that sits behind the distress, fear and uncertainty that triggers suicidality and deliberate self-harm.

- Consider any cultural issues that may impact on the mental state examination (MSE) – including language, behaviour, education level and cultural understandings of mental health/illness.

- Assess risk and safety planning in the context of the unique challenges that refugees and asylum seekers experience that place them at an increased risk of feelings of hopelessness and suicidal behaviour. These challenges include indeterminate uncertainty

about their residence status, separation from family and the experience of multiple traumatic events.
- Focus on strengths and protective factors where possible (without minimising or dismissing the severity and intensity of Nathisan's experiences and feelings); inquire about Nathisan's interests both at school and outside of school, the activities that he enjoys with his peers and the history of these. Identify times when the thoughts of suicide are less intense, what helps to alleviate some distress, and if there are activities or people who help to achieve this.

NURSING ACTIONS AND INTERVENTIONS

- Attempt to engage Nathisan and his family by acknowledging their distress. Speak in a calm and gentle manner.
- Request consent to organise an interpreter, clarify the language and gender of the interpreter preferred. See Box 3.13.1 for recommendations about working with the interpreter. Do not use family members or friends as interpreters.
- Ask Nathisan and his parents if they would like the school counsellor to stay.
- Ensure that Nathisan and his family have been offered a drink and have chairs to sit on. Small gestures of hospitality are appreciated by people from most cultural backgrounds and will assist with engagement and feelings of safety.
- Provide an explanation of the processes and personnel who will attend to Nathisan while he is in the emergency department (ED). Explain all care before it happens, allowing time for Nathisan to respond and ask questions. This is particularly important for people who have lived in immigration detention where their personal decision-making is limited.
- Involve Nathisan's parents in all care provided to reassure them that their son is receiving the right care and to help reduce their anxiety.
- Focus on undertaking basic observations, making sure to quietly describe the procedures. This interaction provides an opportunity to ask about other daily activities, such as appetite, sleep and current comfort level.
- Ask Nathisan if he would like to speak with you alone and whether he would like the interpreter to be there to assist. People who are distressed may find it easier to communicate in their first language despite being proficient in English. Providing Nathisan with choice about these matters will help engagement.
- Contact the mental health team to request a mental health assessment.
- Ensure documentation includes any information that Nathisan, his family or school counsellor have provided, which will be important for the mental health assessment and reduce the need for them to re-tell their story, as this can add to the trauma experienced in a healthcare setting.

Box 3.13.1 Working with interpreters:

- Clarify that the interpreter speaks the right language (for Nathisan's family, Tamil).
- Ask if they have had any contact with the family previously. If they have had contact, check with the family that they are comfortable with this interpreter.
- Provide the interpreter with a pre-briefing, outlining the nature of Nathisan's presentation, and the general issues that will be discussed.
- Introduce the interpreter to the family and reassure them that the interpreter is bound by the same code of confidentiality as you are.
- Look at and speak directly to Nathisan and his family, and not at the interpreter.
- Keep your sentences short and use plain English, providing an explanation of any medical terminology. Leave enough time for the interpreter to respond.

Engagement with family

- Speak with Nathisan's parents about their concerns for their son, demonstrate respect and empathy for their situation. Acknowledge their sense of injustice and the steps they have taken to try and keep their son safe.
- Reassure them that the emergency mental health team will soon be undertaking a full assessment and will support them and Nathisan in making recommendations about further mental health treatment.

RELEVANT TREATMENT MODALITIES AND CONSIDERATIONS

The treatment of young asylum seekers experiencing suicidal ideation and behaviour will be determined by the psychological impact of their traumatic experiences prior to and during the process of seeking asylum in Australia. The goals of the treatment need to be co-constructed with the young person and their family. Some of the goals may include planning for safety, reducing common symptoms of PTSD, such as flashbacks and nightmares, or addressing severely disrupted sleep patterns.

Treatment guidelines for addressing trauma recovery in children and young people are less formalised than those for adults (Kaplan 2020); however, flexibility is recommended in the delivery of such interventions. The use of many creative means to support the young person's expression of their inner world is recommended, such as art, sport, drama and narrative documentation. These interventions need to be age-appropriate and delivered within a culturally respectful milieu.

Safety planning with the young asylum seeker and their family is an essential intervention starting at the point of assessment in the ED. Safety planning is a collaborative process in which the young person and clinician identify the warning signs of a crisis, internal and external supports and coping strategies, including family and friends who may not be with them in Australia, and other services, such as school or mental health services, that can support them at that time (Ferguson et al 2021). Safety planning is a dynamic process that can be adapted to respond to the fluctuations in mental state of the young person.

Other specific treatment modalities include:

- trauma-focused cognitive behaviour therapy (TF-CBT). This involves the cognitive coping and processing of traumatic experiences, and desensitisation to the hyperarousal and distress associated with these experiences (Kaplan 2020).
- KidNET is an adaptation of narrative exposure therapy for young people with refugee experience. This involves the narration of the life timeline using a variety of modalities, with a focus on assisting the young person through graded exposure to the next experience of safety (Kaplan 2020).

Other multi-component approaches include school-based programs such as Foundation House's Rainbow Program and the Kaleidoscope Program, which involve parent and community engagement, psychoeducation and skills development (Foundation House 2021).

SUMMARY

In this chapter we have explored the complexities associated with the refugee and asylum seeker experiences in Australia, and in particular the mental health deterioration associated with prolonged uncertainty about visa status and persistent threats of imminent return to their country of origin experienced by refugees and asylum seekers in Australia during the period from 2013 to 2022. Nurses play an important role in the assessment of young asylum seekers who present to the ED with suicidal ideation and/or behaviours. Establishing rapport with the young person and their family involves consideration of current environmental factors, as well as previous experiences with service providers in immigration detention settings, and creating a safe space in which cultural factors and the family's history of trauma are validated.

Understanding how pervasive refusal syndrome and PTSD are displayed in young people influences how a mental state examination is undertaken, with the principles of trauma-informed care guiding the process in order to avoid the re-traumatisation of the young person.

Reflection

1. How do your own cultural values influence your understanding of the concept of lethal hopelessness in the context of asylum seekers?
2. What barriers exist in your practice in the ED to undertaking a mental health assessment involving young asylum seekers?

Useful websites

Asylum Seeker Resource Centre: asrc.org.au
Foundation House: foundationhouse.org.au
NSW Service for the Treatment and Rehabilitations for Torture and Trauma Survivors (STARTTS): www.startts.org.au/
Refugee Council of Australia: www.refugeecouncil.org.au
Roads to Refuge: www.roads-to-refuge.com.au/whois/whois_government.html

References

Department of Home Affairs 2021. Bridging visa E. Online. Available: https://immi.homeaffairs.gov.au/visas/getting-a-visa/visa-listing/bridging-visa-e-050-051.

Department of Immigration and Border Control 2017. Information about the final departure Bridging E visa. Australian Government. Online. Available: https://refugeelegal.org.au/wp-content/uploads/2017/08/Fact_sheet_-_Final_departure_Bridging_Visa_E-1.pdf.

Ferguson M, Posselt M, McIntyre H et al 2021. Staff perspectives of safety planning as a suicide prevention intervention for people of refugee and asylum-seeker background: A qualitative investigation. The Journal of Crisis Intervention and Suicide Prevention 43(4):331–8.

Foundation House Specialised Programs 2022. Online. Available: https://foundationhouse.org.au/specialised-programs/.

Isobel S, Wilson A, Gill K et al 2021. What is needed for trauma informed mental health services in Australia? Perspectives of clinicians and managers. International Journal of Mental Health Nursing 30:72–82.

Kaplan I 2020. Rebuilding shattered lives: Integrated trauma recovery for people of refugee background. The Victorian Foundation for Survivors of Torture, Brunswick.

Mirabolfathi V, Schweizer S, Moradi A et al 2020. Affective working memory capacity in refugee adolescents. Psychological Trauma: Theory, Research, Practice, and Policy. ResearchGate. https://doi.org/10.1037/tra0000552.

Newman L, O'Connor B, Reynolds V et al 2020. Pervasive refusal syndrome in asylum seekers on Nauru. Australasian Psychiatry 28(5):585–8.

Ngo T, Hodes M 2020. Pervasive refusal syndrome on asylum-seeking children: Review of current evidence. Clinical Child Psychology and Psychiatry 25(1):227–41.

Nickerson A, Byrow Y, O'Donnell M et al 2019. The association between visa insecurity and mental health, disability and social engagement in refugees living in Australia. European Journal of Psychotraumatology, Vol 10. Online publication. www.tandfonline.com/doi/full/10.1080/20008198.2019.1688129.

Nunn KP, Lask B, Owen I 2014. Pervasive refusal syndrome (PRS) 21 years on: A re-conceptualisation and a meaning. European Child and Adolescent Psychiatry 23:162–72.

Operational Data Portal 2022. Refugees fleeing Ukraine (since 24 February 2022). Online. Available: https://data.unhcr.org/en/situations/ukraine/location?secret=unhcrrestricted.

Posselt M, Deans C, Baker A et al 2019. Clinician wellbeing: The impact of supporting refugee and asylum seeker survivors of torture and trauma in the Australian context. Australian Psychologist 54:415–26.

Procter NG, Kenny MA, Eaton H et al 2018. Lethal hopelessness: Understanding and responding to asylum seeker distress and mental deterioration. International Journal of Mental Health Nursing 27:448–54.

Refugee Council of Australia 2022. Our Letter to Prime Minister Anthony Albanese 23 May 2022. Online. Available: www.refugeecouncil.org.au/our-letter-to-prime-minister-anthony-albanese/.

Refugee Council of Australia 2021a. Statistics on people seeking asylum in the community. Available from: www.refugeecouncil.org.au/asylum-community/.

Refugee Council of Australia 2021b. Offshore processing statistics. Online. Available: www.refugeecouncil.org.au/operation-sovereign-borders-offshore-detention-statistics/2/.

Reavell J, Fazil Q 2017. The epidemiology of PTSD and depression in refugee minors who have resettled in developed countries. Journal of Mental Health 26(1):74–83.

United Nations High Commission for Refugees (UNHCR) 2021. Refugee Data Finder 10th November 2021. Update. Online. Available: www.unhcr.org/refugee-statistics/.

Von Werthern M, Robjant K, Chui Z et al 2018. The impact of immigration detention on mental health: a systematic review. BMC Psychiatry 18:382.

Supporting resilience and providing psychological first aid when working in disaster settings as a first responder

Peta Marks, Jamie Ranse and Brent Hayward

KEY POINTS

- Humans are generally resilient and recover from a disaster experience over time through mobilising existing supports and networks, and using existing skills and strategies.
- Nurses and other health professionals have an important role in providing physical and psychological health care in response to disaster.
- A strengths-based approach will support coping and recovery.
- Self-care and clinical supervision are important for health professionals who respond in disaster situations.

LEARNING OUTCOMES

This chapter will assist you to:

- describe the impact of disasters on the mental health of individuals and communities
- understand that mental illnesses can be triggered or exacerbated by a disaster experience, but the majority of persons do not experience mental ill-health
- identify the red flags that may indicate a person affected by disaster is struggling with their emotional wellbeing or mental health
- understand the differences between how children, adolescents and adults can respond to disaster situations from a mental health perspective
- describe the unique challenges and personal impacts of working in disaster settings.

Lived experience comment
by Helena Roennfeldt

VULNERABILITY

The concept of vulnerability in relation to people with a diagnosis of mental illness is multi-layered and complex. Being more vulnerable amid disaster is compounded by experiences of lower socioeconomic status and multiple barriers to supports. It is crucial to consider the need to address added social impacts during disasters, including financial impacts, inability to participate in work or social activities, shortages of resources, inequity, and reduced access to health services. These factors exacerbate stress and affect people unequally. For people with a lived experience of a mental illness, there is also the potential for resilience. Examples have been the use of technology to maintain social networks and provide peer support creatively. People with lived experience themselves are experts in what they need and, with help, will often have the best solutions to navigate additional stress and worry during disasters.

INTRODUCTION

There is no internationally accepted definition of a 'disaster'. The United Nations defines a 'disaster' as 'a serious disruption of the functioning of a community or a society causing widespread human, material, economic or environmental losses which exceed the ability of the affected community or society to cope using its own resources' (United Nations Office for Disaster Risk Reduction (UNDRR) 2009, p. 9). From a health perspective, a disaster requires health assistance from other jurisdictions to ensure that the operational capacity is restored and/or maintained (Ranse & Lenson 2012). A simpler, person-centred description by McFarlane and Norris (2006) is that a disaster is a collectively experienced, potentially traumatic event that has an acute onset and is time-delimited.

Disasters include natural hazards, such as cyclones, tsunamis, earthquakes, fires; events such as military action, terrorism, political unrest, bombings and mass shootings, or industrial accidents such as chemical, biological, nuclear or radiological accidents (Beaglehole et al 2018; Makwana 2019). Fire, flood and cyclone are the most common forms of disaster in Australia causing loss of life, homes and businesses, destroying livestock and habitat, and costing the government and community billions of dollars. For example, the 2019–20 Australian bushfires burnt more than 46 million acres of land across the Northern Territory, over 80% of the Blue Mountains world heritage area in New South Wales and 53% of the remaining Gondwana world heritage rainforests of Queensland. In total, 3500 homes were lost, along with thousands of other buildings. Tragically, 34 people died from direct causes, while 445 died from indirect causes, such as smoke inhalation (Komesaroff & Kerridge 2020; Richards et al 2020).

Whole communities are impacted during and following a disaster through infrastructure damage or loss (e.g. public transport), physical and ecosystem damages that may impinge on local services (e.g. power, water supply), governmental and/or public institutions (e.g. schools, local council services), and the deterioration of social and community resources (e.g. in-home supports, childcare) (Berrebi et al 2020). Positive community effects have also been identified, notably increased community cooperation, improved social cohesion and solidarity. These social changes have been noted both within and outside the affected community (Berrebi et al 2020).

There is a growing understanding of the impact of disasters on individuals within disaster-affected communities. It is clear that disasters can precipitate both acute mental health experiences, such as substance abuse, adjustment disorder, anxiety and increased suicide risk, as well as onset mental illnesses such as post-traumatic stress disorder (PTSD) and depression. The disaster experience may also trigger a relapse of, or exacerbate, a person's pre-existing mental health concerns (Beaglehole et al 2018; Makwana 2018; Warsini et al 2014) and can have long-term effects lasting for years (Usher et al 2020). But only a minority of persons affected by disaster will experience serious psychological harm necessitating treatment (Bonanno et al 2010; La Greca & Silverman 2009), with most people recovering over time without specialist support or intervention (Phoenix Australia 2020).

It is likely that the mental health impacts of disasters, and their management, are unevenly distributed across communities, particularly because they are also influenced by people's individual social and economic circumstances (Fisher et al 2020). Some disasters may be ongoing. The acute risk may have passed for the moment; however, people may still need to be prepared for further periods of risk and threats to property and lives. The psychological impact of disasters will also depend on a person's age and stage of development – behavioural, psychological and emotional impacts will be different for young children, older children and adolescents, than for adults and older adults (Peek 2008; Pfefferbaum et al 2019). Children and adolescents need the support of parents, carers and the broader community to mitigate their stressors they encounter (Dyregrov et al 2018), which may not always be available or sufficient during a disaster.

In a disaster, everyone will be experiencing some impacts on their mental health or psychological wellbeing, but as mentioned above, only a minority will experience serious psychological harm necessitating treatment (Hayward 2020). For many people, the disaster will be their first experience of acute psychological distress. For some, the disaster experience will be 'the straw that breaks the camel's back', particularly if, for example, the disaster has come at the end of other difficulties or traumas (consider the bushfire that demolishes the homes, livestock, fencing and machinery of a farming community that has been struggling through years of drought and financial hardship, or the cyclone that destroys the home of a grieving widow whose grown up children all live away).

People who have been affected by a disaster are known to disclose thoughts, feelings and emotions to nurses that they would not ordinarily disclose to a stranger (Cox 1997; Ranse et al 2021). This is likely to occur when a person presents for the treatment of a minor ailment or injury, or during routine assessment or first aid, as many people who experience psychological distress or mental health concerns after a disaster do not seek formal help for those needs (Beaglehole et al 2018). Nurses working as first responders or in disaster response situations, whether their role is formal or informal, need to be prepared for and understand the potential psychological effects of exposure to disaster and to have the psychological and psychosocial wellbeing of those affected front of mind, regardless of the physical illness or injury that a person might be experiencing. This may represent a significant shift for those who are used to working in a setting where a person's physical health concern is always the primary focus (Ranse 2017).

Government (civilian or defence force) or non-government multidisciplinary disaster medical assistance teams (DMATs) can be deployed to disaster-affected communities. They are tasked with providing a coordinated health response to support, restore and maintain health service capacity (Aitken et al 2014; Van Hoving et al 2010; Watson et al 2019). Nurses can and do respond to disasters independently, outside of formal DMATs, perhaps particularly when a disaster has occurred within (or near to) their own community. They often play a key role in disaster mitigation, preparedness, response and recovery (Deeny & Davies 2018) and there are growing calls for nurses' education to include disaster preparedness content (Ituma et al 2022).

Nurses from a variety of clinical backgrounds participate in disaster response (commonly acute medical, emergency, intensive care, perioperative and mental health) (Ranse et al 2010). Nurses usually deploy in out-of-hospital environments, such as evacuation centres or first aid posts, in makeshift health facilities, such as operating theatres or in resuscitation teams. They undertake a range of activities depending on the situation, the location, the nature of the disaster and their scope of practice – including providing clinical care, such as assessment and first aid, treating minor injuries, monitoring people with chronic conditions, helping people access medicines, undertaking public health surveillance activities, managing communicable diseases and giving opportunistic vaccinations. Nurses can also be involved in command and logistical administration of disaster health services. Importantly, nurses are problem-solvers and coordinators, providing clinical leadership and psychosocial support to disaster relief workers, as well as the affected community (Ranse 2017; Ranse & Lenson 2012).

Providing psychological first aid (PFA) is as important in disaster nursing as physical first aid. PFA is an evidence-informed approach which aims to promote an environment of safety, of self and community efficacy; one that is calm, connected and hopeful (Gispen & Wu 2018). PFA promotes natural recovery by supporting people to reduce their distress, meet their immediate needs, promote flexible coping and encourage adjustment (Hayward 2020). The key elements of PFA are described on p. 234.

Nurses also need to monitor their own personal wellbeing during disaster work, which is invariably physically, emotionally and logistically challenging. Personal and professional growth is a possibility during disaster response work, with nurses and other professionals reporting that they develop a sense of meaning from their work with disaster-affected communities (Berah et al 1984; Hayward 2020; Yang et al 2010). Disaster response requires a significant shift in role for nurses who commonly work in hospital environments. In hospitals, shifts are time-limited and team members constantly change on a shift-by-shift basis; policies, procedures and routines exist; there are clear lines of reporting and responsibility; referral pathways are well established; and support structures are in place for staff. During disaster deployment in the out-of-hospital environment, nurses work extended hours alongside colleagues whom they may also live with – creating a sense of interpersonal closeness and blurring the usual boundaries between work and home life. There may be limited access to equipment, no operating procedures or referral pathways; there may be a lack of clarity around roles, and experiences that are perhaps less common in the hospital setting – for example, the experience of death – may be much more evident (or even emphasised) in a disaster, depending on its magnitude (Ranse 2017). An adjustment in usual coping strategies – both during the disaster and afterwards, when the nurse returns home, will be required (Ranse et al 2021). Nurses who are part of the community under threat may also be experiencing distress due to their personal experience or loss, and whether they are part of the geographical community or not, bearing witness to the emotions of others can be emotionally challenging (Dickerson et al 2002).

Whether in Australia or overseas, participating in disaster response requires that nurses are aware of and consider their personal safety and security, relevant cultural and political issues that may impact on their role, and transport and communication systems which may be impacted by the disaster. A community-focused approach that is culturally aware and underpinned by ethical practice is essential (Deeny & Davis 2018).

SCENARIO 3.14.1
'Reflections from the field'

When I saw people in the disaster-affected area, I didn't know if the person's home was destroyed, if they had lost loved ones or if they were directly affected by the disaster in some other way. I would often just say, 'Hello' or 'How are you going'? Commonly, people would then start to talk about their disaster experience. Most patients who presented for care of their physical injuries and illness displayed some level of psychosocial need (Ranse 2017, p. 168).

I heard stories from people who had lost their children. One woman recounted her disaster experience, which involved her two young children ... She had to let go of her youngest child to save herself and the oldest child ... On another occasion, one mother and father were discussing their five-year-old child with me. Their child was swept away in the water during the disaster ... the child had not spoken a single word since the disaster. One middle-aged woman recounted her experience of being on the roof of her house with her two elderly parents ... a helicopter came past to rescue them ... there was only enough space in the helicopter for one person ... She had the impression that her parents were going to die. I spoke with one man who had lived in his roof space for a week ... Another elderly couple were staying in their home with no electricity or water, cooking on a fire in their backyard and using a hole in their backyard as their toilet. When he came to us, the man was very unwell ... Another elderly man recalled a story of how he became separated from his family in the disaster ... he was told to get on the bus ... his wife had died and other members of his family were missing (Ranse 2017, p. 171).

I was listening to the stories of people who had been in the disaster and I was trying to support these people to the best of my ability. In the Australian hospital environment, I would have many other nurses to share this emotional load. Additionally, I would be able to refer patients to other support services and mental health teams. This is not the case in the disaster environment (Ranse 2017, p. 171).

I now think back to my time in the disaster and ask myself a number of questions: 'Should I still be there helping?' 'Did I do all that I could have done?' 'Did I really make a difference?' I implicitly knew that what I was

Continued

doing was invaluable and making a difference to the disaster-affected community. I know that there was never a day where I did not try my best. Surrounding me there was such a large need for assistance; however, the best I could do was to help one person at a time. Now I am home, I think about particular patients and their situations, their family and their community. There are stories that I heard and situations that I have seen that will stay with me. When comparing my situation to those left behind in the disaster, I had many things; they had nothing (Ranse 2017, p. 173).

RED FLAGS

The following demographics may indicate a person with greater support needs during and following a disaster:

- People (including children) demonstrating an extended distress reaction, persistent hyperarousal, vigilance or fear, having difficulty sleeping or eating, who are withdrawn and/or not utilising services and supports that are available to them beyond the immediate disaster experience (of course, many people also do this so that resources are made available to others who may need them more).
- Relationships between parents and children where there is role reversal; for example, where the child is emotionally supporting the parent, where strong emotion is expressed directly to the child (e.g. rather than to a partner), or where the parent is angry and controlling or overly involved and anxious in relation to their child.
- People who have experienced significant trauma and loss – such as witnessing significant injury or death – both during and prior to the event.
- People with a pre-existing mental health condition or a history of mental illness – particularly mood disorders, anxiety and PTSD.
- People with alcohol and other substance use disorders.
- People with physical, developmental and cognitive disabilities.
- People whose physical safety was directly threatened.
- People who are unable to access their usual medications, services and supports.
- People who are less well educated may find it more difficult to access support services (and need assistance with forms, etc).
- People who are financially disadvantaged and have less financial capacity to cope with the sudden loss of a job, or housing (Gruebner et al 2017; Hayward 2020; SAMHSA 2018).

PROTECTIVE FACTORS

- People with strong social connections and social support, particularly with their community.
- Those engaged in formal interventions, such as participation in support groups or participating in religious/spiritual groups.
- A positive appraisal style (that is, an approach to live that is positive and optimistic) as well as general self-efficacy and good stress response recovery (Veer et al 2020; Woud et al 2018).
- Those who can return to 'normal' life with minimal disruption.
- For people with existing mental illness, engaging with assertive community treatment, peer support services and outreach (SAMHSA 2018).

KNOWLEDGE

- Disasters are experiences that are known to trigger acute symptoms of psychological distress, such as shock, stress and sleep disturbance, and cause feelings of fear, despair, grief and sadness.
- The sudden disruption to a person's routine or functioning can be destabilising – for example, the loss of a job or income, the destruction of one's home and belongings, displacement or death of family members – and will probably challenge a person's feelings of safety and security.
- Some community members may be particularly vulnerable to the psychological impacts of disaster (Hayward 2020; Ranse et al 2014), for example:
  - people who have experienced previous trauma
  - people with existing mental illness, who have different risk and protective factors and whose access to usual support services may be interrupted
  - involvement in the event at peak times or in significantly affected areas of the disaster
  - people who thought that they would die
  - an experience of traumatic bereavement (e.g. watching a loved one die)
  - serious personal impacts – loss of property, community, networks, livelihood (Australian Red Cross 2020; SAMHSA 2018).
- You don't have to be present in a disaster to be significantly impacted by it. Disasters can be experienced vicariously through newspapers, radio, television and social media, and can elicit responses indicative of acute stress reactions – particularly when people feel psychologically connected to the victims of the disaster and when they learn more about them, which leads to feelings of, 'it could have been me' (Jeronimus et al 2019).

The needs of children

The specific needs of children can sometimes be missed in the response to a disaster. Ask parents and carers about their children's affect and behaviour. Has there been a change coinciding with the disaster? Observe the child yourself, as some adults may inadvertently exaggerate or minimise the effect of disaster on children. Observe and interact with children:

- How do they relate to their family members, friends, unknown persons? How are they keeping occupied, or not?
- Are they eating and drinking?
- How are they sleeping?
- Do they ask about other people, especially friends?
- Do they ask about the welfare of pets or livestock?
- Are they candid about their experience? What are they worried about?

Parents and carers can support children by:

- holding them, speaking in a gentle, soothing voice
- asking them how they are feeling, helping them label their emotions. This will not make children upset
- supporting them to express their emotions. Crying and sadness is normal. Not expressing emotions may be a concern, so encouraging children to be 'brave' or 'be good' or 'stop being silly' should be avoided (Schafer et al 2020)
- helping them tell their story if they wish and acknowledging that they and other people in their family are safe, transforming frightening experiences into learning experiences (Lazarus et al 2003)
- providing as much of a stable and familiar environment as possible, this includes remaining with their family
- returning to normal activities and routines as quickly as possible – school is often pivotal to a child/young person's recovery (Schafer et al 2020).

Box 3.14.1 lists common reactions to disaster in children, adolescents and adults.

Box 3.14.1 Common reactions to disaster in children, adolescents and adults.

These are normal and expected responses. It is only when they persist and/or have occupational impacts that they may require more formal evaluation.

Common reactions to disaster in children and adolescents	Common reactions to disaster in adults
• Birth–2 years: being irritable, crying more, wanting to be held. Memories of sights, sounds or smells may endure. How parents cope is the biggest influence. • 3–6 years: intense fear and worry about being separated from their parents/carers. • 7–10 years: may be preoccupied with details of the event, sometimes engaging in play about it; display a range of emotions – sadness, fear, guilt, anger, or fantasies of playing rescuer. • 11–18 years: may be overwhelmed by intense emotions, but unable to discuss them. Feeling that the world is dangerous or unsafe. Risk-taking behaviours like drinking, reckless driving, drug use.	• Sleep disturbance • Feeling numb, sad, depressed, hyperactive, irritable or angry • Lability of mood • Lacking energy or constant exhaustion • Appetite disturbance • Poor concentration, feeling confused • Social withdrawal • Feeling alone – thinking no one else is experiencing the same reactions • Non-specific physical complaints, such as headaches, stomach aches, body pains, tunnel vision, muffled hearing • Misuse of alcohol, tobacco, drugs or prescription medications

Ready 2020; American Psychiatric Association 2022.

ATTITUDES

- Take the lead of affected persons and communities. They know what they need and when (Hayward 2020).
- Remember that people's basic needs must be met as a priority.
- Be prepared to respond to deep levels of distress originating from personal experiences.
- Make unique accommodations for adults and children to participate in events designed to help, for example, offer refreshments, childcare, family-friendly settings, evening scheduling, and make deliberate attempts to encourage the participation of men (Hayward 2020).

MENTAL HEALTH SKILLS

- Be an expert listener, rather than an 'expert'.
- Establish a human connection with the person in a non-intrusive, compassionate way.
- Remaining calm yourself can help to orient someone who is emotionally overwhelmed or distraught.
- Acknowledge the person's strengths and coping efforts, help people realise what they can do in taking an active role in their recovery. A practical, solutions-focused approach is important.

- Consider the needs of children in consultation with parents/carers. 'Counselling' children and young people is not a priority during response and early recovery.
- Be prepared for high levels of expressed emotion and protect children from the emotional overwhelm of their parents – for example, occupy them elsewhere during adult parts of a conversation (Hayward 2020).
- Adjust your approach; for example, ask questions that make it easier for the person to talk about how they are feeling and coping if that's what they want to do.
- The goal is to get people to talk about how they are feeling, but not to repeat what has happened to them. Help people come to a point where the person has told their story, and their story has resolved to the point where they are safe. This is not debriefing. Debriefing is no longer an accepted intervention. This must be guided by what the person wants and by minimising any further distress (Beaglehole et al 2018; Ranse 2017).

NURSING ACTIONS AND INTERVENTIONS

Initially
- Politely observe, don't intrude. Initiate contact only after determining that contact won't be intrusive or disruptive to the person.
- Speak calmly, be patient, be responsive, be sensitive and listen.
- Ask simple respectful questions to find out how you can help. Use simple, concrete terms. Speak slowly and clearly, without jargon.
- Acknowledge what the person has done to keep safe; don't patronise people or focus on helplessness, mistakes or disability.
- Sometimes a calm, supportive physical presence is sufficient. Not everyone wants to talk
- Help to meet the person's immediate needs – the basic necessities. There's no point trying to counsel people who are hungry, ill or unsafe (Deering 2000, p. 14). People might want to tell their story, but they might not, and not everyone exposed to a disaster will be traumatised.
- Provide information that is age-appropriate and directly addresses the person's immediate needs/goals.
  o Matching language to a child's developmental level is important – for example, simple words like mad, sad, scared or worried, rather than extreme words such as terrified or horrified, which may increase distress.
  o Speak to adolescents 'adult-to-adult' so they feel respected in their feelings, concerns and questions.
  o Don't make assumptions based on a person's appearance or age. For example, an older person who is disoriented may not have problems with memory, reasoning or judgement – they may be dehydrated or sleep deprived.
- Clarify with the person that you have understood by repeating answers as required.
- If you are working with an interpreter, make sure you look at and speak to the person, not the interpreter.
- Keep essential aids with the person (e.g. medication, oxygen, wheelchair, respiratory equipment) (NCTSN/NCPTSD 2006).

Then
- Promote and support community events as a component of response to and recovery from disaster. They provide an opportunity for people to come together and share their experiences, which leads to enhanced community bonding (Hayward 2020).
- Be aware of your potential status as an 'outsider'. Some people and communities may be suspicious of or reluctant to engage with you as a clinician or a representative of an organisation that was not already recognised as part of the community.
- When working in a disaster setting, consider the context of the community; for example, people living in rural areas will have very different relationships and sense of connectedness with their community than those in metropolitan areas.

- Help the person identify the natural supports in their life; people who can provide immediate support such as neighbours, school community, friends and family.
- You don't need to have distinct discussions with a person about what's happened to them; do things with other people, have a meal, get kids to play; provide a context for people to feel comfortable to talk.
- If people volunteer that they are already in receipt of psychological support, support them to make contact with their therapist/case manager/treatment professional as required.
- Identify who to contact in a mental health emergency. Refer to the local mental health emergency service. Provide as much detail as you can about the person's history and presenting symptoms, and risk. Do not accept responsibility for the person's ongoing monitoring or safety; this is not the role of a nurse responding to a disaster.

RELEVANT TREATMENT MODALITIES AND CONSIDERATIONS

Many people who have survived a disaster will demonstrate transient distress, then return to their usual level of functioning, using existing coping strategies and support networks. Some people will experience more mild–moderate challenges to their mental health (e.g. dysphoria, stress, disruption to relationships or social functioning), and a small number will develop a mental health disorder (e.g. PTSD, depression, anxiety) (Wade et al 2014). The type of intervention required depends on the needs of the individual, but in all instances a strengths-based approach, focusing on what the person can do (instead of what they can't), supports a 'person's ability to face and deal with adversity and encourages the development of coping mechanisms' (Ogie & Pradhan 2019). Fig. 3.14.1 describes a tiered response to supporting people with psychological symptoms associated with disaster experience.

Psychological first aid

Psychological first aid (PFA) is an evidence-informed approach to supporting people in the immediate aftermath of a disaster. It is designed to reduce the initial distress and foster short- and long-term adaptive functioning and coping (Australian Red Cross 2020).

- PFA helps people to identify their immediate needs and the strengths and abilities that they have to meet those needs

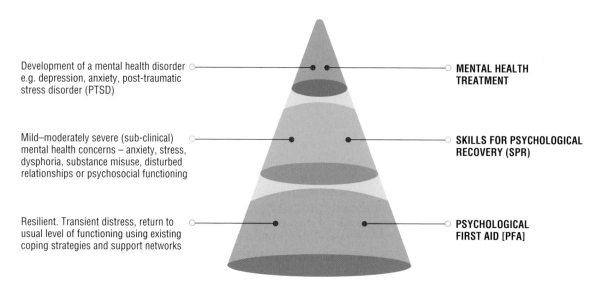

Development of a mental health disorder e.g. depression, anxiety, post-traumatic stress disorder (PTSD) — **MENTAL HEALTH TREATMENT**

Mild–moderately severe (sub-clinical) mental health concerns – anxiety, stress, dysphoria, substance misuse, disturbed relationships or psychosocial functioning — **SKILLS FOR PSYCHOLOGICAL RECOVERY (SPR)**

Resilient. Transient distress, return to usual level of functioning using existing coping strategies and support networks — **PSYCHOLOGICAL FIRST AID [PFA]**

Fig. 3.14.1 A tiered response to psychological support of people impacted by disaster.

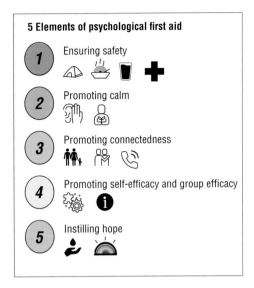

Fig. 3.14.2 The five elements of psychological first aid.
Australian Red Cross 2020.

- The focus is on calming people, listening to them, helping them to feel safe and establishing a human connection that can facilitate belief in their ability to cope.
- See Figure 3.14.2, which outlines the five key elements of psychological first aid.

Skills for psychological recovery

Some people will experience reactions that are distressing and which interfere with adaptive coping. When this occurs, supporting the development of strengths-based skills for psychological recovery (SPR) can help. SPR is an evidence-informed approach to support in the aftermath (weeks/months) of disaster and trauma, delivered by trained providers, for use when PFA has already been utilised. It is designed to help affected people gain the skills that they need to effectively cope with the stressors that arise post-disaster, and to respond to the broad range of reactions that people may experience over time. Research has found that skills-building is more effective than supportive counselling (NCPTSD/NCTSN 2010). The strengths-focused skills included in SPR are:

- problem-solving skills
- skills in planning and undertaking activities that create wellbeing
- managing distressing psychological responses/reactions
- promoting thinking strategies such as self-talk, which are helpful
- rebuilding social connections and accessing practical community supports (Wade et al 2014).

SUMMARY

Disasters disturb healthcare systems, communities and individuals, causing structural and environmental damage, as well as having physical, social and mental health impacts. Nurses and other health professionals are increasingly involved in disaster response, either individually or as part of a disaster response team. There are a range of responses that people can experience, with some people experiencing transient distress and demonstrating psychological resilience, some people experiencing mild–moderate psychological impacts, and some people experiencing significant challenges to their mental health and wellbeing – particularly those with pre-existing mental illness.

Health professionals can help people manage their distress, normalise their stress response, help them achieve physical and psychological safety, mobilise their supports and engage their existing skills and strengths (Schafer et al 2020). Providing emotional support includes acknowledging and empathising with the person's experience, responding in a calm and comforting manner, reassuring the person and supporting them to make sense of their experience. A person-centred, strengths-focused approach is required, and depending on the person's needs, PFA, support to develop skills for psychological recovery, or mental health treatment may be required (this includes referral to, or supporting a person's engagement/re-engagement with existing mental health service providers).

Nurses and other health professionals working in disaster settings also need to ensure sufficient personal and professional self-care, particularly when re-integrating back into 'normal life' and/or where their own community is impacted by the disaster (see Chapter 4 Self Care for Working in Emergency Care Settings for further details). Working with disaster-affected persons requires the deliberate use of alternative and perhaps new nursing practices. It is important that nurses continuously reflect on their practice, seek their own support, and simultaneously consider the needs of individuals, families, and whole communities to effectively support the psychological health and recovery of persons who have been affected by disaster.

Reflection

1. How will you personally and professionally prepare to respond to, and support persons affected by disaster?
2. What mental health nursing skills will you draw on, and how might you need to adapt these in a disaster environment?

Useful websites

Australian bushfires: Psychological preparation and recovery: www.psychology.org.au/Australian-bushfires-2020
Australian Institute for Disaster Resilience: www.aidr.org.au/
Emerging Minds – supporting children and young people following a traumatic event: emergingminds.com.au/
Helping children who have been affected by natural disasters: www.psychology.org.au/getmedia/6245ffaa-14f3-417f-b321-ee862ec2c840/20APS-IS-Helping-children-natural-disasters-P1-(3).pdf
Psychological first aid: www.redcross.org.au/getmedia/dc21542f-16e4-44ba-8e3a-4f6b907bba6f/Psychological-First-Aid-An-Australian-Guide-04-20.pdf.aspx
Skills for Psychological Recovery: www.ptsd.va.gov/professional/treat/type/skills_psych_recovery_manual.asp

References

Aitken P 2015. Developing disaster health preparedness in Australia. PhD thesis. James Cook University. Online. Available: researchonline.jcu.edu.au/43767/1/43767-aitken-2015-thesis.pdf
American Psychiatric Association 2022. Coping after disaster. Online. Available: www.psychiatry.org/patients-families/coping-after-disaster-trauma.

Australian Red Cross 2020. Psychological first aid: Supporting people affected by disaster in Australia. Australian Red Cross and Australian Psychological Society, Melbourne.

Beaglehole B, Mulder RT, Frampton CM et al 2018. Psychological distress and psychiatric disorder after natural disasters: Systematic review and meta-analysis. The British Journal of Psychiatry 213:716–22.

Berah EF, Jones HJ, Valent P 1984. The experience of a mental health team involved in the early phase of a disaster. Australian and New Zealand Journal of Psychiatry 18(4):354–8.

Berrebi C, Karlinsky A, Yonah H 2020. Individual and community behavioral responses to natural disasters. IDEAS. Online. Available: ideas.repec.org/a/spr/nathaz/v105y2021i2d10.1007_s11069-020-04365-2.html.

Bonanno G, Brewin C, Kaniasty K et al 2010. Weighing the costs of disaster. Consequences, risks, and resilience in individuals, families and communities. Psychological Science in the Public Interest 11(1):1–49.

Cox HM 1997. Disaster relief work: Nurses and others in bushfire territory. International Journal of Nursing Practice 3(4):218–23.

Deeny P, Davies K 2018. Nursing in disasters, catastrophes and complex humanitarian emergencies worldwide. In: Veenema TG (ed.) disaster nursing and emergency preparedness, 4th edn. Springer, New York.

Deering CG 2000. A cognitive developmental approach to understanding how children cope with disasters. Journal of Child and Adolescent Psychiatric Nursing 13(1):7–16.

Dickerson SS, Jezewski MA, Nelson-Tuttle C et al 2002. Nursing at ground zero: Experiences during and after September 11 World Trade Center attack. Journal of New York State Nurses Association 33(1):27.

Dyregrov A, Yule W, Olff M 2018. Children and natural disasters. European Journal of Psychotraumatology 9:sup2:1500823.

Fisher JRW, Tran TD, Hammarberg K et al 2020. Mental health of people in Australia in the first month of COVID-19 restrictions: A national survey. Medical Journal Australia 213(10):458–64.

Gruebner O, Lowe SR, Sykora M et al 2017. A novel surveillance approach for disaster mental health. Plos One. Online. Available: https://doi.org/10.1371/journal.pone.0181233.

Hayward BA 2020. Mental health nursing in bushfire-affected communities: An autoethnographic insight. International Journal of Mental Health Nursing 29(6):1262–71.

Ituma OWN, Ranse J, Bail K et al 2022. Disaster education for Australian nursing students: An integrative review of published literature to inform curricula. Collegian 29(1):93–9.

Jeronimus BF, Snippe E, Emerencia AC et al 2019. Acute stress responses after indirect exposure to the MH17 airplane crash. British Journal of Psychology https://doi.org/10.1111/bjop.12358.

Komesaroff P, Kerridge I 2020. A continent aflame: Ethical lessons from the Australian bushfire disaster. Journal of Bioethical Inquiry 17(1):11–14.

La Greca A, Silverman W 2009. Treatment and prevention of posttraumatic stress reactions in children and adolescents exposed to disasters and terrorism: What is the evidence? Child Development Perspectives 3(1):4–10.

Lazarus P, Jimerson S, Brock S 2003. Helping children after a natural disaster: Information for parents and teachers. National Association of School Psychologists, Bethesda, MD.

Makwana N 2019. Disaster and its impact on mental health: A narrative review. Journal of Family Medicine and Primary Care 8(10):3090–5.

McFarlane AC, Norris FH 2006. Definitions and concepts in disaster research. In: FH Norris, S Galea, MJ Friedman et al (eds) Methods for disaster mental health research. Guilford Press.

National Center for PTSD, National Child Traumatic Stress Network 2010. Skills for psychological recovery: Field operations guide. NCPTSD/NCTSN.

National Child Traumatic Stress network and National Centre for PTSD 2006. Psychological First Aid: Field operations guide, 2nd edn. NCTSN/NCPTSD.

Ogie RI, Pradhan B 2019. Natural hazards and social vulnerability of place: The strength-based approach applied to Wollongong. International Journal of Disaster Risk Science 10(3):404–20.

Peek L 2008. Children and disasters: Understanding vulnerability, developing capacities, and promoting resilience – An introduction. Children Youth and Environments 18(1):1–29.

Pfefferbaum B, Nitiéma P, Newman E 2019. A meta-analysis of intervention effects on depression and/or anxiety in youth exposed to political violence or natural disasters. Child Youth Care Forum 48:449–77.

Phoenix Australia 2020. PTSD guidelines. Phoenix Australia. Online. Available: www.phoenixaustralia.org/resources/ptsd-guidelines/.

Ranse J 2017. Australian Civilian Hospital Nurses' Lived Experience of the Out-of-hospital Environment Following a Disaster. Doctoral dissertation, School of Nursing and Midwifery, Flinders University, Adelaide, SA.

Ranse J, Arbon P, Shaban R et al 2021. Phenomenology of Australian civilian hospital nurses' lived experience of the out-of-hospital environment following a disaster. Collegian. DOI: 10.1016/j.colegn.2021.07.009.

Ranse J, Hutton A, Jeeawood B et al 2014. What are the research needs for the field of disaster nursing in the next five years? An international Delphi study. Prehospital Disaster Medicine 29(5):1–7.

Ranse J, Lenson S 2012. Beyond a clinical role: Nurses were psychosocial supporters, coordinators and problem solvers in the Black Saturday and Victorian bushfires in 2009. Australasian Emergency Nursing Journal 15(3):156–63.

Ranse J, Lenson S, Aimers B 2010. Black Saturday and the Victorian bushfires of February 2009: A descriptive survey of nurses who assisted in the pre-hospital setting. Collegian 17(4):153–9.

Ready 2020. Coping with disaster. Online. Available: www.ready.gov/coping-disaster.

Richards L, Brew N, Smith L 2020. 2019–20 Australian bushfires–frequently asked questions: A quick guide. Research Paper Series, 2019–20. Parliamentary Library Information Analysis Advice. Online. Available: https://parlinfo.aph.gov.au/parlInfo/download/library/prspub/7234762/upload_binary/7234762.pdf.

Substance Abuse and Mental Health Services Administration (SAMHSA) 2019. Disaster and Technical Assistance Centre Supplemental Research Bulletin: Disasters and people with serious mental illness. Online. Available: www.samhsa.gov/sites/default/files/disasters-people-with-serious-mental-illness.pdf.

United Nations Office for Disaster Risk Reduction (UNDRR) 2009. UNISDR terminology on disaster risk reduction. (UNISDR-20-2009). Geneva. Online. Available: www.unisdr.org/we/inform/publications/7817.

Usher K, Ranmuthugala G, Maple M et al 2020. The 2019–2020 bushfires and COVID-19: The ongoing impact on the mental health of people living in rural and farming communities. International Journal of Mental Health Nursing (2021)30:3–5.

Van Hoving D, Wallis L, Docrat F et al 2010. Haiti disaster tourism: A medical shame. Prehospital and Disaster Medicine 25(03):201–2.

Veer IM, Riepenhausen A, Zerban M et al 2020. Mental resilience in the Corona lockdown: First empirical insights from Europe. ResearchGate DOI:10.31234/osf.io/4z62t.

Wade D, Crompton D, Howard A et al 2014. Skills for psychological recovery: Evaluation of a post-disaster mental health training program. Disaster Health 2(3–4):138–45.

Warsini S, West C, Mills J et al 2014. The psychosocial impact of natural disasters among adult survivors: An integrative review. Issues in Mental Health Nursing 35(6):420–36.

Watson KE, Singleton JA, Tippett V et al 2019. Defining pharmacists' roles in disasters: A Delphi Study. Plos One. Online. Available: https://doi.org/10.1371/journal.pone.0227132.

Woud ML, Zlomuzica A, Cwik JC et al 2018. Effects of appraisal training on responses to a distressing autobiographical event. Journal of Anxiety Disorders 56:26–34.

Yang YN, Xiao LD, Cheng HY et al 2010. Chinese nurses' experience in the Wenchuan earthquake relief. International Nursing Review 57(2):217–23.

CHAPTER 4
SELF-CARE FOR WORKING IN EMERGENCY CARE SETTINGS

Julia Hunt and Julie Sharrock

KEY POINTS

- Working in an emergency care setting is rewarding, but can also present challenges which have the potential to impact negatively on mental health.
- The emotional labour of emergency work provides meaning and satisfaction, but can also be a significant stressor and factor in the development of compassion fatigue and burnout.
- It is important to understand the personal and systemic factors that may increase vulnerability to workplace stress. Similarly, understanding the protective factors and potential resources that support resilience in the face of emotional adversity and trauma in the workplace is important.
- Resilience encompasses cognitive, emotional and behavioural characteristics, including emotional intelligence, self-awareness and self-efficacy, boundary setting, finding work-life balance, mindfulness, and flexible and creative thinking.

LEARNING OUTCOMES

This chapter will assist you to:
- understand the challenges, workplace stressors and demands of working in an emergency care setting and the associated risks to health and wellbeing
- understand the concepts of, and contributing factors to, secondary traumatic stress, compassion fatigue and burnout
- understand the emotional labour of your role within the emergency care environment and how this may impact on provision of therapeutic care
- acknowledge that all nurses and other health professionals working in emergency care settings are vulnerable to workplace stressors, regardless of years of experience
- develop an understanding of the role of emotional intelligence, self-efficacy and resilience in supporting positive adaptation to adversity and maintenance of a sense of wellbeing in stressful and traumatic situations

Continued

- Self-care is especially important for nurses and health professionals working in emergency care settings. It is fundamental to resilience, optimal physical and mental health, and a positive experience of a workplace that can be demanding and challenging.

- reflect on and develop self-care strategies that support positive physical, emotional, spiritual and social wellbeing and support a sustainable and rewarding career as an emergency care specialist.

INTRODUCTION

Working in an emergency care setting is not only fulfilling and rewarding, but is also emotionally and physically challenging (Yu et al 2021). The emergency department (ED) is a high stimulus environment that can be stressful and unpredictable (McDermid et al 2020). EDs are noisy (Fatovich 2020), bright, sometimes smelly and often chaotic. The work is varied – featuring a breadth of clinical presentations of people with physical and mental health problems, often in high distress, potentially with an altered conscious state, a head injury, the effects of alcohol or drugs, and disturbed behaviour that makes care delivery difficult. People who present to EDs can have different perceptions of health and illness, different levels of health literacy, and will come from diverse backgrounds. As discussed throughout this text, presentation rates of people experiencing mental illness, psychological distress and substance misuse continue to increase (Australian Institute of Health and Welfare (AIHW) 2021), which intensifies the demand on emergency practitioners, who may not be adequately educated in this area (Giandinoto et al 2018).

Quick decision-making is central to emergency work, yet staff experience varying degrees of skill and autonomy in this process, with the less experienced understandably finding autonomous decision-making more challenging (Merrick et al 2021). There is an expectation that staff will communicate effectively, address multiple demands competently, and utilise their experience and skill, simultaneously delivering high-quality compassionate care. These expectations occur in the context of staff being exposed to extreme human distress, trauma, suffering, and critical incidents that may trigger strong emotional reactions (McDermid et al 2020).

The community can have expectations of what services the ED can provide, which might be unrealistic or difficult to meet, and place additional pressure on staff (Alomari et al 2021; Badu et al 2020; O'Callaghan et al 2020). ED nurses have an integral role in communicating with and breaking bad news to families (Trueland 2020). Anxious patients and their relatives are seeking certainty, explanations, reassurance and comfort, which may not be able to be delivered in a timely way, and this can lead to agitation, distress, conflict or violence (Bingöl & İnce 2021). Violent incidents in EDs have been found to be consistently high (Hills et al 2020; Kleissl-Muir et al 2019; McDermid et al 2020; Okoli et al 2020).

Overcrowding, high workloads and under-staffing, coupled with mandated targets such as National Emergency Access Targets (NEAT) are linked to increased stress and low morale

(Forero et al 2020; McDermid et al 2020). EDs are the interface between the hospital and community during disasters, such as bushfires (ANMF 2021; Cameron et al 2009), terrorist and other violent attacks (ANMF 2017; De Stefano et al 2018), and during the recent COVID-19 pandemic (Hesselink et al 2021).

There can be a perception by other nursing specialties, disciplines, the public in general and sometimes ourselves, that ED nurses are somehow more able to process and respond to stress and distress, that they are more tenacious, resilient and capable (Li et al 2018; O'Callaghan et al 2020). However, the ED milieu can be overwhelming at times for both recent graduates and experienced clinicians (Hesselink et al 2021). It can be easy to feel overwhelmed, which may be especially challenging when it appears that everyone else is competent and coping.

The previously described challenges of working in an ED, while often exciting and stimulating, can also have negative consequences for the health and wellbeing of ED nurses (Badu et al 2020; Peters 2018; Wang et al 2020).

It is possible to provide effective care and experience ED nursing work as fulfilling and meaningful. Regardless of years of experience, it is important that we all recognise and attend to our own physical and mental health. This includes:
- understanding the factors that may negatively impact on our health
- increasing self-awareness of personal vulnerabilities
- strengthening responses to stress
- developing emotional intelligence and resilience
- learning how to implement professional boundaries
- incorporating self-care strategies into both personal and professional practice.

In the first section of this chapter, the concepts of anxiety and stress, secondary traumatic stress, emotional labour, compassion fatigue and burnout are described. In the second section, protective factors and self-care strategies that can be strengthened to manage the demands of working in an emergency environment will be explored. Brief vignettes are interspersed in the chapter to stimulate reflection and consideration of issues that commonly occur in the emergency setting.

ANXIETY AND STRESS

Anxiety and *stress* are often used interchangeably as the physical manifestations are similar, with a pounding heart, increased heart rate and a churning stomach, and they are often triggered by instances where ' . . . the brain fails to distinguish the difference between a perceived and a real threat' (Giannakakis et al 2017, p. 90). Both anxiety and stress are normal experiences and are not necessarily negative. Anxiety helps us avoid danger as it gives us a physiological and emotional stimulus to escape potentially dangerous situations. In addition, anxiety and stress can be catalysts for change or stimulate positive action. However, excessive anxiety can lead to poor physical and mental health (Giannakakis et al 2017; Schneiderman et al 2005), and chronic stress can impact negatively on health and wellbeing, and if unchecked, can lead to burnout (Hesselink et al 2021; Maslach & Leiter 2017; Soto-Rubio et al 2020).

It is significant that most Australian nurses experience moderate-to-high levels of stress, and experience psychological detachment or emotional disconnection at work (Badu et al

2020). These experiences of psychological distress are predominantly associated with emotional dissonance; that is, the tension between the emotional expectations of a role and the experienced emotions. The physical manifestations of stress are associated with illness, injury and physical exhaustion, and increased work absences or sick leave (Badu et al 2020). The psychological work required to manage consistent exposure to distress and trauma, at the same time as maintaining competent and compassionate care, not only impact on mental and physical health, but also the ongoing capacity to provide therapeutic care to the recipients of the services we provide.

SECONDARY TRAUMATIC STRESS

Secondary traumatic stress is considered an occupational hazard for nurses because of their regular exposure to extremely stressful or traumatic events (Wang et al 2020). Those working in emergency care settings are particularly vulnerable to secondary traumatic stress when exposed to violence, the death or sexual abuse of children, and interpersonal conflict with staff, families, carers and patients (Duffy et al 2015). The incidence of secondary traumatic stress has been estimated to range from 39.0% to 77.9% among nurses (Wang et al 2020), and is especially prevalent in those working in emergency, psychiatric and paediatric departments (Morrison & Joy 2016). The effects of secondary traumatic stress may manifest as irritability, poor concentration, anger and sleep disturbance, as well as intrusive or recurrent disturbing thoughts and rumination (Hinderer et al 2014).

EMOTIONAL LABOUR

Recognising the emotional 'work' required of emergency care professionals is important if we are to understand both the stressors and sources of job satisfaction. This concept, known as *emotional labour*, has been applied to nursing and is considered a form of workplace stress (Theodosius 2008). In managing emotions to meet the expectations of the role, nurses 'supress or create feelings to present an outward appearance that will give another person . . . a sense of being cared for' (Sharrock 2020, p. 89). The concept of emotional labour helps us to understand factors that increase vulnerability to burnout and compassion fatigue, and are integral in supporting resilience, self-reflection, emotional intelligence and, subsequently, the development of self-care strategies and skills to support working in an emergency care setting.

There are two components of emotional labour: surface acting and deep acting (Hochschild 2012). *Surface acting* is the active suppression of actual emotion and/or simulating a more appropriate emotion. The key is that the nurse appears to experience an emotion that is not genuinely experienced. In contrast, *deep acting* is where the nurse feels genuine emotions that are appropriate to the situation. It appears that *surface acting* has a greater negative impact on the nurse than *deep acting* (Delgado et al 2017), in that the sense of loss of the 'authentic self' (Humphrey et al 2015) can result in discomfort, emotional exhaustion and burnout (Soto-Rubio et al 2020).

> *Paradoxically, emotional labour in nursing work can also be experienced as a source of satisfaction. The emotional work of nursing has been described as 'emotionful' work and a 'gift' (Bolton 2000). Demonstrating compassion, using oneself as the therapeutic tool and dealing with emotionally charged*

interpersonal interactions are all sources of both satisfaction and labour (Edward et al 2017). This view is consistent with the evidence that there is a 'bright side of emotional labour' (Humphrey et al 2015), in that deep acting, as well as the expression of naturally felt emotions, have positive impacts on clinicians (Sharrock 2020, p. 89).

Aspects and realities of working in an emergency care setting that have been identified as emotionally labour-intensive include:

- bearing witness to human distress and suffering
- feeling and expressing compassion
- managing one's own emotions at the same time as managing the emotions (particularly anxiety and distress) of others
- engaging in interactions that are intense and that trigger a range of emotions
- interactions that require a significant degree of effort, such as working with patients who are difficult to engage or not cooperative with treatment and interventions
- interactions where higher levels of stress and a strong sense of responsibility for patient outcomes is perceived
- managing crisis situations, promoting adherence with treatment and navigating the power structure within the therapeutic relationship
- conflict between professional identity (professionalism) and personal identity (authenticity), for example, in ethical dilemmas or threats that challenge the physical or psychological safety of the nurse
- feeling blamed
- feeling burdened by or unprepared for what is expected
- interpersonal difficulties and conflict with other staff (Delgado et al 2017; Edward et al 2017).

Practice Example

Deen is a 22-year-old nurse working in an Aboriginal Medical Service as their first post-registration job. Every day they see the impacts of colonisation on the physical and mental health of Aboriginal and Torres Strait Islander clients to the service, who present in crisis or in response to an emergency. Today they heard of yet another client who has died by suicide. They feel angry and sometimes overwhelmed by the stories they hear each day. Deen's flatmate has commented that they do not seem to be enjoying their job.

Reflection

1. What do you think is happening for Deen?
2. What strategies do you think would be helpful?
3. How can Deen effectively establish boundaries around their workplace experiences to support emotional resilience and wellbeing?

COMPASSION FATIGUE

Compassion fatigue is a significant concern in healthcare and has been referred to as the cost of caring (Wang et al 2020). First examined in ED nurses in 2010 (Hooper et al 2010), compassion fatigue is a combination of physical, cognitive, emotional, spiritual and behavioural responses to providing care. It is:

> *a preventable state of holistic exhaustion that manifests as a physical decline in energy and endurance, an emotional decline in empathetic ability and emotional exhaustion, and a spiritual decline as one feels hopeless or helpless to recover that results from chronic exposure to others' suffering, compassion, high stress exposure, and high occupational use of self in the absence of boundary setting and self-care measures (Peters 2018, p. 70).*

The antecedents to compassion fatigue are:
- chronic exposure to the suffering of others
- lack of self-care measures
- inability to maintain professional boundaries
- high stress exposure
- high occupational use of self
- compassion (Peters 2018, p. 473).

Compassion fatigue 'evolves when rescue-caretaking strategies are unsuccessful, leading to caregiver feelings of distress and guilt' (Boyle 2011, p. 3). It affects the clinician's ability to provide compassionate care to patients, effectively restore themselves, and cognitively process the work of nursing in an emergency care setting (Peters 2018; Yu et al 2021).

Practice Example

Toni is working on the ICU ward with COVID-19 patients – all are seriously ill and some have died. They have held the person's hand and the iPad as their loved ones have said goodbye. It is heart-breaking. Toni feels distressed and increasingly emotional at work and at home, and is feeling worried about passing the illness onto family members who are vulnerable.

Reflection

1. How would you describe what Toni is experiencing?
2. What are the potential risks of constant exposure to suffering, distress and trauma to nurses and other health professionals working in settings where managing crisis and intense human (physical and emotional) suffering is part of routine practice?
3. What strategies would be useful to support resilience, clinical boundaries and self-care for Toni?
4. If you were working with Toni, what could you do to support their wellbeing?

The symptoms of compassion fatigue have been categorised as work-related, physical and emotional (Lombardo & Eyre 2011) and are presented in Table 4.1.

Practice Example

Dani is feeling frustrated with Cathie, who has presented to the ED for the fourth time in two weeks with self-inflicted lacerations to her arms and legs. She rolls her eyes when she sees Cathie's name next to hers on the whiteboard.

TABLE 4.1 Symptoms of compassion fatigue

Work-related	Physical	Emotional
• Avoidance or dread of working with certain patients • Reduced ability to feel empathy towards patients or families • Inability to share in suffering • Poor judgement • Frequent use of sick days • Loss of interest at work, lack of joyfulness and diminished job satisfaction • Self-doubt • Cynicism or a sense of futility • Diminished performance and inefficiency	• Increased physical complaints • Fatigue • Headaches • Digestive problems: diarrhoea, constipation, upset stomach • Muscle tension • Sleep disturbances: inability to sleep, insomnia, too much sleep • Fatigue • Cardiac symptoms: chest pain/pressure, palpitations, tachycardia	• Emotional exhaustion • Mood swings • Restlessness • Irritability • Oversensitivity • Anxiety • Excessive use of substances: nicotine, alcohol, illicit drugs • Depression • Anger and resentment • Loss of objectivity • Memory issues, poor concentration, loss of focus, and diminished judgement

Cross 2019; Lombardo & Eyre 2011; Soto-Rubio et al 2020.

Reflection

1. What do you think is underlying Dani's response?
2. What aspects of emotional labour are evident in this vignette?
3. How does compassion fatigue and burnout affect the care that Dani may provide to Cathie? What are the therapeutic risks here for Cathie?
4. Does this reflect some of the experiences you have had in working with people who repeatedly present with self-harm?
5. What strategies would be helpful for Dani to understand her response and to develop effective skills in working with individuals that self-harm?

BURNOUT

The psychological syndrome of *burnout* is associated with compassion fatigue. It has a slower onset and is longer lasting than compassion fatigue (Lombardo & Eyre 2011). It has three dimensions:

- overwhelming feelings of physical and emotional exhaustion, a sense of depletion and over-extension without seeing a source of replenishment or getting a chance to recover
- feelings of detachment from the job and from others, negative perceptions and attitudes towards others, negative or harsh responses without interest in the other, cynicism and a loss of ideals
- a loss of self-efficacy and productivity, a lack of a sense of accomplishment, and disillusionment with work, the caring role, the organisation and the health system (Maslach & Leiter 2017).

Burnout is not a personal failing, and it is not the sole responsibility of the individual to prevent. The high rates of burnout in health professionals signal that it is more accurate to consider burnout as an organisational issue where an employee reacts to the work and the workplace (Maslach & Leiter 2017).

Staff working in emergency settings are at increased risk of burnout (Gómez-Urquiza et al 2017; Yu et al 2021). A recent review found that 40.5% of ED nurses experienced high emotional exhaustion, 44.3% experienced depersonalisation (feeling detached), and 42.7% experienced low personal accomplishment (Li et al 2018). An older study found that approximately 82% of ED nurses had 'moderate-to-high' levels of burnout, and nearly 86% had 'moderate-to-high compassion fatigue' (Hooper et al 2010, pp. 424–5). Given this, nurses and organisations both have a role in reducing the impact of workplace stressors of the ED and adopting practices that support staff rather than contribute to stress and burnout (Maslach 2017).

PROTECTIVE STRATEGIES AND SELF-CARE

Secondary traumatic stress, compassion fatigue and burnout all have the capacity to negatively impact on the mental and physical health of emergency nurses and detrimentally affect their capacity to provide optimal and therapeutic care, utilise professional judgement, and experience job satisfaction and strong professional identity. Given the potential psychological and physical risks that working in an emergency care setting poses, it is essential that we understand the nature of the work, risk factors for compassion fatigue and burnout, and strategies and resources that are available to mitigate the potential negative impact of the setting. This is important, not only for recent graduates, but also experienced clinicians. The next section of this chapter will provide an overview of the concepts of resilience and emotional intelligence, as well as self-care strategies and resources that can not only reduce the detrimental effects of stress, but support a sense of wellbeing and work satisfaction.

RESILIENCE

Resilience is a personal attribute or set of internal skills that supports nurses to manage and cope with workplace adversity, the challenges and demands of bearing witness to high levels of suffering and distress, and interpersonal difficulties and conflict (Badu et al 2020; Foster et al 2019). Through the management of thoughts, emotions and behaviours, resilience supports the nurse to adapt positively to adversity, regain a sense of wellbeing after difficult or stressful situations. It has also been associated with improved wellbeing by moderating the potentially harmful aspects of the work of nursing (Craigie et al 2016; Delgado et al 2017; Foster, Schochet et al 2018).

Some of the cognitive, emotional, and behavioural characteristics found in resilient individuals are:
- flexible and creative thinking
- honesty
- optimism
- tenacity
- self-control or the ability to restrain impulsive action
- interpersonal connectedness
- decisive action organising and structuring work
- finding a work–life balance
- mindfulness
- self-reliance mechanisms including positive thinking
- emotional intelligence (Badu et al 2020; Tubbert 2016).

It is becoming increasingly apparent that resilience can be learnt. A program for mental health nurses, called Promoting Adult Resilience, has been found to have a promising impact on the health and wellbeing of the participants (Foster, Cuzzillo et al 2018; Foster, Shochet et al 2018). The program aims to promote 'self and affect/emotion regulation in the face of stress', utilises the strengths of the participants, and integrates cognitive, emotional, behavioural and interpersonal concepts (Foster, Shochet et al 2018, p. 1472). A nurse in this study described resilience as where:

> *you grow and you learn and excel through hardship. That doesn't mean that you can't be affected by something, but that in time you use that positively, or to improve yourself, or improve your practice in some way as you go on (Foster, Cuzzillo et al 2018, p. 342).*

Importantly, resilience should be considered as an interaction between an individual and their environment. This way of thinking highlights that the individual needs to consider internal resources, as well as resources from their environment and workplace. In addition, it places some of the responsibility for promoting resilience and wellbeing on the organisation. A summary of internal and external resources and supports that are available and which enable and enhance wellbeing is provided in Figure 4.1.

Emotional intelligence

Emotional intelligence is the ability to experience and recognise our own emotions, make connections between our emotions and our thoughts, and regulate our emotions and subsequent actions. This requires a level of self-awareness of our individual reactions and interpersonal response to environments, events and the behaviours of others. The capacity for self-awareness is intrinsic to emotional intelligence and supports an understanding of complex emotional and

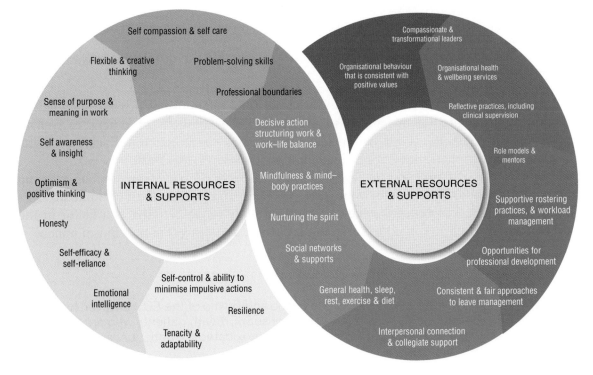

Fig. 4.1 Internal and external resources and supports that enable and enhance wellbeing.

physiological responses to challenging work environments, trauma and distress. This skill of coping with one's own emotions, as well as those of others, enables clinicians to manage stress more effectively, which subsequently positively supports their own health, as well as the individuals for whom they are providing care (Soto-Rubio et al 2020). This is especially relevant in emergency care with the high emotional work or burden of caring for patients with high levels of suffering, pain, trauma and emotional distress. The concept of emotional intelligence also includes the ability to recognise the emotional states of others (Dugué et al 2021).

Emotional intelligence is integral to nursing, in the context of addressing risks to mental health, as well as the genesis of core skills – including effective communication, sensitivity and creativity, self-discipline, assertiveness and awareness of self (Soto-Rubio et al 2020).

It can be considered a component of resilience (Foster, Cuzzillo et al 2018), in that it can diminish the psychological impacts of stressors and psychological distress and encompasses the ability to regulate responses to adversity, maintain a sense of control, and deal with external stressors, as well as integrate and make sense of experiences (Cleary et al 2018).

Practice Example

Mika recently started a clinical rotation in the ED. She feels really anxious about going back to work after a particularly stressful shift, where a young man who was intoxicated with methamphetamine trashed a cubicle and security was called. Everyone else seemed to just get on with their day, so she feels worried she will not be a good nurse.

Reflection

1. Can you identify with Mika's experience?
2. What factors, both individual to Mika as well as external, are relevant to her experience and emotional response?
3. Consider strategies and resources that could support Mika in developing resilience and supporting self-care.

Effective therapeutic relationships and interpersonal relationships are also founded on emotional intelligence, as the ability to understand the emotions of others, as well as knowledge and regulation of our own emotional response, is the foundation of acknowledging the experience of others, thus supporting empathy (Hofmeyer et al 2020).

Higher levels of emotional intelligence equate to higher levels of emotional wellbeing and support the ability to manage patient care effectively and therapeutically despite stressors (Badu et al 2020). Emotional intelligence is consistently recommended as a factor in the development of resilience in addressing trauma, stress, and distress in the clinical milieu.

Practice Example

James is a recent graduate who enjoys the hustle and bustle of the ED. However, he finds it particularly stressful when he is often called for support with patients who are presenting with acute mental health concerns or who are intoxicated (or both), because he is not sure what the best approach is.

Reflection

1. What strategies or resources are available to James to support develop his confidence and confidence in these situations?
2. What role could emotional intelligence play?

Self-efficacy

Self-efficacy has a role in influencing the acquisition, initiation and sustenance of positive, health promoting behaviours while suppressing behaviours that result in damaging practices (Bandura 1977). Strategies that support self-efficacy are those that nurture the self and support self-management, such as exercising self-control, taking on new challenges, building self-confidence, assertive communication, and increased autonomy that supports greater control over work, work routine and choice of roles (Badu et al 2020; McDonald et al 2016; Slatyer et al 2018).

Being able to reflect on practice is linked with self-efficacy. This includes being able to identify stressors, question and validate one's actions, think differently about problems, develop insight into practice, grow through adversity, and ultimately maintain positivity, optimism and pride and passion in the work (Abraham et al 2018; Badu et al 2020; Cope et al 2016; Slatyer et al 2018). Badu (2020) conceptualised self-reliance, positive thinking, emotional intelligence and having passion and interest in one's work as strategies to support 'self-efficacy strategy'.

Practice Example

Enid has worked in the ED of a regional hospital for the past 15 years. She recognises that she is feeling increasingly frustrated by people who present when intoxicated. Having grown up with her father who was an alcoholic, Enid wonders whether her own life experience may be impacting on her feelings towards this particular patient group and impacting on her practice.

Reflection

1. Consider how Enid's self-awareness and level of emotional intelligence may be beneficial as self-care strategies.

BOUNDARIES

The skill of maintaining emotional and professional boundaries is valuable for nurses and other health professionals. Maintaining a balance between work, rest and leisure has become more difficult over time as employment outside the home became part of people's daily lives. Achieving and maintaining 'work–life balance' is now a major social and health issue requiring attention (Köse et al 2021). A successful balance in work and life mean ' . . . having enough time and energy to meet the requirements of work and non-work life' (Köse et al 2021, p. 316).

Work–life balance is especially challenging for nurses who are shift workers and working unsociable hours (Leyva-Vela et al 2018). Consciously creating a boundary between work and home, such as by using the commute to unwind from work or taking a bath to metaphorically wash away the workplace stress (Mills 2018), can be effective self-care strategies. Establishing and maintaining boundaries has been associated with increased resilience (Brown et al 2018). This includes avoiding excessive overtime, arriving early or leaving late, taking work home or checking and responding to work emails out of hours (Badu et al 2020). Organisations can support work–life balance through flexibility in rostering, supporting a reduction in working hours, monitoring overtime (Perry et al 2017), decreasing exposure to heavy physical work and being mindful of clinical workloads. They can also undertake initiatives that focus on supporting clinicians to structure adequate rest and relaxation outside of working hours (Badu et al 2020).

Building self-awareness, becoming familiar with the types of patients or events that affect us (and why) and understanding our motivations for doing the work that we do, all assist in supporting our boundary-setting (Sharrock 2020). Resisting over-involvement with patients and engaging in processes that support closure following a death or traumatic event, also assist in building resilience (Cope et al 2016).

Practice Example

Ramesh works in the ED on the night shift and assesses a woman who is 37 weeks pregnant and presents with spotting and UTI symptoms. On ultrasound, it is confirmed that the baby has died. Ramesh feels devastated for the woman and worried about his own partner who is expecting their first child next month. He feels embarrassed at how emotional he feels as he cries in the staff toilets.

Reflection

1. The emotional labour of working with trauma and loss can be especially difficult when the circumstances of others resonate with our own experience. What may be helpful in supporting you in a situation similar to that of Ramesh?
2. Why would the capacity to recognise personal vulnerabilities be helpful in this scenario?
3. What organisational supports are available for Ramesh?
4. What is the role of professional boundaries here?
5. What other strategies could support Ramesh to make sense of his experience and emotional response?

REFLECTIVE PRACTICE

As nurses we often 'do' our work rather than take time to reflect on our work; to consider our emotional processes, the personal impact of clinical experiences, the theoretical knowledge we use, or other influences on our reactions to our work. Workplace demands and high workloads, shift work, long working hours, and the perceived expectation that we should cope and 'get on with it' often leave little opportunity for reflection and evaluation of the potential impacts of our work on our health and wellbeing.

Practice Example

Aminah is a 24-year-old nurse working in a busy metropolitan ED. Today she worked with the team on a 4-year-old child who died after sustaining significant internal injuries during a motor vehicle accident on the way home from daycare. The father, who was driving, died at the scene. On the way home, Aminah felt overwhelmed with sadness and exhaustion.

Reflection

1. Do you consider Aminah's response to be 'normal' in the context of a traumatic and challenging shift at work?
2. What strategies may be helpful to support Aminah to reflect, make sense of and acknowledge her response in a manner that supports development of resilience?
3. How would you know if Aminah was not coping effectively with this workplace experience?

Reflective learning is an educational modality proposed in the 1930s (Dewey 1933), and is used in a range of educative endeavours in nursing. The capacity to reflect on practice is a desired aspect of nursing (Freshwater 2008), and has been identified as a core characteristic of the expert nurse (Benner 1984).

> *Reflective practice is an active and deliberate process of critically examining practice where an individual is challenged and enabled to undertake the process of self-enquiry to empower the practitioner to realize desirable and effective practice within a reflexive spiral of personal transformation (Duffy 2007, p. 1405).*

Nurses are encouraged to engage in formal regular reflecting processes to support the development of their expertise. One of these practices is clinical supervision.

Clinical supervision

The material discussed in Box 4.1 clinical supervision is related to the work of the supervisee. This includes clinical care, therapeutic relationships, and interactions between the nurse and consumers. Clinical supervision can also provide an opportunity for nurses to reflect upon the subjective experience of their work. In order to develop the nurse's capacity for empathy, acceptance, nurturing and honest reflection, the clinical supervisor needs to be able to model these capacities in their relationship with the supervisee. Clinical supervision can occur in one-to-one sessions or in groups. In both settings the establishment of a safe, confidential non-blaming environment in which nurses feel able to share their clinical experiences is paramount (ACMHN, ACM & ACN 2019; Buus et al 2013; Sharrock 2020, pp. 95–6).

Practice Example

Lee does not understand why so many teenagers are coming in with self-harm and suicidal ideation, and the teenagers with eating disorders are particularly mystifying. She wonders, what is wrong with kids these days?! It seems like such a waste of time when there are people waiting who are really sick.

Box 4.1 Clinical Supervision

Clinical Supervision is a professional development opportunity and an effective forum to reflect on practice after the event as opposed to point of care learning which is in the clinical area and very likely occur at the time of a practice event.

> *Clinical Supervision is a formally structured professional arrangement between a supervisor and one or more supervisees. It is a purposely constructed regular meeting that provides for critical reflection on the work issues brought to that space by the supervisee(s). It is a confidential relationship within the ethical and legal parameters of practice. Clinical Supervision facilitates development of reflective practice and the professional skills of the supervisee(s) through increased awareness and understanding of the complex human and ethical issues within their workplace (ACMHN, ACM & ACN 2019, p. 2).*

Reflection

1. Consider how Lee's attitude and perceptions may impact on her provision of therapeutic care?
2. What role do you think emotional intelligence and self-awareness may play in supporting Lee to work more effectively with these particular patient groups?
3. How could clinical supervision help Lee to develop her critical reflection skills and understand more effectively her response to young people presenting with behaviours that she finds confronting and confusing?

Self-awareness, meaning making and self-compassion

Essential to self-care are the concepts of nurturing yourself to be able to nurture others, and of *self-compassion*. Before we can address the needs of others, we must be able to understand and be aware of our own needs (Hofmeyer et al 2020). Developing compassion towards oneself can increase our capacity to care for ourselves and for others (Reyes 2012).

Self-awareness means to understand our subjective view of the world and how it is influenced by our cultural, social, and family background and life experiences. It has been argued that:

> *. . . developing awareness and understanding of what brings us to take up a helping role is important. If we do not do this, we can fall into the trap of compulsive helping which results in metaphorically 'giving ourselves away' with nothing left for ourselves or anyone else. Self-care is vital for nurses in order to mitigate against workplace stressors and challenges and to maintain our health and wellbeing (Sharrock 2020, p. 91).*

Reflecting on the work we do, why we do it and the effect it has on us supports the development of self-awareness. Part of this is understanding our motivation to work in an emergency care setting and accepting that the desire to help others in some way underpins this. Understanding the attraction to the challenging and fast-paced setting of ED is also an important component of self-awareness. Exposure to trauma, loss, grief and violence will, most likely, affect us personally at some point in our careers. An acknowledgement of our emotional vulnerabilities (which at other points in time may be our emotional strengths), and the capacity to explore and understand the meaning of our responses, are important skills in self-care and maintaining emotional wellbeing. Having the opportunity to explore, normalise, share and make sense of experiences is valuable for personal and professional development.

Believing the work we do to be valid and important, and identifying meaning in it, supports our ongoing energy and passion for our work and also impacts positively on colleagues and the organisation (Lee 2015):

> *Meaning making that leads to adaptive behaviours help us manage our expectations, sit with the suffering of others and maintain the passion of our work, and is also a key part of resilience (Sharrock 2020, p. 92).*

Making meaning out of work experiences, especially stressful and potentially traumatic events, supports the development of adaptive behaviours and growth, and mitigates against burnout (Hamama-Raz et al 2020). Examples of cognitive processes that lead to adaptive behaviours are reframing adverse events (Prosser et al 2017) or making sense of challenging situations or recognising when a positive contribution has been made (Foster et al 2019). This latter strategy can be hard, especially if you are someone who has a harsh internal critic that goes into overdrive after a major incident. This is where self-compassion and self-kindness can be useful.

MIND–BODY PRACTICES

It can be easy to think of our body as the vehicle through which we deliver our care and skill to others. Focusing on the issues at hand, continually assessing, considering how to respond, and deciding how to intervene, can cause us to ignore the needs of our body and neglect self-care. Engaging in practices that bring the mind and body together can be useful in promoting health and managing workplace stress (Mills et al 2018). Some examples come from Eastern cultures and are centuries old, including yoga, meditation, mindfulness, tai chi and qi gong. Engaging the mind at the same time as focusing on breath, alongside gentle movements or specific postures, engages the whole person and are thought to reduce the psychological and physiological stress response:

> *Meditation is a simple yet powerful tool that takes us to a state of profound relaxation that dissolves fatigue and the accumulated stress that accelerates the aging process. During meditation, our breathing slows, our blood pressure and heart rate decrease, and stress hormone levels fall. By its very nature, meditation calms the mind, and when the mind is in a state of restful awareness, the body relaxes too. Research shows that people who meditate regularly develop less hypertension, heart disease, insomnia, anxiety, and other stress-related illnesses (Chopra 2021).*

Meditation is associated with mindfulness practice where the qualities of awareness, careful attention, discernment and memory can be cultivated and developed. Through mindful practice, awareness emerges through intentionally paying attention, without judgement, in the present moment, and as the experience unfolds, moment by moment (Shapiro & Carlson 2017).

Mindfulness is particularly important and relevant for nurses and other health professionals working in emergency care settings as a means of organising and detaching from situations that are highly emotive, reflecting on the experience, learning from it, and identifying what can be done to move on from it (Cusack et al 2016). Badu (2020) conceptualised consciously and intentionally organising work and work–life balance as a 'mindful strategy'.

SLEEP, REST, EXERCISE, DIET AND GENERAL HEALTH

Restful and restorative sleep is essential to physical and mental health and it assists us to approach stressful situations with more calm (Chopra 2021). There are some fundamental principles of sleep hygiene:

- listen to and obey your body clock
- ensure your sleeping environment is conducive to sleep
- minimise exposure to electronic devices (e.g. phones and computers) before going to bed
- avoid drugs, alcohol, stimulants, stimulating activity and heavy meals before sleep, and
- relax your mind (Chopra 2021).

However, it can be impossible to obey your body clock during shift work; for example, when your eyes want to close at four o'clock in the morning, or when on a busy shift you grab a meal when you can, rather than when you are hungry. We know that shift work impacts negatively on health, so it essential that shift workers attend to sleep hygiene, diet, exercise and fitness as much as possible (Wilson & Brooks 2018). Maintaining a healthy body weight, engaging in exercise and ensuring adequate intake of all food groups are key areas for nurses to consider (Torquati et al 2018).

Nurses can also neglect their bodies by not attending to their healthcare needs (Perry et al 2018), such as regular health screening, including Pap smears, breast and prostate checks, and regular general practitioner reviews. Most organisations offer physical and mental health programs for staff through staff clinics, immunisation programs and psychological services to support the emotional, mental and general psychological wellbeing of their employees, as well as critical incident stress debriefing after traumatic events or disturbing experiences. Some organisations offer self-care education, such as resilience or mindfulness training. External organisations such as the Nurse and Midwife Support Service and the Nursing and Midwifery Health Program Victoria (see Useful websites at the end of this chapter) are also available.

SPIRITUAL CARE

Holding sustaining belief systems that include religious and cultural dimensions (Prosser et al 2017) can be important aspects of self-care. However, spiritual care does not only refer to religious practices, but those activities that are 'our life force that gives us the will to live, love and endure' (Lloyd 2019, p. 23). Engaging with nature, singing, dancing and engaging in mind-body practices are some of the activities that can energise our life force.

SUMMARY

The focus of this chapter is on the importance of self-care and strategies to support resilience for nurses and other health professionals working in emergency care settings, such as the emergency department. The emotional labour experienced by emergency care professionals in their daily work in the context of an often challenging, chaotic and confronting clinical milieu presents particular risks to both mental and physical wellbeing, as well as impacting on the quality and sometimes the capacity to provide compassionate and therapeutic care. These risks are relevant to all emergency care professionals, from new graduates to those with a wealth of experience.

This chapter has described the factors that increase vulnerability to compassion fatigue, burnout and secondary traumatic stress. Understanding and making sense of our daily work, recognising our emotional responses and reactions, as well as the capacity to regulate our emotions and associated actions are important facets of emotional intelligence, itself a component of resilience. Self-awareness, the ability to reflect on practice, self-efficacy, mindfulness, work–life balance and cognitive flexibility, are all important components of resilience and skills that can be developed and refined throughout our professional lives.

The second half of the chapter focused on protective strategies and self-care, as well as the internal and external resources inherent in supporting physical and mental wellbeing. Reflection on the concepts discussed and the strategies described should provide a framework to develop the skills, resilience and self-awareness to not only enhance current experiences of clinical work, but also support meaning, satisfaction and optimism across the breadth of your career as a nurse or health professional in a dynamic emergency care environment.

Useful websites

Heads Up Better Mental Health in the Workplace: www.headsup.org.au/
Healthcare worker wellbeing, Safer Care Victoria: www.bettersafercare.vic.gov.au/support-and-training/hcw-wellbeing
Nurse and Midwife Support: www.nmsupport.org.au
Nursing and Midwifery Health Service: www.nmhp.org.au

References

Abraham LJ, Thom O et al 2018. Morale, stress and coping strategies of staff working in the emergency department: A comparison of two different-sized departments. Emergency Medicine Australasia 30(3):375–81.

Alomari AH, Collison J, Hunt L et al 2021. Stressors for emergency department nurses: Insights from a cross-sectional survey. Journal of Clinical Nursing 30(7/8):975–85.

Australian College of Mental Health Nurses (ACMHN), Australian College of Midwives (ACM) and Australian College of Nursing (ACN) 2019. Position statement: Clinical supervision for nurses and midwives. Online. Available: members.acmhn.org/about-clinical-supervision.

Australian Institute of Health and Welfare (AIHW) 2021. Mental health services provided in emergency departments. Online. Available: www.aihw.gov.au/getmedia/e33fb012-0ec6-4fd2-b182-c9e78cc5c6cf/Mental-health-services-provided-in-emergency-departments-2019-20.pdf.aspx.

Australian Nursing and Midwifery Federation 2021. Short-term health impacts of 2019–20 bushfires examined. Australian Nursing and Midwifery Journal 27(2):5.

Australian Nursing and Midwifery Federation 2017. How nurses rallied in the aftermath of the Bourke Street tragedy. Australian Nursing and Midwifery Journal 24(9):8.

Badu E, O'Brien AP, Mitchell R et al 2020. Workplace stress and resilience in the Australian nursing workforce: A comprehensive integrative review. International Journal of Mental Health Nursing 29(1):5–34.

Bandura A 1977. Self-efficacy: Toward a unifying theory of behavioral change. Psychological Review 84(2):191.

Benner P 1984. From novice to expert. Addison-Wesley, Menlo Park, CA.

Bingöl S, İnce S 2021. Factors influencing violence at emergency departments: Patients' relatives perspectives. International Emergency Nursing 54: DOI 10.1016/j.ienj.2020.100942.

Boyle DA 2011. Countering compassion fatigue: a requisite nursing agenda. Online Journal of Issues in Nursing 16(1):2.

Brown S, Whichello R, Price S 2018. The impact of resiliency on nurse burnout: An integrative literature review. Medical–Surgical Nursing 27(6):349.

Buus N, Cassedy P, Gonge H 2013. Developing a manual for strengthening mental health nurses clinical supervision. Issues in Mental Health Nursing 34(5):344–9.

Cameron PA, Mitra B, Fitzgerald M et al 2009. Black Saturday: The immediate impact of the February 2009. bushfires in Victoria, Australia. Medical Journal of Australia 191(1):11–16.

Chopra D 2021. Seven mind–body practices to transform your relationship with stress. Online. Available: chopra.com/articles/7-mind-body-practices-to-transform-your-relationship-with-stress.

Cleary M, Kornhaber R, Thapa DK et al 2018. The effectiveness of interventions to improve resilience among health professionals: A systematic review. Nurse Education Today 71:247–63.

Cope V, Jones B, Hendricks J 2016. Why nurses chose to remain in the workforce: Portraits of resilience. Collegian 23(1):87–95.

Craigie M, Slatyer S, Hegney D et al 2016. A pilot evaluation of a mindful self-care and resiliency (MSCR) intervention for nurses. Mindfulness 7(3):764–74.

Cross LA 2019. Compassion fatigue in palliative care nursing: A concept analysis. Journal of Hospice and Palliative Nursing 21(1):21–8.

Cusack L, Smith M, Hegney D et al 2016. Exploring environmental factors in nursing workplaces that promote psychological resilience: Constructing a unified theoretical model. Frontiers in Psychology 7:600.

De Stefano C, Orri M, Agostinucci JM et al 2018. Early psychological impact of Paris terrorist attacks on healthcare emergency staff: A cross-sectional study. Depression and Anxiety 35(3):275–82.

Delgado C, Upton D, Ranse K et al 2017. Nurses' resilience and the emotional labour of nursing work: An integrative review of empirical literature. International Journal of Nursing Studies 70:71–88.

Dewey J 1933. How we think. JC Heath, Boston.

Duffy A 2007. A concept analysis of reflective practice: Determining its value to nurses. British Journal of Nursing 16(22):1400–7.

Duffy E, Avalos G, Dowling M 2015. Secondary traumatic stress among emergency nurses: A cross-sectional study. International Emergency Nursing 23(2):53–8.

Dugué M, Sirost O, Dosseville F 2021. A literature review of emotional intelligence and nursing education. Nurse Education in Practice 54:103124.

Edward K.-l, Hercelinskyj G, Giandinoto J-A 2017. Emotional labour in mental health nursing: An integrative systematic review. International Journal of Mental Health Nursing 26(3):215–5.

Fatovich DM 2020. The signal is clear: Its noisy in the emergency department. Emergency Medicine Australasia 32(2):354–6.

Forero R, Man N, Nahidi S et al 2020. When a health policy cuts both ways: Impact of the National Emergency Access Target policy on staff and emergency department performance. Emergency Medicine Australasia 32(2):228–39.

Foster K, Cuzzillo C, Furness T 2018. Strengthening mental health nurses resilience through a workplace resilience programme: A qualitative inquiry. Journal of Psychiatric and Mental Health Nursing 25(5–6):338–48.

Foster K, Roche M, Delgado C et al 2019. Resilience and mental health nursing: An integrative review of international literature. International Journal of Mental Health Nursing 28(1):71–85.

Foster K, Shochet I, Wurfl A et al 2018. On PAR: A feasibility study of the Promoting Adult Resilience programme with mental health nurses. International Journal of Mental Health Nursing 27(5):1470–80.

Freshwater D 2008. Reflective practice: The state of the art. In: Freshwater D, Taylor B, Sherwood G (eds) International textbook of reflective practice in nursing. Wiley-Blackwell, Oxford.

Giandinoto J-A, Stephenson J, Edward K-L 2018. General hospital health professionals attitudes and perceived dangerousness towards patients with comorbid mental and physical health conditions: Systematic review and meta-analysis. International Journal of Mental Health Nursing 27(3):942–55.

Giannakakis G, Pediaditis M, Manousos D et al 2017. Stress and anxiety detection using facial cues from videos. Biomedical Signal Processing and Control 31:89–101.

Gómez-Urquiza JL, De la Fuente-Solana EI, Albendín-García L 2017. Prevalence of burnout syndrome in emergency nurses: A meta-analysis. Critical Care Nurse 37(5):e1–e9.

Hamama-Raz Y, Hamama L, Pat-Horenczyk R et al 2020. Posttraumatic growth and burnout in pediatric nurses: The mediating role of secondary traumatization and the moderating role of meaning in work. Stress and Health 37(3):1–20.

Hesselink G, Straten L, Gallée L et al 2021. Holding the frontline: A cross-sectional survey of emergency department staff wellbeing and psychological distress in the course of the COVID-19 outbreak. BMC Health Services Research 21(1):525.

Hills S, Crawford K, Lam L et al 2020. The way we do things around here. A qualitative study of the workplace aggression experiences of Victorian nurses, midwives and care personnel, Collegian, Elsevier 28(2021):18–26.

Hinderer KA, VonRueden KT, Friedmann E et al 2014. Burnout, compassion fatigue, compassion satisfaction, and secondary traumatic stress in trauma nurses. Journal of Trauma Nursing 21(4):160–9.

Hochschild AR 2012. The managed heart: Commercialization of human feeling. University of California Press, Berkeley.

Hofmeyer A, Taylor R, Kennedy K 2020. Knowledge for nurses to better care for themselves so they can better care for others during the COVID-19 pandemic and beyond. Nurse Education Today 94:104503.

Hooper C, Craig J, Janvrin DR et al 2010. Compassion satisfaction, burnout, and compassion fatigue among emergency nurses compared with nurses in other selected inpatient specialties. Journal of Emergency Nursing 36(5):420–7.

Humphrey RH, Ashforth BE, Diefendorff JM 2015. The bright side of emotional labor. Journal of Organizational Behavior 36(6):749–69.

Kleissl-Muir S, Raymond A, Rahman MA 2019. Analysis of patient related violence in a regional emergency department in Victoria, Australia. Australasian Emergency Care 22(2):126–31.

Köse S, Baykal B, Bayat İK 2021. Mediator role of resilience in the relationship between social support and work life balance. Australian Journal of Psychology 73:316–25.

Lee S 2015. A concept analysis of Meaning in work and its implications for nursing. Journal of Advanced Nursing 71(10):2258–67.

Leyva-Vela B, Henarejos-Alarcón S, Llorente-Cantarero FJ et al 2018. Psychosocial and physiological risks of shift work in nurses: A cross-sectional study. Central European Journal of Public Health 26(3):183–9.

Li H, Cheng B, Zhu XP 2018. Quantification of burnout in emergency nurses: A systematic review and meta-analysis. International Emergency Nursing 39:46–54.

Lloyd J 2019. A hospital is the place to heal a ravaged body, but what about a wounded spirit? Australian Nursing and Midwifery Journal 26(6):23.

Lombardo B, Eyre C 2011. Compassion fatigue: A nurse's primer. Online Journal of Issues in Nursing 16(1):3.

Maslach C 2017. Finding solutions to the problem of burnout. Consulting Psychology Journal: Practice and Research 69(2):143–52.

Maslach C, Leiter MP 2017. New insights into burnout and health care: Strategies for improving civility and alleviating burnout. Medical Teacher 39(2):160–3.

McDermid F, Judy M, Peters K 2020. Factors contributing to high turnover rates of emergency nurses: A review of the literature. Australian Critical Care 33(4):390–6.

McDonald G, Jackson D, Vickers MH et al 2016. Surviving workplace adversity: a qualitative study of nurses and midwives and their strategies to increase personal resilience. Journal of Nursing Management 24(1):123–31.

Merrick E, Busby Grant J, McKune A et al 2021. Measuring psychological and physiological stress in emergency clinicians. Australasian Emergency Care 24(1):43–8.

Mills J 2018. Examining self-care, self-compassion and compassion for others: A cross-sectional survey of palliative care nurses and doctors. International Journal of Palliative Nursing 24(1):4–11.

Mills J, Wand T, Fraser JA 2018. Exploring the meaning and practice of self-care among palliative care nurses and doctors: a qualitative study. BMC Palliative Care 17(1):1–12.

Morrison LE, Joy JP 2016. Secondary traumatic stress in the emergency department. Journal of Advanced Nursing 72(11):2894–906.

O'Callaghan EL, Lam L, Cant R et al 2020. Compassion satisfaction and compassion fatigue in Australian emergency nurses: A descriptive cross-sectional study. International Emergency Nursing 48:100785.

Okoli CT, Seng S, Otachi JK et al 2020. A cross-sectional examination of factors associated with compassion satisfaction and compassion fatigue across healthcare workers in an academic medical centre. International Journal of Mental Health Nursing 29(3):476–87.

Perry L, Nicholls R, Duffield C et al 2017. Building expert agreement on the importance and feasibility of workplace health promotion interventions for nurses and midwives: A modified Delphi consultation. Journal of Advanced Nursing 73(11):2587–99.

Perry L, Xu X, Gallagher R et al 2018. Lifestyle health behaviors of nurses and midwives: The fit for the future study. International Journal of Environmental Research and Public Health 15(5):945.

Peters E 2018. Compassion fatigue in nursing: A concept analysis. Nursing Forum 53(4):466–80.

Prosser SJ, Metzger M, Gulbransen K 2017. Don't just survive, thrive: Understanding how acute psychiatric nurses develop resilience. Archives of Psychiatric Nursing 31(2):171–6.

Reyes D 2012. Self-compassion: A concept analysis. Journal of Holistic Nursing 30(2):81–9.

Schneiderman N, Ironson G, Siegel SD 2005. Stress and health: Psychological, behavioral and biological determinants. Annual Review of Clinical Psychology 1:607–28.

Shapiro SL, Carlson LE 2017. What is mindfulness? The art and science of mindfulness: integrating mindfulness into psychology and the helping professions, 2nd edn. American Psychological Association, Washington DC.

Sharrock J 2020. Professional self care. In: O'Brien A, Foster K, Marks P et al (eds) Mental health in nursing: Theory and practice for clinical settings. 5th edn. Elsevier Australia, Sydney.

Slatyer S, Craigie M, Rees C et al 2018. Nurse experience of participation in a mindfulness-based self-care and resiliency intervention. Mindfulness 9(2):610–17.

Soto-Rubio A, Giménez-Espert MDC, Prado-Gascó V 2020. Effect of emotional intelligence and psychosocial risks on burnout, job satisfaction, and nurses health during the COVID-19 pandemic. International Journal of Environmental Research and Public Health 17(21):7998.

Theodosius C 2008. Emotional labour in health care: The unmanaged heart of nursing. Routledge, London.

Torquati L, Kolbe-Alexander T, Pavey T et al 2018. Changing diet and physical activity in nurses: A pilot study and process evaluation highlighting challenges in workplace health promotion. Journal of Nutrition Education and Behavior 50(10):1015–25.

Trueland J 2020. Breaking bad news: What you need to know: Informing patients and their families is never easy, but it is part of emergency department life. Emergency Nurse 28(6):8–10.

Tubbert SJ 2016. Resiliency in emergency nurses. Journal of Emergency Nursing 42(1):47–52.

Wang J, Okoli CTC, He H et al 2020. Factors associated with compassion satisfaction, burnout, and secondary traumatic stress among Chinese nurses in tertiary hospitals: A cross-sectional study. International Journal of Nursing Studies 102:103472.

Wilson DR, Brooks EJ 2018. Sleep and immune function: Nurse self-care and teaching sleep hygiene. Beginnings 38(1):6–23.

Yu H, Qiao A, Gui L 2021. Predictors of compassion fatigue, burnout, and compassion satisfaction among emergency nurses: A cross-sectional survey. International Emergency Nursing 55:100961.

INDEX